Alpena General Hospital

202558

 W9-CLC-491

Property of
AGH
Health Resource
Center

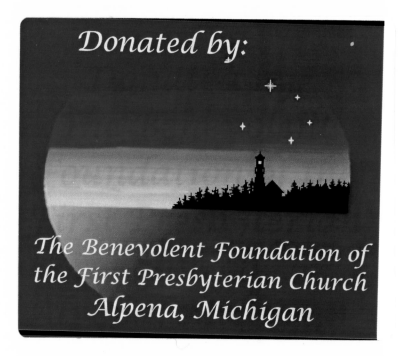

Donated by:

The Benevolent Foundation of
the First Presbyterian Church
Alpena, Michigan

Caregiving
SOURCEBOOK

Health Reference Series

First Edition

Caregiving
SOURCEBOOK

*Basic Consumer Health Information
for Caregivers, Including a Profile of
Caregivers, Caregiving Responsibilities and
Concerns, Tips for Specific Conditions, Care
Environments, and the Effects of Caregiving*

*Along with Facts about Legal Issues,
Financial Information, and Future
Planning, a Glossary, and a Listing of
Additional Resources*

Edited by
Joyce Brennfleck Shannon

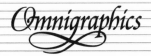

Omnigraphics

615 Griswold Street • Detroit, MI 48226

Bibliographic Note

Because this page cannot legibly accommodate all the copyright notices, the Bibliographic Note portion of the Preface constitutes an extension of the copyright notice.

Each new volume of the *Health Reference Series* is individually titled and called a "First Edition." Subsequent updates will carry sequential edition numbers. To help avoid confusion and to provide maximum flexibility in our ability to respond to informational needs, the practice of consecutively numbering each volume has been discontinued.

Edited by Joyce Brennfleck Shannon

Health Reference Series

Karen Bellenir, *Managing Editor*
Maria Franklin, *Permissions Assistant*
Joan Margeson, *Research Associate*
Dawn Matthews, *Verification Assistant*
Carol Munson, *Permissions Assistant*
Jenifer Swanson, *Research Associate*

EdIndex, Services for Publishers, *Indexers*

Omnigraphics, Inc.

Matthew P. Barbour, *Vice President, Operations*
Laurie Lanzen Harris, *Vice President, Editorial Director*
Kevin Hayes, *Production Coordinator*
Thomas J. Murphy, *Vice President, Finance and Controller*
Peter E. Ruffner, *Senior Vice President*
Jane J. Steele, *Marketing Coordinator*

Frederick G. Ruffner, Jr., *Publisher*

© 2001, Omnigraphics, Inc.

All rights reserved. No part of this publication may be reproduced or transmitted in any form or by any means, electronic or mechanical, including photocopy, recording, or any information retrieval system, without permission in writing from the publisher.

Library of Congress Cataloging-in-Publication Data

Caregiving sourcebook: basic consumer health information for caregivers, including a profile of caregivers, caregiving responsibilities and concerns, tips for specific conditions, care environments, and the effects of caregiving; along with facts about legal issues, financial information, and future planning, a glossary, and a listing of additional resources / edited by Joyce Brennfleck Shannon.-- 1st ed.
    p. cm. -- (Health reference series)
  Includes bibliographical references and index.
  ISBN 0-7808-0331-0 (lib. bdg. : alk. paper)
  1. Caregivers. 2. Care of the sick. 3. Home care services. 4. Helping behavior. 5. Consumer education. I. Shannon, Joyce Brennfleck. II. Series.

RA645.35 .C37 2001
362.1--dc21

                                                    2001033129

∞

This book is printed on acid-free paper meeting the ANSI Z39.48 Standard. The infinity symbol that appears above indicates that the paper in this book meets that standard.

Printed in the United States

Table of Contents

Part III: Caregiving for Specific Conditions and Diseases

Part IV: Care Environments

Part V: Legal and Financial Information

Part VI: Additional Help and Information

Preface

About This Book

There are nearly 27 million family caregivers in the United States. They provide 80% of home care services for an estimated 10.4 million individuals who require care outside of residential institutions. Many of these caregivers have a willing spirit, but often they lack the information and support needed to help with the challenges of caring for a loved one who is ill or disabled.

Research has affirmed that caregiving is stressful and costly. For example:

- Sixty-one percent of "intense" family caregivers (those providing at least 21 hours of care a week) have suffered from depression. Some studies have shown that caregiver stress inhibits healing.

- American businesses lose between $11 billion and $29 billion each year due to employees' need to care for loved ones 50 years of age and older.

- The value of the services family caregivers provide for "free" is estimated to be $196 billion a year.

(Source: "Family Caregiving Statistics," National Family Caregivers Association.)

This *Sourcebook* has information for the novice and the entrenched caregiver. It provides encouragement and support, including tips for the physical, mental, financial, legal, and spiritual concerns of both the patient and caregiver. A glossary of terms and a directory of resources provide additional help and information.

How to Use This Book

This book is divided into parts and chapters. Parts focus on broad areas of interest. Chapters are devoted to single topics within a part.

Part I: Compassion in Action: A Look at Caregiving in America identifies caregivers in the United States, presents the stages of caregiving, and examines the related costs and impacts of caregiving.

Part II: Caregiving Responsibilities and Concerns explains the day-to-day issues involved in caregiving, including activities of daily living (ADLs), health care issues, creating safe environments, and transportation needs. It also addresses caregiver stress, future planning, and grief.

Part III: Caregiving for Specific Conditions and Diseases explains the unique needs and problems caregivers may experience as they care for patients with Alzheimer's disease and dementia, brain injuries, cancer, cerebral palsy, multiple sclerosis, Parkinson's disease, and physical disabilities.

Part IV: Care Environments provides information about community services, respite care, and hospice care. Evaluation tools and resources are included to assist when transitions from home to residential care are required.

Part V: Legal and Financial Information offers basic information on financial planning, advance directives and other legal documents that can assure appropriate care, and government and private insurance choices.

Part VI: Additional Help and Information includes a glossary of caregiving terms, a description of federal support programs, and a directory of organizations able to provide additional information.

Bibliographic Note

This volume contains documents and excerpts from publications issued by the following U.S. government agencies: Administration on

Aging (AoA); Agency for Health Care Research and Quality (AHRQ); Corporation for National Service; Federal Trade Commission (FTC); Food and Drug Administration (FDA); Health Care Financing Administration (HCFA); National Cancer Institute (NCI); National Center for Chronic Disease Prevention and Health Promotion; National Information Center for Children and Youth with Disabilities (NICHCY); National Institute on Aging (NIA); and the Women's Bureau of the U.S. Department of Labor.

In addition, this volume contains copyrighted documents from the following organizations and individuals: American College of Physicians (ACP); The American Parkinson Disease Association, Inc.; Denise M. Brown; Beverly Evans; *The Healthy Caregiver Magazine*; Kenneth Hepburn, Ph.D.; Land-of-Sky Regional Council, NC Area Agency on Aging; National Alliance for Caregiving (NAC); National Council on the Aging, Inc.; National Family Caregivers Association (NFCA); North Carolina Cooperative Extension Service at North Carolina State University; North Carolina Division of Aging; Carolyn Rocchio; Ellen Warner, M.Ed.; and Mark Warner A.I.A., NCARB.

Full citation information is provided on the first page of each chapter. Every effort has been made to secure all necessary rights to reprint the copyrighted material. If any omissions have been made, please contact Omnigraphics to make corrections for future editions.

Acknowledgements

Special thanks to the many organizations, agencies, and individuals who have contributed materials for this *Sourcebook* and to the managing editor Karen Bellenir, permissions specialists Maria Franklin and Carol Munson, verification assistant Dawn Matthews, indexer Edward J. Prucha, and document engineer Bruce Bellenir.

Note from the Editor

This book is part of Omnigraphics' *Health Reference Series*. The series provides basic information about a broad range of medical concerns. It is not intended to serve as a tool for diagnosing illness, in prescribing treatments, or as a substitute for the physician/patient relationship. All persons concerned about medical symptoms or the possibility of disease are encouraged to seek professional care from an appropriate Health Care provider.

Our Advisory Board

The *Health Reference Series* is reviewed by an Advisory Board comprised of librarians from public, academic, and medical libraries. We would like to thank the following board members for providing guidance to the development of this series:

Dr. Lynda Baker, Associate Professor of Library and Information Science, Wayne State University, Detroit, MI

Nancy Bulgarelli, William Beaumont Hospital Library, Royal Oak, MI

Karen Imarasio, Bloomfield Township Public Library, Bloomfield Township, MI

Karen Morgan, Mardigian Library, University of Michigan-Dearborn, Dearborn, MI

Rosemary Orlando, St. Clair Shores Public Library, St. Clair Shores, MI

Health Reference Series *Update Policy*

The inaugural book in the *Health Reference Series* was the first edition of *Cancer Sourcebook* published in 1990. Since then, the Series has been enthusiastically received by librarians and in the medical community. In order to maintain the standard of providing high-quality health information for the layperson the editorial staff at Omnigraphics felt it was necessary to implement a policy of updating volumes when warranted.

Medical researchers have been making tremendous strides, and it is the purpose of the *Health Reference Series* to stay current with the most recent advances. Each decision to update a volume will be made on an individual basis. Some of the considerations will include how much new information is available and the feedback we receive from people who use the books. If there is a topic you would like to see added to the update list, or an area of medical concern you feel has not been adequately addressed, please write to:

Editor
Health Reference Series
Omnigraphics, Inc.
615 Griswold Street
Detroit, MI 48226

The commitment to providing on-going coverage of important medical developments has also led to some format changes in the *Health Reference Series*. Each new volume on a topic is individually titled and called a "First Edition." Subsequent updates will carry sequential edition numbers. To help avoid confusion and to provide maximum flexibility in our ability to respond to informational needs, the practice of consecutively numbering each volume has been discontinued.

Part One

Compassion in Action: A Look at Caregiving in America

Chapter 1

The Invisible Caregiver: A Visible Problem

Caregivers are everywhere. Surveys show that 265 out of 1,000 adults recognize they are family caregivers—when you ask them a direct question—do you care for a spouse, child, parent, or other...? And even Americans who are not currently caregivers are aware of others who are. Forty-three percent say they know someone who is a family caregiver. But caregivers are also invisible.

"So much of caregiving is invisible to the outside world. Much of what goes on in bedrooms and in bathrooms deals with issues that the able-bodied and mentally-competent world take for granted: showering, toileting, dressing, moving, in some cases even breathing. And because of that, caregiving can be very isolating," NFCA president Suzanne Mintz said in a September press conference announcing the Caregiving Agenda for Action.

If You Don't Ask, Most Don't Tell

If you don't ask, very few people identify themselves as caregivers without some definition or prompting. That's why NFCA proposes even more caregiver outreach and self-identification projects in the years ahead.

This chapter includes the following copyrighted excerpts reprinted from "A National Report on the Status of Caregiving in America, November 1999," pp. 10-15 with permission of the National Family Caregivers Association, Kensington, MD, the nation's only organization for all family caregivers, 800-896-3650; www.nfcacares.org.

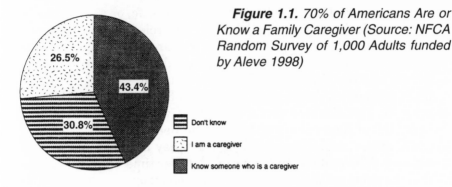

Figure 1.1. *70% of Americans Are or Know a Family Caregiver (Source: NFCA Random Survey of 1,000 Adults funded by Aleve 1998)*

Don't know

I am a caregiver

Know someone who is a caregiver

Figure 1.2. *59% of Americans Are or Expect to Be a Family Caregiver (Source: NFCA Random Survey of 1,000 Adults funded by Aleve 1998)*

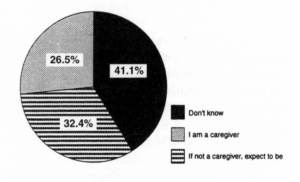

Don't know

I am a caregiver

If not a caregiver, expect to be

Figure 1.3. *Many Felt a Strong Sense of Isolation and Loss of Personal Time (Source: NFCA/ Fortis Report* Caregiving Across the Life Cycle *1998)*

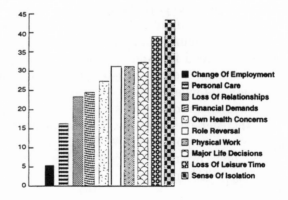

- Change Of Employment
- Personal Care
- Loss Of Relationships
- Financial Demands
- Own Health Concerns
- Role Reversal
- Physical Work
- Major Life Decisions
- Loss Of Leisure Time
- Sense Of Isolation

"You see yourself as a good mom, or a good wife, or a good daughter, and you don't realize you have this other role," Lauren Agoratus of Hamilton, mother of a special needs 7-year-old daughter and the New Jersey area coordinator for the National Family Caregivers Association, told the *Newark Star Ledger* in August.

Most of America's more-than-25-million family caregivers for the elderly, ill, and disabled at home—collectively providing approximately 80% of America's long-term home health care—are so busy juggling duties, schedules, and finances, they never realize they're caregivers. "The realization dawns on you over time," Suzanne Mintz said in the same article. "We caregivers often struggle alone for years thinking: This is just part of our responsibility, as a parent, adult child, spouse, or sibling before we reach out for help. Realizing one is a caregiver can be the beginning of regaining a sense of balance and well-being."

Donna Wagner, director of gerontology at Towson University in Maryland, thinks one reason caregivers don't self-identify is that caregiving tends to be either intermittent or all consuming. When intermittent, it doesn't pack an overwhelming punch and so doesn't generate the passionate concern needed to propel a movement—and when all consuming, it is so overwhelming and isolating that many caregivers don't have the time or energy to stand up and be counted.

Caregivers Want a Voice

But despite these barriers—or perhaps because of them—caregivers do want a voice—they do want to be heard and when presented with a message that promotes caregiver self-advocacy, caregiver self-worth, caregiver value, they begin to become empowered and this is the first step in building a grassroots caregiver movement. But empowerment doesn't come right away—it requires time and a repetition of the message.

In its 1999 Member Impact Survey, the National Family Caregivers Association found that caregivers believe that NFCA can accomplish the most good for America's family caregivers by being their advocate—telling their stories, promoting awareness of caregiver concerns, broadening awareness of meaningful statistics about caregiving and its impacts on individuals and society, and advocating for their rights.

NFCA's particular message of caregiver self-advocacy is viewed as extremely important (95%) and a message that should be communicated more broadly. Support for this message of self-advocacy, at least among NFCA members, the majority of who are providing intensive

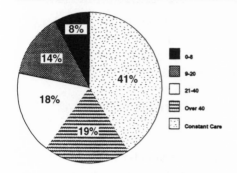

Figure 1.4. For Most Caregivers, Caregiving Is Equivalent to a Full Time Job (Source: NFCA/Fortis Report Caregiving Across the Life Cycle 1998)

Figure 1.5. 76% Get No Help from Other Family Members (Source: NFCA/Fortis Report Caregiving Across the Life Cycle 1998)

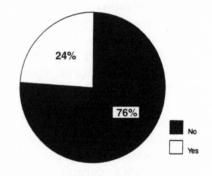

Figure 1.6. Most Caregivers Wait 4-5 Years before Reaching Out for Help and Support (Source: NFCA 1999 Impact Study)

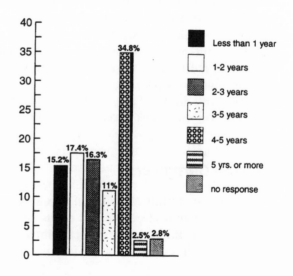

levels of care, is universal and cuts across categories of age, length of time being a caregiver, and relationship to care recipient. It can serve as a good model for empowering caregivers in a broad range of circumstances and has already empowered 55% of NFCA members.

Caregivers Want Information but Don't Easily Reach Out for Help

As much as caregivers want a voice to impact change over the long haul, on a day to day level they are hungry for information to help them cope and to lessen their isolation. But that doesn't mean that caregivers easily reach out for information and support. Many caregivers cope quietly on their own for years before seeking outside assistance. Caregivers want information, but caregiving breeds isolation and creates a tug of war between need and the ability to satisfy the need. Whether caregivers aren't asking or others aren't seriously offering is not clear, but most caregivers are going it alone. Seventy-six percent of NFCA caregivers don't get consistent help from other family members. Spouses get the least at 16%.

What Is of Concern to Caregivers

As much as caregivers want a voice and need information, one of their primary concerns is being a good caregiver. This is particularly true among caregivers between the ages of 25-64, who are also concerned about the stress and anxiety that accompanies the caregiving role. Older caregivers are understandably concerned about their own health. When you realize that in this day and age of increasing numbers of octogenarians, we have an unheard of phenomenon of the old caring for the even older, this is not surprising.

Although finances play a significant role in caregiving, when it comes to what caregivers worry about most, it isn't money. If there was ever any doubt about the widespread existence of strong family values in America, NFCA's Aleve-funded survey should put that question to rest.

Rallying Caregivers

Building a caregiver movement is not an easy endeavor, but it is obviously a worthwhile, and in today's world, a necessary one. The barriers are formidable but the message is clear—caregivers do want to be heard, they want change for themselves and their loved ones, and as many studies have shown when provided with information and support, when empowered, they are better able to take on the challenge of both their caregiving role and their own defense.

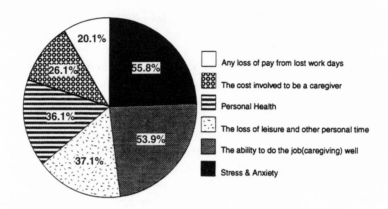

Figure 1.7. *Major Concerns of Caregivers of All Ages (Source: NFCA Random Survey of 1,000 Adults funded by Aleve 1998)*

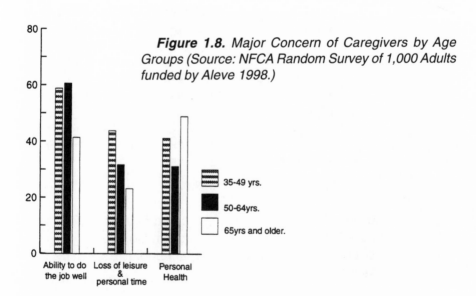

Figure 1.8. *Major Concern of Caregivers by Age Groups (Source: NFCA Random Survey of 1,000 Adults funded by Aleve 1998.)*

Table 1.1. The 25 States with the Largest Population of Caregivers*

States	Value (Millions of Dollars)	Number of Caregivers	Caregiving Hours (Millions)
California	22,914.3	3,009,523	2,801.3
Texas	13,636.0	1,790,931	1,667.0
New York	13,525.3	1,776,382	1,653.5
Florida	11,214.6	1,472,899	1,371.0
Pennsylvania	9,155.1	1,202,411	1,119.2
Illinois	8,651,4	1,136,260	1,057.6
Ohio	8,298.3	1,089,878	1,014.5
Michigan	7,207.8	946,663	881.2
New Jersey	6,059.2	795,802	740.7
North Carolina	5,508.7	723,498	673.4
Georgia	5,422.7	712,203	662.9
Virginia	5,033.5	661,094	615.3
Massachusetts	4,645.9	610,184	468.0
Indiana	4,327.1	568,307	529.0
Washington	4,113.6	540,272	502.9
Tennessee	4,021.2	428,142	491.6
Missouri	3,974.1	521,950	485.8
Maryland	3,803.5	499,539	465.0
Wisconsin	3,791.8	498,009	463.5
Minnesota	3,403.7	447,037	416.1
Arizona	3,243.4	425,977	396.5
Alabama	3,221.8	423,143	393.9
Louisiana	3,119.2	409,665	381.3
Kentucky	2,921.3	383,673	357.1

*Source: Study conducted by Peter S. Arno and Margaret Memmott of the Montefiore Medical Center/Albert Einstein College of Medicine and Carol Levine of the United Hospital Fund. Prepared for the Alzheimer's Association.

Chapter 2

The Caregiving Years

Six Stages to a Meaningful Journey

When you expect a child, the community (your family, friends, co-workers) rally around you and your spouse. When you expect your first child, you receive gifts, well wishes and the encouragement that you are entering a wonderful, albeit challenging, chapter in your life. As you prepare to welcome your child, you feel pride at the thought of your role as parent: How you will shape the mind of a youngster, impacting him or her with your wisdom, insights, and knowledge.

Now think about a similar life experience, just one on the other end of the spectrum. An aging relative, a spouse, a parent, a grandparent, needs your help. And, you want to help—you believe in making the most of the years you have left together. But, when you tell your friends, your colleagues, even other family members, the comments you may hear are a far cry from well-wishes. "I could never do that! Why do you?" Or, the more common response: "Why don't you just put your mother (or your wife, or your grandfather) in a nursing home? That way you won't be so stressed out."

With support like that, no wonder you might find yourself fighting self-doubts during your caregiving journey, asking yourself, "Why me? Why am I the one to do this?" These self-doubts can erode your

Reprinted with permission, "The Caregiving Years," © 1998 Denise M. Brown, *Caregiving Newsletter*.

ability to handle your caregiving responsibilities effectively and efficiently. Even worse, these self-doubts cloud your ability to understand how important this caregiving journey is to your care recipient, your family, and yourself.

This chapter describes what to expect throughout the caregiving journey. By having information about your role as caregiver—understanding what information to gather and the actions to take—you can spend more time making this experience meaningful, for your care recipient, your family, and yourself.

This topic is separated into six stages, each stage defined by the number of years spent as a caregiver. But these definitions were created to use only as a guide. Your care recipient's illness and diagnosis will determine how quickly or slowly you pass through the stages. While the length of time spent in each stage may differ for each caregiver, the emotions and experiences felt will remain constant.

Stage I: The Expectant Caregiver

Who are you? You have a growing concern that within the next 12 to 18 months or so, your aging relative will need more and more of your assistance and time. You're concerned because of your relative's age, past and present medical condition, and current living condition.

Your purpose: You expect to become a caregiver; this is your time to prepare. You should research options, gather information, and provide the opportunity for your care recipient to share his or her feelings and values. This is also your time to concentrate on taking care of yourself—keeping up with family and friends, enjoying your hobbies and interests, pursing your career goals, taking trips you've always dreamed of.

Although an immediate crisis may not face you, the threat of one seems to hang in the horizon. Rather than closing your eyes to avoid seeing that horizon, you can take some proactive steps now that will make your future caregiving days easier.

What You Can Do as an "Expectant Caregiver"

1. **Consult with a good lawyer familiar with eldercare issues**. Find out about durable powers of attorney for health care and living wills; start the process to ensure that the necessary legal papers in order.

2. **Determine financial situations.** Knowing the financial status can help determine future health care choices. Determine monthly income from pensions and social security; learn about annuities, stock investments, and bank accounts.

3. **Investigate community health care options.** What home health care agencies in the area offer quality, affordable home care? What housing options are available: retirement communities, assisted living centers? Contact community organizations to request brochures and pamphlets.

   In addition, consider your aging relative's current living condition. Will your aging relative be able to reside safely in her home if she uses a wheelchair, becomes bed-bound? What changes can you make today that will prevent future barriers to providing care in her home? Or, are the necessary changes almost an impossibility? If so, what other options do you have: your home, an assisted living facility, a retirement community?

4. **Determine the current health care providers.** Who are the physicians, and what is the diagnosis? In addition, learn about medications and why the medications have been prescribed.

5. **Concentrate on the reality of the situations.** Keep a realistic view of the situation. What's the worst that could happen? What's the best possible outcome? Then, determine what options are available for each of these outcomes.

6. **Start a journal; chronicle your feelings, your concerns, and your actions**. You may be surprised at your feelings of loss. Your preparation of the future allows you to see what your care recipient and you might lose. You both will experience changes in your relationship, your schedules, and your amount of freedom. Write down your thoughts about the potential losses and how you might be able to hang on to them, through minor adjustments and changes, for a little longer.

Stage II: "The Freshman Caregiver"

Who are you? You have been caring for an aging relative for six months to 18 months. Your duties range from running errands and paying bills to hands-on care.

Your purpose: This is your entry into the caregiving role. This is your time to experiment, to get your feet wet and see what works. This is your opportunity to learn how the health care industry works with, or in some cases, against you. Now is the time to shape your caregiving personality: What duties are you comfortable with? What duties make you uncomfortable? How well are you and your care recipient getting along? What situations would create overwhelming stress for both of you? What situations should you try to avoid because you know they will lead to nasty fights and bitter arguments?

You'll get a feel for the present and future budgets needed to provide the care your care recipient requires. In addition, keep up with your hobbies and interests (you may be able only to keep the ones that you enjoy most), ensuring you have made a habit of spending time on your own, enjoying yourself.

What You Can Do as a "Freshman Caregiver"

1. Learn as much as you can about your care recipient's illness, disease, or condition. Consult the local branches or chapters of national organizations such as the Arthritis Foundation, the Alzheimer's Association, the Cancer Society. What does the future hold for you and your care recipient?

2. Learn how to provide proper care from health care professionals or from health care videos, manuals, or books. If your care recipient is hospitalized or receives short-term therapy at a nursing home, ask the staff to show you proper caregiving techniques: lifting, transfers, bathing. Or, search the Internet for hands-on care information. It's very difficult to provide care when you are unsure of what you're doing. You'll feel much better when you're confident of your skills.

3. Join a support group—online or in your community. It's so isolating to be a caregiver! Support groups will hook you up with others in similar situations; often, you'll learn of community resources and options from other caregivers of which you were not aware.

4. Count on regular breaks from caregiving. You can't be a good caregiver to someone else if you don't take care of yourself. Plan for regular breaks—an hour daily, an afternoon weekly, or a day monthly—whatever you can manage. Enlist the help of relatives and community services (such as a volunteer group at your local

church) so you can take time off regularly. Relatives can help in many ways through financial support, social support (calling the care recipient regularly just "to talk"), as well as respite support.

5. Rely on help from community organizations. Meals on Wheels, home care agencies, and day care centers, to name just a few, may offer services that your care recipient needs.

   Contact your local Area Agency on Aging for a listing of services and organizations in your community. Visit your local medical equipment supply store to find devices and gadgets that enhance your care recipient's abilities and independence from you. Remember, allowing the help of others is a sign of strength!

   In addition, ask about local, state, or federal programs that might provide financial assistance for you and/or your care recipient. As your care recipient's care needs increase, so will the costs associated with his or her care. Understanding what programs can help, in addition to understanding what your care recipient can afford, will help you plan appropriately for the future.

6. Keep in mind what your care recipient's wishes are. If appropriate, ask for his or her input and ideas. Does your care recipient still feel good about living at home? What does your care recipient fear or dread? (These are also good questions to ask yourself!)

7. Reflect the changes in your journal. How do you feel now? What are your concerns? Fears? What outcomes are you working toward? What losses have you noticed during this period? What changes in the relationship cause you to feel sad? What changes have given you comfort?

Stage III: "The Entrenched Caregiver"

Who are you? You've been involved in your care recipient's care for two to five years. Your involvement is almost daily—if not constant. Your care recipient may live with you or your involvement means that your day is structured to be available to your care recipient. You begin to wonder, how much longer can you live this way? Your mood is sometimes upbeat—you're proud you've been able to provide such wonderful care and make decisions that support your care recipient's best wishes—and sometimes melancholy—why you? You've been mourning the loss of your care recipient's abilities and functions and often long for the days before caregiving. And, you're tired.

Your purpose: To develop a routine, create a familiar schedule for both yourself and your care recipient. A routine will help you deal with the overwhelming stresses and responsibilities that wear you out. A routine will provide comfort for you and your care recipient. This stage may be the most difficult for both of you. The changes you prepared for in Stage I and II are now a reality—you have become something of a lifeline to a family member or friend.

What You Can Do as an "Entrenched Caregiver"

1. **Determine your limits.** How long can your care recipient remain at home? What's your comfort level in providing care in your home? For instance, some caregivers feel uncomfortable providing care when their care recipients become incontinent. Others determine they can provide care at home as long as Medicare or insurance benefits offset some of the home care expenses. Others feel that can provide care as long as their other family members, like spouses and adult children, will put up with it. Everyone has a limit. What is yours?

2. **Continue regular breaks.** Consider annual weekly breaks. Investigate short-term respite stays in your community's nursing homes. Or, ask relatives to take over the caregiving role for a week or two every year or every two years. Continue to take daily, weekly, and monthly breaks. Keep up with your own interests and hobbies as best you can.

3. **Keep up with a support system**. Join a caregiver's support group and nurture empathetic and understanding family members and friends.

4. **Continue to learn** about your care recipient's illness or condition. What's next for your care recipient? Are you up to the next steps in his or her illness?

5. **Start a second journal** that you use to detail your care recipient's needs and your caregiving responsibilities. Note any changes in your care recipient's health and condition so that you can confidently discuss your concerns during physician appointments. Continue to chronicle your caregiving journey in your first journal. What causes you to mourn?

Stage IV: "The Pragmatic Caregiver"

Who are you? You've been caregiver for more than five years. You've been through it all: hospital admission and discharges; short-term rehab stays in nursing homes; and a vast array of community services. You may appear to doubt the advice given by health care professionals; you've just been through the health care system long enough to know that sometimes health care professionals may not seem to have your best interest in mind.

Some family members and health care professionals worry about your ability to find humor in situations they find offensive. They view your attitude as "calloused" and "uncaring." Far from it, you have a very practical, very realistic approach toward your caregiving role—and your sense of humor has been a critical tool for your survival. Without your sense of humor, you would have given up a long time ago.

Your Purpose: To gain a better understanding of yourself and your care recipient. You've settled into your role and your routine; now is your opportunity to step back and reflect. The first three stages laid the groundwork for this stage, your period of personal growth.

What You Can Do as a "Pragmatic Caregiver"

1. **Work on finding joy in your relationship** with your care recipient. The biggest joy-killers are your hands-on duties: bathing, dressing, incontinence care. But these duties bring you together, this is your time together. Add some fun to your hands-on care: sing songs, tell jokes, share goals and dreams.

2. **Work on forgiving your care recipient** for past hurts. Resentment toward past wrong and injustices will make your present caregiving role very difficult. Let go of what was and concentrate on making what is healthy and productive.

3. **Develop a habit of enjoying shared activities.** Develop a routine of time shared as husband-wife, mother-daughter, father-son rather than as just caregiver and care recipient. Releasing the roles of caregiver and care recipient allows you to enjoy each other.

4. **Begin to think about your future**. What goals have you yet to achieve? How can you achieve them? Can your care recipient help you achieve them?

Stage V: "The Transitioning Caregiver"

Who are you? You've been a caregiver over a period of several years and have recently made a decision about your role as caregiver. Or, your care recipient's condition has taken a turn for the worse and you know his time is very limited. As a result, you've changed your role—or are just about to change your role.

Your purpose: To walk with your care recipient during his last months and weeks, implementing his or her decisions about end-of-life care that you both discussed during Stage I. This stage is about loving and feeling good about the shared journey. As you both feel the journey end, this is also a time to mourn and grief. As you mourn, you might find yourself questioning what will be the next chapter in your life. You've been a caregiver for so long, can you possibly do anything else?

What You Can Do as a "Transitioning Caregiver"

1. **Allow yourself time to mourn and grief.** This is a time of experiencing and feeling tremendous losses. For caregivers facing the nursing home decision, this may be a time of greater mourning than when your care recipient dies.

2. **Remember your care recipient.** You don't have to give away clothes or remove pictures until you want to. When family and friends seem hesitant to talk about your care recipient (they worry they will upset you), assure them that sharing memories, laughs, and stories brings you great comfort.

3. **Reflect back** on your caregiving responsibilities and decisions with pride. Find comfort in knowing that you did the best you could.

4. **Review your journal.** How are you different today than you were on the day you first started writing in your journal? How will you use this experience to enhance your future relationships?

Stage VI: "The Godspeed Caregiver"

Who are you? Your role as caregiver ended more than two years ago. You find yourself compelled to make a difference in the lives of other caregivers. You share information readily with caregivers in the earlier stages, you start a business dedicated to helping family caregivers or you find a job in which you assist family caregivers. And, you treasure each relationship you have in your life, recognizing that each day, and your health, should never be taken for granted.

Your Purpose: To implement your lessons learned from your role as caregiver, from your care recipient, and from your family members and friends. During this stage, which can last as long you wish—even your lifetime—you reap the benefits of your efforts.

What You Can Do as a "Godspeed Caregiver"

1. **Follow your dreams**. Make your goals your achievements.

2. **Share.** Family caregivers will look to you as a mentor and leader. Allow caregivers in earlier stages the same freedom to stumble and steady themselves that you had. Share your experiences with expectant caregivers, freshman caregivers, entrenched caregivers and pragmatic caregivers. They can learn from you!

3. **Treasure the memories** you have of your care recipient. Continue to remember your care recipient regularly through rituals, such as enjoying an ice cream cone in her honor on her birthday, or by planting trees in her name. Reading and reviewing your diary will be a great way to remember.

Your best memorial to your care recipient's memory is a life you build for yourself filled with healthy relationships, productive careers, joy, and laughter.

—Denise M. Brown

Denise M. Brown is the editor and publisher of *Caregiving Newsletter.*

Caregiving Newsletter
Tad Publishing Co.
P.O. Box 224
Park Ridge, IL 60068
Tel: 847-823-0639
Website: http://www.caregiving.com

Chapter 3

Who Provides Care?

Introduction

The field of research on family caregiving extends back forty years, evolving from early studies of the 1950s and 1960s looking at the family unit in general; to studies in the 1980s and early 1990s focusing on specific caregiving activities, roles and responsibilities; to the current emphasis on understanding the processes and impacts of caregiving across different physical and mental conditions and ethnically diverse populations. We have progressed from small descriptive studies of available caregiving populations—usually service utilizing—to larger local area and national studies of random samples. Methodology and instrumentation have similarly improved, with current study designs and analyses being more sophisticated and comprehensive. The result is that we have considerable knowledge about who needs care, who receives care, who provides this care, what care is provided, the costs of care, and the impacts of this care on the caregiver. This chapter summarizes what we have learned from many studies on informal caregiving, identifies issues in need of further study, and discusses the implications of empirical data for selected policy and practice issues regarding long-term care for frail older individuals.

"Family Caregiving in an Aging Society," by Sharon Tennstedt, Ph.D., presented at the U.S. Administration on Aging Symposium: Longevity in the New American Century, Baltimore, MD, March 29, 1999, Administration on Aging (AoA).

Who Needs Care

Nearly one-quarter (22.9%) of all people aged 65 and over in this country are functionally disabled or currently in need of some form of long-term care (American Academy of Actuaries, 1999; Doty, 1986; NCHS, 1987). According to a monograph recently released by the American Academy of Actuaries (1999), the best care scenario projects that by the year 2040 the population of severely disabled (i.e., >3 ADLs) elderly will increase by 90%. This means that they need help with personal activities of daily living (bathing, eating, dressing, toileting), with instrumental activities of daily living (cooking, cleaning, laundry, transportation, etc.), with transfer or mobility, or they require skilled care of the sort provided by home health care agencies or nursing homes. Data have revealed that 1.2 million fewer older adults in 1994 were disabled than had been expected based on previous rates, but the actual scenario takes this recent trend into consideration. However, although the rates are lower, persons turning 65 (in 1996) can expect 5.3 years of dysfunction characterized by acute or chronic illness.

Who Receives Care

To be distinguished from who needs care is who receives care. Whether some older people are more likely than others to receive informal care at all, or to receive greater amounts of assistance, has implications for appropriate targeting of services to subgroups with unmet need, or with patterns for service delivery to certain subgroups. Looking first at the likelihood of receiving informal care, noteworthy differences emerged when those people who rely on formal services for most of their care are compared with those who receive all of their help from informal caregivers. We have found that those who were not married, lived alone, and lived in public housing were less likely to have informal caregivers available for assistance and therefore more likely to rely on formal services for assistance. This describes the typical senior housing resident (McKinlay and Tennstedt, 1986).

Turning to variations in the levels or amounts of informal care provided, differences have been associated with the degree of disability, the gender of the elder, as well as with the elder's living arrangement. Most studies report a direct relationship between the elder's degree of functional disability and receipt of informal care (Sherwood et al., 1981; Horowitz and Dobrof, 1982; Branch and Jette, 1983). That is, those elders with the most impairment receive significantly more informal care than those who are minimally or moderately impaired (McKinlay and Tennstedt, 1986). It is interesting, however, that an expected simple linear relationship between level of frailty and receipt of care, where moderately impaired elders receive more care than minimally impaired elders, was not apparent in this study conducted in Massachusetts (Table 3.1). Minimally and moderately impaired elders received similar amounts of informal care, indicating a possible threshold of impairment, at which the amount of such care increases substantially. This apparent threshold may be related to:

- an increase in the number and scope of needs, necessitating a wider variety of help and more intensive care;

- a preference by elders for care by their families;

- the family's sense of responsibility for providing care;

- the greater ability of informal care to meet specific needs (e.g., flexibility in response, intimate knowledge of elder); and/or

- problems with access, availability, or limitations of formal services (e.g., restricted hours/functions, staff shortages, reimbursement issues).

Further, the receipt of informal care increases far more dramatically than the use of formal services with an increase in disability. These data underscore the predominance of informal care even at a point when use of more formal services might be expected.

Table 3.1. Average Hours Per Week of Care from Informal and Formal Sources by Level of Frailty

Frailty Level	Informal	Formal
Minimal	33	8
Moderate	27	6
Severe	60	9

Gender clearly influences the type and amount of informal care received. While women are more likely than men to receive help from informal caregivers, it does not appear that they also receive more such care. Consistent with other findings (Branch and Jette, 1983), our Massachusetts data indicate that, controlling for functional status, men receive more care than women (Tennstedt and McKinlay, 1989). This finding may be a function of the time required to perform gender specific types of care received. Older men are more likely to receive help with personal care, housekeeping tasks, and meals, activities which may require more time than the assistance with transportation, shopping, and home repairs which were more frequently received by women. In addition, while men receive more care, on average they are likely to get that help from only one person, usually their spouse. Older women, on the other hand, have larger numbers of caregivers, typically two to four.

These differences in types and related amounts of assistance received are probably related to both traditional gender/social role behavior, as well as the influence of gender/social role stereotypes on perception of need for help. Older people most likely continue to do those tasks of daily living with which they feel familiar, and for which they have skills, and to receive help in those areas with which they are unfamiliar or less skilled. Conceptual models of utilization behavior (e.g., Anderson and Newman, 1973; Mechanic, 1962) have often related use of services to perceived need, as distinguished from objective need determined by functional assessment of health indicators. Older men and women appear to perceive their need for assistance differently. One male respondent who was physically able to perform household tasks, yet received substantial help, told us that he would rather starve than learn to cook his own meals! Similarly, caregivers' expectations of the elder may differ according to the elder's gender, and therefore be an additional determinant of the type of informal care provided. For example, caregivers may be more likely to provide meals for older men because they do not expect them to cook for themselves.

Finally, our data and that of others indicate that an elder's living arrangement is an important predictor of the level of care received (Tennstedt and McKinlay, 1989). Elders living with a spouse (78 hours/week) or others (66 hours/week) were likely to receive substantially more care than those who lived alone (9 hours/week). Our data also indicate that those living alone are nearly twice as likely to use paid formal help (Tennstedt et al., 1993a). It should be noted that living alone has consistently emerged in studies as a major predictor of institutionalization of the elderly (Shanas, 1979; Kahana and Kiyak, 1980; Prohaska and McAuley, 1983), having important implications for identification of subgroups most in need of community services.

Who Provides Care

Families have always been and continue to be the primary source of help to disabled elders. It is estimated nationally that family and friends are the sole source of assistance for nearly three-quarters of impaired older adults in the community (Doty, 1986). They are also the preferred source of help for most elders (Shanas et al., 1968; Comptroller General of the U.S., 1977; Eggert et al., 1977; U.S. DHEW, 1978; Cantor and Johnson, 1978; Community Council of N.Y., 1978; Branch and Jette, 1983; McAuley and Arling, 1984; McKinlay and Tennstedt, 1986; Stone et al., 1987). In 1996, the National Alliance for Caregiving and AARP conducted a nationwide telephone survey to identify and profile the experiences of caregiving (National Alliance for Caregiving and American Association for Retired Persons, 1997). This survey provides the most recent national data on a random sample of households in the U.S. The sampling strategies ensured the inclusion of minorities and enabled the identification of caregivers for persons age 50 and over with a variety of disabling conditions. This data set provides our most current prevalence estimates of caregiving—the experiences and impacts. Based on results of this survey, nearly one in four U.S. households with a telephone contained at least one caregiver (defined as currently or previously providing care within the last 12 months to a relative or friend at least 50 years old). This translates into 22.4 million caregiving households nationwide during the 12-month period of study.

The findings of the NAC/AARP study are overwhelmingly consistent with data from earlier studies. The majority of caregivers are women. The NAC/AARP study reports that 72.5% of the national sample of caregivers were female. Any small differences in gender in other studies is likely related to the age inclusion criterion for the care recipient. Average age of caregivers is similarly influenced by the age of care recipients—the older the care recipient, the older the caregiver.

Consistently across all studies of caregiving and as has been reported in the NAC/AARP study, spouses are the first source of caregiving assistance. Likely related to the nature of the marital relationship, spouses are often the sole caregiver (Stone, Cafferata, and Sangl, 1987; Tennstedt, McKinlay, and Sullivan, 1989) and provide the most extensive and comprehensive care (Cantor, 1983; Horowitz, 1985; Johnson, 1983; McKinlay and Tennstedt, 1986; Shanas 1979; Soldo and Myllyuoma, 1983; Stephens and Christianson, 1986; Stone, Cafferata, and Sangl, 1987). This holds true for caregivers of elders with dementia or with functional disabilities only. Offspring are usually the next source of informal care, also for both groups, with daughters more likely than sons to be in this role. Friends and neighbors are mobilized in the absence of family caregivers, or as supplemental sources of assistance (Cantor and Johnson, 1978; Sherwood et al., 1981; Shuval et al., 1982; Stoller and Earl, 1983; McKinlay and Tennstedt, 1986). However, caregiving for elders with dementia is less frequent among extended kin or non-kin, likely because of the greater commitment and involvement required.

An important point about gender and relationship of caregivers. While females predominate in the role, our longitudinal study in Massachusetts has reported that spousal caregivers are just as likely to be male as female (Tennstedt et al., 1993a). Further, these men were more likely to be the sole caregiver, with no assistance from others (Tennstedt et al., 1989). That is, male spousal caregivers are similar to female spousal caregivers.

Data have shown that generally caregiving is not a shared activity. Consistent with several other studies (Horowitz, 1978; Frankfather, Smith, and Caro, 1981; Horowitz and Dobrof, 1982; Johnson, 1983; Stoller and Earl, 1983; National Alliance for Caregiving and American Association for Retired Persons, 1997), we found that one person tends to provide the majority of informal care. Secondary caregivers are often few in number and provide much less care, and then on an intermittent basis. Further, our data indicate that women—usually daughters—caregivers are more likely than men to receive assistance from others in caring for the older person and that these secondary caregivers are often the caregiver's spouse and children (Tennstedt et al., 1989). This focusing of caregiving responsibilities on a nuclear family unit has obvious implications for potential negative impact, which may, in turn, contribute to increased risk of institutionalization of the elder.

Caregivers typically live in close proximity to the care recipient. The NAC/AARP survey (1997) reports that 20% share a household and another 55% live less than 20 minutes from the care recipient. This proximity clearly facilitates the provision of care. A decision to co-reside is often related to the elder's need for care. However, residential proximity likely also influences who in an extended family assumes the primary caregiving role. If there is a choice, the adult child who lives close by and has few competing responsibilities (not employed, not married, few or no children) is the likely candidate.

In the last 10 years, there has been increasing attention to differences in caregiving across ethnic groups. The early comparative studies focused primarily on comparisons of African-Americans and Whites.

More recently, researchers have studied Hispanic and Asian sub-groups as well. The NAC/AARP survey (1997) included Whites, Blacks, Hispanics, and Asians. They reported higher incidence of caregiving among Asian-American (31.7%), African-American (29.4%), and Hispanic (26.8%) households than in the general population. The larger and modified extended families of African-Americans and Hispanics are thought to increase the informal care resources of older persons in these two groups (Chatters et al., 1985, 1986; Montgomery and Hirshorn, 1990; Delgado and Humm, 1982). In fact, caregivers in these three minority groups are more likely than in the general population to provide care for more than one person. They were also more likely than White caregivers to live with the care recipient and to have help from other persons (National Alliance for Caregiving, 1998).

Types and Amounts of Informal Care

Studies have shown that informal caregivers provide a wide variety of assistance, with emotional support often cited as the most common activity (Horowitz and Dobrof, 1982; Shuval et al., 1982; McKinlay and Tennstedt, 1986; Stone et al., 1987). As displayed in Table 3.2, caregivers in the NAC/AARP study provided help with many instrumental tasks. Data in Table 3.2, however, indicate that help with personal care is less frequent. Although sometimes mentioned, generally financial contributions are not an important type of assistance, although out-of-pocket expenses may be incurred in providing

Table 3.2. Assistance with Instrumental ADLs

Instrumental Activity of Daily Living	Percent Receiving Assistance
Transportation	79%
Grocery Shopping	77%
Housework	74%
Meal Preparation	60%
Managing Finances	56%
Arranging/Supervising Outside Services	54%
Medications	37%
No IADL Assistance	2%

Source: National Alliance for Caregiving and AARP, 1997

care. It appears that families are more inclined to provide services directly than to purchase them for the elder (Horowitz and Dobrof, 1982; McKinlay and Tennstedt, 1986). However, recent data from the NAC/AARP survey (1997) show that caregivers in higher income categories are more likely than those with less income to purchase in-home services.

The type of care provided by a specific caregiver appears related to gender-expected activity. Female caregivers typically provide personal care, housekeeping tasks, and meals, while male caregivers provide assistance with home repairs, transportation, and financial management (Treas, 1977; Horowitz and Dobrof, 1982; Stoller and Earl, 1983).

However, one cannot assume that because women are more likely to provide care, that they also provide larger amounts of care. Only a few studies have explored whether the actual amount of care varies by the caregiver's gender, and the results of these studies are less consistent (Stoller and Earl, 1983; McKinlay and Tennstedt, 1986; Stone et al., 1987). In our sample (Tennstedt et al., 1993a), we found that male and female spousal caregivers provided similar amounts of care. However, all other female caregivers were found to provide considerably more help than male caregivers. Similar results were found in the National Long Term Care Survey (Stone et al, 1987) and in the National Alliance on Caregiving/AARP Study (1997). However, while observing these gender differences, it should be noted that both groups provide substantial amounts of care. According to the nationwide NAC/AARP Survey (1997), on average caregivers spend 18 hours per week on caregiving, with almost one-fifth (18.6%) of caregivers providing constant care for 40 or more hours per week. The difference

Table 3.3. Assistance with Personal ADLs

Transfer in/out of chairs	37%
Dressing	31%
Bathing	27%
Toileting	26%
Feeding	19%
No PADL Assistance	49%

Source: National Alliance for Caregiving and AARP, 1997

in hours may well be a function of the time and frequency of contact required to provide different types of care (e.g., meals vs. home repairs). This underscores the importance of considering both type and amount of care when examining differential impact of helping activities on the caregiver.

Differences in amounts and types of care are directly influenced by the type and extent of the care recipient's impairment. The care recipient's profile of need for care can be based on duration (acute vs. chronic) or type of impairment (physical vs. cognitive vs. combined). Most acute situations involve physical conditions and require care provision at potentially high levels for time-limited periods. Sometimes these situations do not even get defined as caregiving by those providing assistance because of the short duration. They are considered similar to care of any illness or injury of a family member of any age. The situations defined as caregiving usually involve chronic conditions necessitating long-term care, including both physical and cognitive impairments. A distinction between dementia care and non-dementia care has been made by researchers recently to study differences in the caregiving experiences. According to NAC/AARP (1997) data, 22% of caregivers report that their care recipients suffer from dementia. As would be expected, dementia caregivers provide more hours of care (19.0 vs. 12.5 hrs), more types of care, and were more likely to help with personal ADLs than were non-dementia caregivers (National Alliance on Caregiving and Alzheimer's Association, 1999).

The proximity of the caregiver to the care recipient is a critical factor in determining the pattern of care. In particular, if the caregiver and care recipient co-reside, there will be greater caregiving involvement and less use of formal services (Chappell, 1991; Diwan, 1997; Tennstedt et al., 1993a), regardless of caregiver relationship (Tennstedt et al., 1993a). Co-residence is more likely for dementia caregivers, especially at later stages of disease, which likely accounts for the greater caregiving involvement when compared to all non-dementia caregivers. Yet, the relationship between co-residence and lower use of selected dementia services has also been reported (Gill et al., 1998). Proximity to the care recipient is less of an issue in the provision of short-term or "crisis" care. Himes and colleagues (1996) have reported no difference in amount of care by those living with or very near the care recipient and by those caregivers more distant when the care was for a time-limited period. This is less relevant for primary caregivers in the care of elders with dementia, underscoring the importance of proximity or co-residence in the provision of care.

The employment status—a competing responsibility—of the caregiver has been related to the level of care provided, but results across studies have been quite inconsistent. However, most studies including the NAC/AARP survey (1997) report that employment has no effect on the amount of care provided. Instead, it appears that employed caregivers make accommodations in their work schedule or arrangements in order to meet caregiving responsibilities.

Ethnic or racial differences in types and amounts of care have also been studied. At the bivariate level, many studies (National Alliance on Caregiving and American Association for Retired Persons, 1997; Hays and Mindel, 1973; Cantor, 1979; Mitchell and Register, 1984; Tennstedt et al., 1998) have reported that minority caregivers provide more care than do White caregivers. Typically, cultural differences (e.g., greater familial reciprocity) have been assumed to account for this. Others assert that the increased disability of minority elders accounts for higher levels of caregiving. In our cross-cultural comparative study, we found that even when controlling for disability, caregivers in the two minority groups provided more care than did White caregivers (Tennstedt and Chang, 1998).

It is commonly thought that the size and composition of the caregiving network influences the organization and provision of care. Larger networks of caregivers, closely related and/or very committed to providing care, are thought to result in sharing of caregiving responsibilities. This would seem particularly relevant in care for elders with dementing illness for whom needs for care are frequently great. The composition of the caregiving network evolves over time, influenced by the age, gender, and race of the care recipient, but is generally stable (Peek et al., 1997). Burton and colleagues (1995) have reported that the number of caregivers does not differ by race although others have reported that minority elders have more caregivers due to the involvement of modified extended families (Chatters et al., 1985, 1986; Miller et al., 1994; Hatch, 1991; Cox and Monk, 1990).

Yet in light of these data, it has been reported consistently that the primary caregiver provides most of the care. In a study by Stommel et al. (1995), which included both dementia and non-dementia caregivers, the primary caregiver provided assistance with IADLs almost exclusively, but help with ADLs was shared with others. Data from this study revealed no specific threshold at which secondary caregivers are involved, but involvement was more likely when a high frequency of care was needed. The primary pattern of division of labor was one of supplementation, i.e., that secondary caregivers shared the responsibility for specific tasks with the primary caregiver rather than a splitting up of tasks (or specialization) among the caregivers. Other data reported by these investigators (Stommel et al., 1998) indicate that division of labor is influenced by race. Consistent with the larger caregiving networks of African-Americans, these caregivers are more likely than White caregivers to share care with secondary helpers but again remain involved in most activities.

Interface of Informal and Formal Care

Division of labor also extends to the involvement of formal service providers. This interface between the informal and formal sources of care has been of public policy interest in response to the concern that changing social trends—smaller family size, increased geographic mobility, greater participation of women in the work force, and rising rates of marital disruption—will decrease the availability or willingness of family members to provide care to a disabled elder. Division of formal and informal labor is of concern from a clinical perspective in terms of timely and appropriate use of formal services to ensure the well-being of both care recipient and caregiver.

To address the first question, longitudinal data from the Massachusetts Elder Health Project (Tennstedt et al., 1993) were analyzed to determine if formal services ever replaced or substituted for informal care. We did find evidence of replacement of informal care by formal services in <20% of cases. This occurred when there was a change in the informal caregiving arrangement, particularly loss or change in the primary caregiver. It was also more likely if the primary caregiver had not been a close relative. Typically, the change or loss in caregiver was due to illness or death (an involuntary situation) of the caregiver rather than to competing demands as had been speculated. The data also indicated that this substitution of formal services for informal care was temporary and that informal care was again in place by the next contact. The data from this study show that service substitution is not a major trend and support the fact that formal services are being used as intended. This study was conducted in a state with a well-established, publicly funded home care program, which would have made substitution of formal services for informal care easier. However, the fact that service substitution was temporary and related to availability of the primary caregiver suggests that public funding for home care does not result in widespread and undesired service substitution. There were no data to suggest that large numbers of families were voluntarily withdrawing their help in favor of formal service use. Rather, these publicly funded services appear to be doing what they are intended to do: supporting and sustaining the informal caregiving arrangement or providing care during the disruption of this arrangement to keep the elder in the community.

More recently, data from the HCFA-funded Medicine Alzheimer's Disease Demonstration show consistent results for dementia caregiving situation (Yordi et al., 1997). This three-year study investigated the effects of expansion of community-based services and case management to over 5000 caregivers of dementia clients to test the effect of service expansion on levels of informal care. In a randomized trial, caregivers in the treatment group used slightly more care over time. However, there were no differences in primary caregiver hours or in the number of tasks by primary or secondary caregivers between caregivers in the treatment group vs. control group. An important finding in this study is the value of case management. That is, a decrease in the number of unmet needs and a better match between assistance needed and services received in the treatment group suggests that case management was beneficial.

In general, formal services are used by relatively few caregivers and care recipients. National data from both the *Supplement on Aging to the National Health Interview Survey* and the *1982 Long Term Care Survey* show that only a small proportion (9% and 5% respectively) receive all their care from formal, community-based providers (Doty, 1986). Further, only 26% of this formal community care is government financed. The remainder is privately paid by older people themselves and their families (U.S. Bureau of the Census, 1983; Soldo, 1983; Liu, Manton, and Liu, 1986). Clearly, the vast majority of long-term care is provided informally, and privately, at no public cost.

The involvement of a co-residing caregiver consistently has been related to lower use of formal services by elders with (Gill et al., 1998) and without dementing illness (Tennstedt et al., 1993a, 1996). Initial use, or increased use, of formal services usually occurs in the presence of informal care but when care needs increase or when there is a change in the primary caregiver (Tennstedt et al., 1993b, 1996). The use of formal services is more likely when the elder has ADL deficits (Diwan et al., 1997). There are no published longitudinal data about these transitions in dementia care. Similar to findings for elders with physical disabilities, cross-sectional data indicate that use of formal services is greater by elders with dementia who have greater functional impairment, live alone, and have higher incomes (Bass et al., 1992; Caserta et al., 1987; Gill et al., 1998; Mullan, 1993; Penning, 1995). Finally, use of services is lower among minority elders and caregivers than for White caregiving dyads (Tennstedt et al., 1998).

Costs of Care

Costs of care for elders with and without dementia have also been studied, with estimates made of the value of the informal care provided. Several years ago, Massachusetts Elder Health Project (MEHP) data were used to estimate costs of care for community-residing disabled elders (Harrow et al., 1995). The cost of informal caregiving hours was calculated using a market value approach. The costs of formal services were calculated using actual hourly rates for each type of service used. The total economic costs of community care (both informal care and formal services) were estimated at $9,552/year (in 1991 dollars). About 80% of these costs were for informal care, representing no expenditure of real dollars by individuals or by the government. As might be expected, cost estimates for informal care of elders with Alzheimer's disease are substantially higher, estimated by others in 1991-1992 to be between $43,600 (Max et al., 1995; Rice et al., 1993) and $38,900 (Weinberger et al., 1993). Similarly, from 80-90% of these costs were for informal care.

The MEHP cost estimates for type of care provide an interesting picture of how resources, both informal and formal, are being spent on community care. There is a consistent pattern over time, and for both informal care and formal services, for the majority of resources to be spent on housekeeping, personal care, and meals, in that order. Of interest here is that the majority of both informal and formal resources are expended in these areas of care. In other words, formal services are used to supplement care provided informally rather than to complement the informal care. This suggests that formal services are used where needs are greatest rather than to provide care for which services are best suited as proposed by Litwak (1985). These results also suggest that demand for services, particularly if the availability of informal care is diminished in the future, will be the greatest for home health aides, homemakers, and home delivered meal services.

MEHP data were also used to compare cost of community care to that of nursing home care. Two scenarios were compared to nursing home costs:

1. total actual costs of informal care and formal services, and
2. a simulation of all care provided by formal services only.

Average cost of nursing home care in Massachusetts in 1991 was $35,522. As previously stated, actual total costs of community care (both informal and formal) was $9,552. However, if all of this care were provided by formal services, the cost would be $13,799. While these costs for formal services are almost 50% higher than for combined informal care and formal services, the costs for meeting all of the elder's needs with formal services was less than half the cost of nursing home care. Even adding $7,200 for out-of-pocket expenditures on food and shelter, as taken from the Consumer Expenditure Survey (U.S. Bureau of the Census, 1992), community care was still less expensive than nursing home care for most disabled elders. It was only when an older person was severely disabled and required about 40 hours of care per week (equivalent to a full-time job for a caregiver) did the cost of community care plus living expenses approach or exceed the cost of nursing home care.

Most recently, the NAC/AARP data were used to develop a national estimate of the economic value of informal care (Arno et al., 1999). Using a market wage approach and a single wage rate, they developed three estimates—low, mid-range, and high—of the value of care (Table 3.4). Based on 17.9 weekly hours of care at $8.18 hourly wage and 25.8 million caregivers, the mid-range national estimate of the economic value of informal care in 1997 was $196 billion. Comparing it to available national spending for home care ($32 billion), nursing home care ($83 billion), and total health care ($1,092 billion), we see that the economic value of informal care is equivalent to approximately 18% of national health care spending and exceeds spending for home care and nursing home care combined.

Table 3.4. Economic Value of Informal Care Compared to National Expenditures (1997)

Home Care	$32 billion
Nursing Home Care	$83 billion
Informal Care	$196 billion
Total Health Care	$1,092 billion

Source: Arno et al, Health Affairs, 1999

Impacts of Care

For many years, researchers have focused on documenting burden among caregivers, and then on identification of which caregivers were most likely to be burdened. The personal, social, and health impacts of caregiving have now been well documented. However, it is critical to look separately at caregivers for elders with and without dementing illness. Their experiences are different. We must be careful not to generalize to all caregivers what we have learned about dementia caregivers. Most of the early studies of caregiver burden were of dementia caregivers. These early studies were often of non-representative samples identified through service agencies—caregivers who were more likely to be stressed. Measurement was less sophisticated in these early studies. The rates of burden reported from these studies were alarming and unfortunately were generalized to all caregivers. Questions were developed for these studies that asked directly about the stresses of caregiving. Measures in more recent studies include general physical and emotional health indicators of stress, such as depression, sick days, and health care utilization.

Given these multidimensional issues, what has been reported consistently across studies, including the recent NAC/AARP survey, is the constraints or restrictions of caregiving on time for leisure, social, and personal activities (National Alliance for Caregiving and Alzheimer's Association, 1999; McKinlay et al., 1995). Table 3.5 displays negative impacts for dementia and non-dementia caregivers. Overall, 55% of caregivers reported less time for other family members and giving up vacations, leisure time, or hobbies. This personal time restriction is greater when needs for care—as in dementia care—are greater (National Alliance for Caregiving and Alzheimer's Association, 1999). This makes ultimate sense—the more time one spends

Table 3.5. Impacts of Care

Impact	Dementia Caregivers	Non-Dementia Caregivers
Less time for families	56%	40%
Had to give up vacations, hobbies, own activities	53%	40%
Physical or mental health problems	23%	12%
Changes in Work Schedule	57%	47%
Change in Employment	Up to 13%	Up to 11%

Source: National Alliance for Caregiving and Alzheimer's Association, 1999

on caregiving, the less time one has for oneself. Other types of negative impacts are less frequently reported. In the NAC/AARP study (National Alliance for Caregiving and Alzheimer's Association, 1999), less than one-quarter reported physical or mental health problems as a result of caregiving. Again, however, these problems were more likely for dementia than for non-dementia caregivers. Accommodations to employment have been reported for up to one-fifth of caregivers. Also, more likely for dementia caregivers than non-dementia caregivers were decisions to change work schedules, turn down a promotion, and terminate employment entirely (Ory et al., 1999). Of important note, few caregivers in ethnic groups reported financial hardships as a result of their provision of care.

There has been considerable attention directed toward mental health impacts of caregiving. Depression and anxiety are the outcomes most frequently studied. Prevalence rates of depression among dementia caregivers have been as high as 43%-46% (Haley et al., 1987; Gallagher et al., 1989), nearly three-times the rates found among representative middle-aged and older populations (Eaton and Keisler, 1981; Frerichs et al., 1981). While rates of depression across studies of dementia caregivers vary, the consistent finding is that dementia care is psychologically distressing. The MEHP examined depression among non-dementia caregivers and found a rate of 35.2% or twice that in the general population. A comprehensive review by Schulz and colleagues (1995) has pointed out the bias in such findings introduced by the non-representative samples of most dementia caregiving studies, but also the robustness of the finding that caregiving is psychologically stressful.

The data regarding physical health effects of caregiving, however, are less strong. Caregivers often report their health to be worse than do non-caregivers. However, the results across studies are inconsistent (Schulz et al., 1995). We cannot draw clear conclusions from these data for any subgroup of caregivers. However, those caregivers reporting high psychological distress often also report health problems, alerting us to a potentially high risk group in need of intervention.

No clear conclusions can be drawn about ethnic differences in psychological or physical distress of caregivers. Again, there are inconsistent findings across studies with some reporting no differences in psychological or physical health outcomes and others reporting that White caregivers report more distress and burden (c.f. Calderon and Tennstedt, 1998; Ory et al., 1999). Given that minority elders are more disabled and receive more care, it is reasonable to expect that caregiver burden or distress would be higher. However, research to date does not generally support this. I would caution against quickly assuming that cultural differences (e.g., increased familism or reciprocity) mediate the negative effect of care on caregivers well-being. A recent qualitative analysis in NERI's cross-cultural comparative study raises the possibility that these lower levels of burden in minority caregivers are a product of the measures used in previous studies—measures developed with White populations. This analysis (Calderon and Tennstedt, 1998) reveals that minority caregivers express their distress differently than do White caregivers—using anger, frustration, and somatic complaints—which are not captured in the common measures of caregiver burden. It is incumbent upon researchers to develop culturally sensitive measures of caregiver distress.

This brings us to an area of increasing interest to researchers and one with important implications for service providers. Caregiving is not universally distressing. There are a great many caregivers who report minimal or no untoward effects of their helping role (McKinlay et al., 1995) and describe caregiving in positive terms (National Alliance for Caregiving, 1997). Researchers are now interested in factors that cause distress and, perhaps even more important, factors that mediate distress. It has been commonly assumed that caregiving distress is related to caregiving tasks—the more care provided, the more burden for the caregiver. More recent sophisticated analytical models have shown this not to be true (Schulz et al., 1995; Yates et al., 1999). Neither the disability status or the amount and type of care provided are related to caregiver burden. However, the manifestations of problem behaviors (wandering, hitting, disrobing) associated with AD or other dementias has been consistently related to greater caregiver burden and likely account for the differences between dementia caregivers and non-dementia caregivers in perceived burden.

Because the amount of care provided does not result in caregiver burden, the caregivers perception or appraisal of the caregiving demands has been of recent research interest. The MEHP measured this appraisal using a scale of role overload (Pearlin et al., 1990), which indicates how much an individual feels overwhelmed by the tasks of caregiving, specifically perceptions of exhaustion, having enough time for oneself and to do required tasks of caregiving, and perceived progress in terms of caregiving. The results of the path analysis model show that role overload was greater if the caregiver provided more hours of care and cared for an elder who exhibited problem behaviors. Further, a caregiver who reported role overload was also more likely to be depressed (Yates et al., 1999). We were interested in what resources available to a caregiver might mediate or buffer the effect of amount of care on role overload and risk of depression. We found that a better quality of caregiver/care recipient relationship, a sense of mastery, and emotional support decreased the likelihood of role overload and, in turn, depression.

A recent qualitative study regarding the experience of control in caregiving (Szabo and Strang, 1999) supports these findings. Control is seen as a factor that influences a caregiver's ability to manage stress and burden associated with the caregiving role. Maintaining control in this study was indicated by identifying internal resources, recognizing a need for help and asking for it, anticipating the future, and taking corrective action when impending loss of control was felt. Lack of control, on the other hand, was reflected by inability to recognize their need or ask for help, not anticipating the future, and identifying negative internal resources, i.e., lacking confidence in their caregiving abilities.

Several studies, including our work, have taken a more salutogenic approach and investigated how caregivers cope with the daily demands of caregiving. This work offers useful data to inform the development of supportive interventions. Caregivers use a variety of private, personal, or informal methods to cope with stress. The NAC/AARP Survey (National Alliance for Caregiving and American Association for Retired Persons, 1997) reported the following common methods of coping: prayer (74%), talking with friends or relatives (66%), exercise (38%), and hobbies (36%). Sixteen percent had sought professional help or counseling. Most caregivers used multiple coping mechanisms, and, not surprisingly, the number of coping mechanisms increased as the level of care increased and was higher in dementia care.

An important point—with clear implications for intervention—is the degree to which caregivers anticipate and plan for the future. Many studies have found that people do not plan for how and when they will assume a caregiving role (Horowitz, 1985). Instead, it happens to them. Montgomery and Koslowski have conceptualized stages or markers of the caregiving career. For many, this emergent stage is a gradual process in which an adult child provides some assistance (e.g., shopping or home maintenance) before it is essential. As the parent develops functional disabilities, more tasks are taken on. For others, there is an acute or defining event (e.g., a CVA or hip fracture) that thrusts them suddenly and unexpectedly into the caregiving role. This latter situation is more stressful. For some time I have thought that caregiving in a stable situation, while demanding of time and energy, is not necessarily stressful because the caregiver establishes a routine and adapts to it. However, an acute event, whether it is the initial event or an event superimposed on a chronic situation, upsets the routine, requires additional time and energy resources, and therefore is more stressful. An early study by Zarit et al. (1986) showed that caregiver burden diminished over time as caregivers likely adapted to the demands of caring. A more recent study by Given et al. (1999) investigated the effect of new demands for assistance on caregiver well-being. They found that caregivers who experienced high numbers of new demands for care following a hospitalization were more likely than those who did not to experience increased levels of depression. These findings are particularly relevant in the current health care environment in which patients are discharged earlier, once intensive therapy is completed, which increases the complexity of care needed in the home. Limits on Medicare home health visits resulting from the 1997 Balanced Budget Act place more demands on family caregivers. While some policy makers remain concerned with the availability and willingness of families to provide care, concern should be directed toward their ability and skills to do so.

An important point here again is that increased involvement of family caregivers has long been associated with lower use of formal care services. Data from the NAC/AARP survey (National Alliance for Caregiving and Alzheimer's Association, 1999) are consistent with that of other studies. On average, two services of a possible 10 services were used by caregivers in that study. Service use increases with level of care needed and is higher for dementia care than non-dementia care. However, while it is plausible that use of formal services would alleviate the caregiver's sense of role overload, the MEHP data (Yates et al., 1999) indicate that this is not the case. Service use appeared to have little or no effect on caregiver well-being.

Studies of caregiver interventions, particularly respite care, have shown inconsistent results (Knight et al., 1993; Zarit et al., 1998). Respite care can be provided through in-home services, adult day care, volunteer programs, and brief residential care often in nursing homes. Adult day care has been the form of respite most frequently studied. Caregiver outcomes investigated in these studies include stress, anxiety, somatic complaints, depression, and psychological well-being. Results of early studies showed limited therapeutic benefit (e.g., Strain et al., 1988; Guttman, 1991; Gottlieb and Johnson, 1995; Henry and Capitman, 1995) and results across these studies were inconsistent. However, as described by Zarit et al. (1998), limitations in study design and measurement might have obscured the value of adult day care as respite. The well-designed study by Zarit and his colleagues (1998) demonstrated both short-term (3 months) and long-term (12 months) benefits of adult day care use in decreasing caregiver stress and enhancing psychological well-being. This study also focused on the caregiver's appraisal of the situation (using the same measure of role overload discussed previously), underscoring the subjective experience of caregiving as an important target of intervention.

Another intervention approach—support and counseling—was studied by Mittelman and colleagues (1996). They provided individual and family counseling followed by support groups for spouse-caregivers of elders with dementia to see if it resulted in delaying nursing home admission. The intervention was successful in prolonging the time that these caregivers provided care at home, particularly during the early to middle stages of dementia.

These recent data support an upstream approach (McKinlay, 1975, 1996), in which one attempts to intervene before an issue becomes a problem too difficult to solve, would focus on the contributors to overload and attempt to intervene in a way that prevents stress rather than simply relieving it. If we consider the recent findings regarding a caregiver's appraisal of their situation, upstream interventions might address issues of evaluating the elder's needs, coming to terms with the needs of the elder versus the caregiver's ability and willingness to provide care, and developing strategies to prevent overload, by training caregivers in technical skills or in obtaining emotional support before they actually need it. The challenge here is to identify caregivers and intervene perhaps before they identify themselves as caregivers, or perceive the need for outside intervention.

Finally, we turn to cessation of the caregiving role. Very few studies have investigated why caregivers voluntarily leave the caregiving role (i.e., for reasons other than institutionalization). Using national data from the National Long-Term Care Survey, Kasper et al. (1994) found that ending caregiving occurred for only 5% of cases and was related to higher levels of care, need for constant supervision, caregiving for less than one year, and a sense that good feelings did not outweigh caregiving stress. It was also more common in caregivers who were not closely related to the elder. Analysis of this question in the MEHP data revealed that cessation of caregiving was related to manifestation of problem behaviors, not having a good relationship with the care recipient, lack of confidence in ability to provide more care, and not being a close relative.

Implications for Policy and Practice

Major findings with important policy and practice implications include the following:

Patterns of Care

While family care is very common, most of the care is provided by one person.

Contrary to common assumption, there is little sharing of care. Even in cases where multiple caregivers are involved, they tend to supplement the care provided by the primary caregiver. We see little division of labor. Given that restrictions on personal and leisure time is the most frequently reported caregiving impact, working with the primary caregiver to identify both other informal and formal sources of care to provide respite in a timely manner is indicated. A second point is that we should not take for granted that minority elders have larger caregiving networks. Hispanic elders are a case in point. As the largest growing minority group and the most disabled in later years, Hispanic elders face social situations that could diminish caregiving resources— smaller family size, increased employment of women, and the economic necessity of living at a distance from adult children. Given a strong sense of familism, these adult children face considerable challenges if trying to provide care in light of these social circumstances.

Family care is generally stable. Few families voluntarily abandon their role in favor of community services or institutional care.

Research data do not support the policy concern that families will stop caring if more publicly funded services are available. Yet we do see disruptions in the informal care arrangements which result in increased service use on a temporary basis. I would argue that this is an appropriate and effective use of community services. Agencies should be sensitive to and prepared to respond in order to divert an undesirable nursing home admission. Research data can be used to develop client profiles to target service to at-risk elders.

Most caregivers are women. However, in the case of spousal caregiving arrangements, men are highly involved.

More attention should be directed to situations in which the primary caregiver is male, particularly if the care recipient requires extensive

41

and personal care. Male caregivers in these situations are usually older. This current cohort of older men is least likely to be prepared and skilled to provide a range of help. They might also be challenged by their own health conditions or physical disability. These situations merit special attention. Men want to care for their wives but may need skill training or supportive services (especially personal care) in order to do so.

Impacts of Care

The care of disabled older adults can be burdensome, but caregiving stress is not universal.

For many caregivers of elders with dementia, caregiving is emotionally and physically stressful. Yet, data from studies of caregivers of elders with functional disabilities indicate that, other than the shared restrictions on personal and leisure time, caregiving is not generally perceived as stressful by most caregivers. From a policy perspective, it is important not to generalize the findings from studies of dementia caregivers to non-dementia caregivers and vice versa. Doing so would likely result in over- or under-estimates respectively of the need for support and services. The strains and needs of both groups of caregivers should be acknowledged yet clearly distinguished for at least two reasons:

1. to accurately identify how best to assist caregivers in each group since their stressors, perceived stress, and resulting needs may differ; and

2. to more accurately estimate the demand for long-term care and caregiver support services, both types and amount.

A second point—I strongly caution about accepting research findings to date that minority caregivers are less burdened than White caregivers, that they are more resilient and have more resources to meet caregiving demands. Researchers must evaluate the sensitivity and cultural appropriateness of commonly used measures of caregiver distress to ensure that these measures are not underestimating the stress experienced by minority caregivers.

Physical and emotional well-being of caregivers is influenced not by the type and amount of care they provide but rather by their appraisal of that care.

If caregivers feel overwhelmed or overloaded by their caregiving responsibilities, they are more likely to experience physical and especially emotional problems. It should not be assumed that all caregivers providing extensive care to severely disabled elders are burdened, or that services to offer respite are the only answer. The assessment of at-risk caregivers should be directed at their feelings about their caregiving responsibilities—their ability to manage multiple demands, their confidence in their caregiving skills, their organizational and time management skills—rather than on what they do.

Caregiver well-being is enhanced by a sense of mastery, the quality of the relationship with the care recipient, and feeling supported in the role.

Caregivers use a wide variety of coping mechanisms. Interventions that take a salutogenic approach—develop caregiving and coping skills and mobilize sources of informal support—are likely to show more therapeutic benefit than ones taking a pathogenic approach of trying to relieve burden.

Dementia caregiving should be distinguished from non-dementia caregiving.

Dementia care, particularly at advanced stages of disease, is undoubtedly stressful. The manifestation of problem or disruptive behaviors is particularly stressful. Developing interventions to specifically address these behaviors by changing the elder's behavior or by developing the caregiver's skills to manage the behaviors is indicated (Schulz et al., 1995). Intervention protocols, some of which are now underway and being evaluated, include skills training, education, and counseling. As pointed out by Schulz et al. (1995), since the dementia patient is usually the contact person with the service system, patient assessments offer an opportunity for assessment of the caregiver's status as well.

Formal services are used infrequently.

Although economic constraints have limited service availability in recent years, even when services were more widely available in the early 1980s, they were not widely used. In general, services are targeted on the basis of extent of need for care and availability of informal sources of care. Assessments typically are care recipient focused.

Research data support more attention to assessment of the caregiver's status. Again, assessment is better directed at the caregiver's appraisal of the caregiving arrangement rather than at the caregiver's availability and physical ability to provide care.

In the case of dementia care, use of formal services is not only appropriate but also clinically indicated as severity increases. From a practice perspective, it is important to determine the optimal mix of formal services and informal care in order to ensure the well being of both care recipient and caregiver. Transition to a special care environment is another important juncture in this regard. Assistance with appropriate timing and with negotiating a role for continued involvement of the caregiver(s) will facilitate what might be interpreted as another in a series of losses by a caregiver who sees this transition as loss of an important role.

From a policy perspective, the issue of eligibility criteria for services is important. For both publicly and privately (i.e., third party payer) funded services, eligibility typically is based on functional disability in the performance of specified ADLs. The Advisory Panel on Alzheimer's Disease (1989) has advocated for the expansion of eligibility criteria to provide services in situations where the degree of cognitive impairment interferes with the person's ability to complete either IADLs or ADLs without substantial supervision. The cost analyses performed by Paveza et al. (1998) "suggest that changes in cognitive impairment are independent factors affecting cost regardless of the magnitude of ADL/IADL impairment" (p. 79). Similar findings from the National Long-Term Care Channeling Demonstration Project in the 1980s were reported by Liu et al. (1990). These findings support the notion of applying a cognitive weighting factor to the degree of ADL/IADL impairment in establishing eligibility for services.

Most caregivers do not plan for the future. Unexpected acute events are stressful.

Not only do most adults not plan how they will provide care for their parents or other relatives, most caregivers also do not plan for changes in caregiving needs. A common coping strategy is to "take one day at a time." This works as long as the situation is stable, or changes gradually. A major acute health event which suddenly increases the need for care is an appropriate time for formal intervention. This may be organizationally challenging for service providers since services might be needed quickly and at times when services are not normally provided. However, all the research data on well-being of both care

44

recipient and caregiver indicate that these services are needed and will likely have a beneficial effect.

An alternative approach is to engage a caregiver in mutual planning for handling of such situations. This is challenging, as most people will not seek out information until they need it. General information sessions about community services are frequently not well attended. The most effective strategy might be to engage a caregiver in planning shortly after experiencing an acute event. The recent experience might sensitize them to the need and increase their receptivity to new information.

Finally, the challenges we face include:

- The widely recognized changing sociodemographics of the older population—the aging baby boomers;

- Projected changes in active life expectancy and the compression of disability, meaning higher needs for care but perhaps for shorter periods of time at advanced ages;

- The availability and ability of families—which will be smaller and older—to care for very old and perhaps severely disabled elders; and

- The increased ethnic diversity of the population, underscoring the need for culturally sensitive and appropriate services and service delivery mechanisms.

In closing, we should not lose sight of the fact that caregiving is imbedded in the family experience, history, and values. How caregivers respond to the presenting needs for care, how they perceive the personal impact of that care, and how they interface with the formal service system will be shaped by their personal situation. As we have argued for recognition of the heterogeneity of older adults, in all that we do as researchers, practitioners, and policy makers, we must recognize the heterogeneity of their caregivers.

References

Advisory Panel on Alzheimer's Disease. (1989). *Report of the Advisory Panel on Alzheimer's Disease.* DHHS Pub. No. (ADM) 89-1644. Washington, DC: Supt. of Docs., U.S. Government Printing Office.

Anderson, R, and Newman J. (1973). Societal and individual determinants of medical care utilization in the United States. *Milbank Memorial Fund Quarterly, 51*, 95-124.

Arno, P.S., Levine, C., and Memmott, M.M. (1999). The economic value of informal caregiving. *Health Affairs, 18*(2), 182-188.

Branch, L. and Jette A. (1983). Elders' use of informal long-term care assistance. *The Gerontologist 23*, 51-56.

Burton, L., Kasper, J., Shore, A., Cagney, K., LaVesit, T., Cubbin, C. and German, P. (1995). The structure of informal care: are there differences by race? *The Gerontologist, 35*, 744-752.

Calderon, V., and Tennstedt, S. (1999). Ethnic differences in expression of caregiver burden. *Journal of Gerontological Social Work, 30*(1/2). Reprinted in M. Delgado (Ed.). 1998. *Latino Elders in the Twenty-First Century: Issues and Challenges for Culturally Competent Research and Practice.* New York: Hayworth Press.

Cantor, M. (1980). The informal support system: its relevance in the lives of the elderly. In E. Borgotta and N. McCulsky (Eds.), *Aging and Society.* Beverly Hills, CA: Sage.

Cantor, M. (1983). Strain among caregivers: a study of experience in the United States. *The Gerontologist, 23*, 597-604.

Cantor, M., and Johnson, J. (1978). The informal support system of the "familyless" elderly—who takes over? Proceedings of the 31st Annual Meeting of the Gerontological Society of America. Dallas, Texas.

Cantor, M.A. (1979). The informal support system of New York's inner city elderly: Is ethnicity a factor? In D. Gelfand and A. Kutzik (Eds.). *Ethnicity and aging: Theory, Research, and Policy.* New York: Springer.

Chappell, N. (1991). Living arrangement and sources of caregiving. *Journal of Gerontology: Social Sciences, 46* S1-S8.

Chatters, L.M., Taylor, R.J., and Jackson, J.S. (1985). Size and composition of the informal helper networks of elderly blacks. *Journal of Gerontology, 40*, 605-614.

Chatters, L.M. Taylor, R.J., and Jackson, J.S. (1986). Aged blacks' choice for an informal helper network. *Journal of Gerontology, 41*, 94-100.

Community Council of Greater New York (1978). *Dependency in the Elderly of New York City.* New York: Community Council of Greater New York.

Comptroller General of the United States (1977). Report to Congress: *The Well-Being of Older People in Cleveland*, Ohio. Washington, D.C.: General Accounting Office.

Cox, C., and Monk, A. (1990). Minority caregivers of dementia victims: A comparison of Black and Hispanic families. *Journal of Applied Gerontology*, 9, 340-354.

Cox, C. (1997). Findings from a statewide program of respite care: A comparison of service users, stoppers, and non users. *The Gerontologist, 37*, 511-517.

Delgado, M., and Humm-Delgado, D. (1982). National support systems: Source of strength in Hispanic communities. *Social Work*, 83-89.

Diwan, S., Berger, C., and Manns, E.K. (1977). Composition of the home care service package: predictors of type, volume, and mix of services provided to poor and frail older people. *The Gerontologist, 37*, 169-181.

Doty, P. (1986). Family care of the elderly: the role of public policy. *Milbank Memorial Fund Quarterly, 64*, 34-75.

Eaton, W.W., and Kessler, L.G. (1981). Rates of symptoms of depression in a national sample. *American Journal of Epidemiology*, 114, 528-538.

Eggert, G., Granger, C. Morris, R. and Pendleton, S. (1977). Caring for the patient with long-term disability. *Geriatrics, 32*, 102-19.

Frankfather, D., Smith, M., and Caro, F. (1981*). Family care of the elderly*. Lexington, MA: D.C. Heath and Co.

Frerichs, R.R., Aneshensel, C.S., and Clark, V.A. (1981). Prevalence of depression in Los Angeles County. *American Journal of Epidemiology*, 113, 691-699.

Gatz, M., Bengtson, V.L., and Blum, M.J. (1990). Caregiving families. In J.E. Birren and J.W. Schaie (Eds.). *Handbook of the psychology of aging. 3rd edition*. San Diego: Academic Press, Inc.

Given, C.W., Given, B.A., Stommel, M., and Azzouz, F. (1999). The impact of new demands for assistance on caregiver depression: tests using an inception cohort. *The Gerontologist, 39*(1), 76-85.

Gottlieb, B.H., and Johnson, J. (1995). *Impact of day care programs on family caregivers of persons with dementia*. Guelph, Ontario: Gerontology Research Centre, University of Guelph.

Guttman, R. (1991). *Adult day care for Alzheimer's patients: Impact on family caregivers.* New York: Garland.

Hatch, L. (1991). Informed support patterns of older African-American and white women. *Research on Aging,* 13, 144-170.

Harrow, B., Tennstedt, S., and McKinlay, J. (1995). How costly is it to care for disabled elders in the community? *The Gerontologist, 35*(6), 803-813.

Hays, W., and Mindel, C. (1973). Extended kinship relations in black and white families. *Journal of Marriage and the Family,* Feb, 51-57.

Henry, M.E., and Capitman, J.A. (1995). Finding satisfaction in adult day care: Analysis of a national demonstration of dementia care and respite services. *Journal of Applied Gerontology,* 14, 302-320.

Himes, C.L., Jordan, A.K., and Farkas, J.I. (1996). Factors influencing parental caregiving by adult women. *Research on Aging,* 18, 349-370.

Horowitz, A. (1978). Families who care: a study of natural support systems of the elderly. Proceedings of the 31st Annual Meeting of the Gerontological Society of America. Dallas, Texas.

Horowitz, A. (1985). Family caregiving to the frail elderly. In M.P. Lawton and G. Maddox (Eds.), *Annual Review of Gerontology and Geriatrics,* Vol 5. New York: Springer.

Horowitz, A., and Dobrof, R. (1982). The role of families in providing long-term care to the frail and chronically ill elderly living in the community. Final report submitted to Health Care Financing Administration, USDHHS, Grant No. 18-P-97541/2-02.

Johnson, C. (1983). Dyadic family relations and social support. *Gerontologist 23,* 377-83.

Kahana, E., and Kiyak, H. (1980). The older woman: impact of widowhood and living arrangements on service needs. *Journal of Gerontological Social Work,* 3, 17-29.

Kasper, J.D., Steinbach, U., and Andrews, J. (1994). Caregiver role appraisal and caregiver tasks as factors in ending caregiving. *Journal of Aging and Health,* 6(3), 397-414.

Max, W., Webber, P., and Fox, P. (1995). Alzheimer's disease: The unpaid burden of caring. *Journal of Aging and Health,* 7, 179-199.

McAuley, W., and Arling, G. (1984). Use of in-home care by very old people. *Journal of Health and Social Behavior, 25,* 54-65.

McKinlay, J. (1975). A case for refocusing upstream —the political economy of sickness. In A. Enelow et al. (Eds.), *Behavioral aspects of prevention.* American Heart Association.

McKinlay, J.B., and Tennstedt, S.L. (1986). Social networks and the care of frail elders. Final Report to the National Institute on Aging, Grant No. AG03869. Boston: Boston University.

McKinlay, J.B., Crawford, S., and Tennstedt, S. (1995). The everyday impacts of providing care to dependent elders and their consequences for the care recipients. *Journal of Aging and Health, 7*(4): 497-528.

McKinlay, J. (1996). Some contributions from the social system to gender inequalities in heart disease. *Journal of Health and Social Behavior, 37* (March), 1-26.

Mechanic, D. (1962). The concept of illness behavior. *Journal of Chronic Diseases,* 15, 189-194.

Miller, B., McFall, S., and Campbell, R.T. (1994). Changes in sources of community long-term care among African-American and white frail older persons. *Journal of Gerontology: Social Sciences, 49,* S14-S24.

Mitchell, J., and Register, J.C. (1984). An exploration of family interaction with the elderly by race, socioeconomic status, and residence. *The Gerontologist, 24,* 48-54.

Mittelman, M.S., Ferris, S.H, Shulman, E., Steinberg, G., and Levin, B. (1996). A family intervention to delay nursing home placement of patients with Alzheimer disease: A randomized controlled trial. *JAMA, 276*(21), 1725-1731.

Montgomery, R.V., and Hirshorn, B.A. (1991). Current and future family help with long-term care needs of the elderly. *Research on Aging,* 13(2), 171-204.

Montgomery, R. (1992). Examining respite: Its promise and limits. In M.G. Ory and A.P. Duncker (Eds.). *In-home care for older people* (pp. 75-96). Newburg Park, CA: Sage Publications, Inc.

National Alliance for Caregiving and the American Association of Retired Persons. (1997). *Family Caregiving in the U.S.: Findings from a National Survey.* Bethesda, MD.

National Alliance for Caregiving and the Alzheimer's Association. (1999). *Who Cares? Families Caring for Persons with Alzheimer's Disease*. Bethesda, MD.

Ory, M.G., Hoffman, R.R., Yee, J., Tennstedt, S., and Schulz, R. (1999). Prevalence and impact of caregiving: a detailed comparison between dementia and non-dementia caregivers. *The Gerontologist*, 39(2), 177-186.

Paveza, G.J., Mensah, E., Cohen, D., Williams, S., Jankowski, L. (1998). Costs of community-based long-term care services to the cognitively impaired aged. *Journal of Mental Health and Aging*, 4, 69-82.

Peek, C.W., Zsembik, B.A., and Coward, R.T. (1997). The changing caregiving networks of older adults. *Research on Aging*, 19, 333-361.

Prohaska, T., and McAuley, W. (1983). The role of family care and living arrangements in acute care discharge recommendations. *Journal of Gerontological Social Work*, 5, 67-80.

Rice, D., Fox, P., Webber, P., Lindeman, D., Hauck, W., and Segura, E. (1993). The economic burden of Alzheimer's disease. *Health Affairs*, 12, 164-176.

Schulz, R., O'Brien, A.T., Bookwala, J., and Fleissner, K. (1995). Psychiatric and physical morbidity effects of dementia caregiving: prevalence, correlates, and causes. *The Gerontologist*, 35(6), 771-791.

Shanas, E. (1979). The family as a social support system in old age. *Gerontologist*, 19, 169-174.

Shanas, E., Townsend, P., Wedderburn, D., Friis, H., Milhoj, P., and Stehouwer, J. (1986). *Old people in three industrial societies*. New York: Atherton.

Sherwood, S., Morris, J., and Gutkin, C. (1981). Meeting the needs of the impaired elderly: the power and resiliency of the informal support system. Final report to the Administration on Aging Grant No. 90-A-1294. Boston, MA: Hebrew Rehabilitation Center for the Aged.

Shuval, J.T., Fleishman, R. and Shueli, A. (1982). Informal support for the elderly: social networks in a Jerusalem neighborhood. Jerusalem: Brookdale Institute of Gerontology and Adult Human Development in Israel.

Soldo, B., and Myllyluoma, J. (1983). Caregivers who live with dependent elderly. *The Gerontologist*, 23, 605-11.

Stephens, S., and Christianson, J. (1986). *Informal care of the elderly.* Lexington, MA: Lexington Books.

Strain, L.A., Chapell, N.L., and Blandford, A.A. (1988). Changes in life satisfaction among participants of adult day care and their informal caregivers. *Journal of Gerontological Social Work, 11*(3/4), 115-129.

Stoller, E.P., and Earl, L.L. (1983). Help with activities of everyday life: sources of support for the noninstitutionalized elderly. *The Gerontologist, 23,* 64-70.

Stommel, M., Given, B.A., Given, C.W., and Collins, C. (1995). The impact of frequency of care activities on the division of labor between primary caregivers and other care providers. *Research on Aging, 17,* 412-433.

Stommel, M., Given, B.A., and Given, C.W. (1998). Racial differences in the division of labor between primary and secondary caregivers. *Research on Aging, 20* 199-217.

Stone, R., Cafferata, G.L., and Sangl, J. (1987). Caregivers of the frail and elderly: a national profile. *The Gerontologist, 27,* 677-683.

Szabo, V., and Strang,,V.R. (1999). Experiencing control in caregiving. *Journal of Nursing Scholarship, 31*(1), 71-75.

Tennstedt, S. and McKinlay, J. (1989). Informal care for frail older persons. In M. Ory and N. Bond (Eds.). *Aging and Health Care: Social Science and Policy Perspectives.* London Routledge.

Tennstedt, S., McKinlay, J., and Sullivan, L. (1989). Predictors of informal care for frail elders: the role of secondary caregivers. *The Gerontologist, 29*(5), 677-683.

Tennstedt, S., Cafferata, G., and Sullivan, L. (1992). Depression among caregivers of impaired elders. *Journal of Aging and Health, 4*(1), 58-76.

Tennstedt, S., Crawford, S., and McKinlay, J. (1993a). Determining the pattern of community care: is coresidence more important than caregiver relationship? *Journal of Gerontology: Social Sciences, 48*(2), S74-S83.

Tennstedt, S., Crawford, S., and McKinlay, J. (1993b). Is family care on the decline? A longitudinal investigation of the substitution of formal long-term care services for informal care. *Milbank Quarterly, 71*(4), 601-624.

Tennstedt, S., and Chang, B. (1998). The relative contribution of ethnicity vs. socioeconomic status in explaining differences in disability and receipt of national care. *Journal of Gerontology: Social Sciences, 53B*(2), 861-870.

Tennstedt, S., and Chang, B., and Delgado, M. (1999). Patterns of long-term care: a comparison of Puerto Rican, African-American and non-Latino White elders. *Journal of Gerontological Social Work, 30*(1/2).

Treas, J. (1977). Family support systems for the aged: some social and demographic considerations. *The Gerontologist, 17*, 486-91.

U.S. Bureau of the Census. (1992). Table 692: Average annual income and expenditure of all consumer units: 1990. In *Statistical abstract of the United States: 1992* (pp. 442-443). Washington, DC: U.S. Government Printing Office.

U.S. Department of Health, Education and Welfare (1978). HEW task force report on long-term care. Washington, D.C.: Office of the Secretary, Special Assistant to the Secretary.

Weinberger, M., Gold, D., Divine, G.W., Cowper, P.A., Hodgson, L.G., Schreiner, P.J., and George, L.N. (1993). Expenditures in caring for patients with dementia who live at home. *American Journal of Public Health, 83*, 338-341.

Yates, M.E., Tennstedt, S., and Chang, B.H. (1999). Contributors to and mediators of psychological well-being for informal caregivers. *Journal of Gerontology: Psychological Sciences, 54B*(1), P12-P22.

Yordi, C., DuNah, R., Bostrom, A., Fox, P., Wilkinson, A., and Newcomer, R. (1997). Caregiver supports: Outcomes from the Medicare Alzheimer's disease demonstration. *Health Care Financing Review, 19*(2), 97-117.

Zarit, S., Reever, K., Bach-Peterson, J. (1980). Relatives of the impaired elderly: correlates of feelings of burden. *Journal of Gerontology, 20*, 649-55.

Zarit, S.H., Todd, P.A., and Zarit, J.M. (1986). Subjective burden of husbands and wives as caregivers: A longitudinal study. *The Gerontologist, 26*, 260-266.

Zarit, S.H., Stephens, M.P., Townsend, A., and Greene, R. (1998). Stress reduction for family caregivers: Effects of adult day care use. *Journal of Gerontology, 53B*(5), S267-S277.

Chapter 4

Caregiver Profile

Introduction and Background

Numerous studies have been conducted on various aspects of informal (unpaid) or family caregiving of older adults. Nationwide information on the magnitude, intensity, and types of informal caregiving provided, however, together with its physical, emotional, and financial repercussions, has been lacking. In particular, similarities and differences among racial/ethnic groups with respect to caregiving practices and the impact of informal caregiving on caregivers' lives have not been systematically studied on a nationwide basis.

This study attempts to identify and profile the various impacts of family caregiving in today's society. Using a broad definition of caregiving, the survey documents for corporate America, policy makers, and the general public the experiences and attitudes of persons who provide care to older Americans. A broad definition was used in order to determine the type of care family and friends provide to older persons, ranging from light, occasional tasks to round-the-clock care, including care provided from a distance.

The present study is the first of its kind to address these issues systematically, using survey methodology, across four racial/ethnic groups within the United States: Whites, Blacks, Hispanics, and Asians.[1] It was sponsored and designed by the National Alliance for Caregiving (NAC) and the American Association of Retired Persons

"Family Caregiving in the U.S.–Final Report," © June 1997, National Alliance for Caregiving, reprinted with permission.

53

(AARP), with funding provided by a grant from Glaxo Wellcome, Inc.[2] Additional funding was provided by the Archstone Foundation, ManorCare Health Services, and Metropolitan Life Insurance Company.[4]

Overview of Methodology

The study was designed as a telephone survey to be used with a nationwide random sample of caregivers aged 18 and over, with oversamples of Black, Hispanic, and Asian caregivers to ensure adequate numbers of each of these groups for analytic purposes. NAC contracted with the ICR Survey Research Group, Inc., of Media, PA, to generate the samples, conduct the survey, and prepare a topline report.

The survey was conducted between August 13 and September 20, 1996 with respondents capable of answering questions in English by telephone. (Funds were not available to conduct the survey in languages other than English.) See the Appendix at the end of the chapter for a detailed description of the methodology used to generate the samples.

A total of 1,509 English-speaking family caregivers participated in this telephone survey: 623 Whites, 306 Blacks, 307 Hispanics, and 264 Asians.

Limitations of This Study

Although this is the first U.S. study of its kind to include large enough oversamples of caregivers drawn from three racial/ethnic minority groups, these samples under-represent recent immigrant or first generation caregivers who speak little or no English, such as Hispanics who are fluent only in Spanish or Portuguese, or Asians who speak only Chinese, Japanese, Korean, or Vietnamese, or other Far Eastern languages. It is also possible that the respondents, being of diverse cultural and linguistic backgrounds, may not have interpreted all questions identically.

Additionally, because this was a survey conducted by telephone, it under-represents households that do not have a telephone (6% of households nationwide).

Caregiving, Caregiver: Definitions Used for This Study

What is informal or family caregiving, and who is an informal or family caregiver? These terms are used inconsistently in the literature;

there are no universally accepted criteria for designating an activity as caregiving or a person as a caregiver among scholars, policymakers, or advocates.

Informal or family caregiving is typically performed by relatives and close friends for a person who is no longer able to manage all aspects of his or her daily life and/or personal care. It generally involves everyday activities related to managing a household, or to performing personal care, such as dressing, bathing, toileting, and feeding. By providing unpaid assistance and support to older family members or friends who need it, informal or family caregivers may help avoid or delay institutional placement of the older person, or the need for paid caregiving services.

For purposes of this study, the term caregiving was defined to prospective respondents in the following words:

> By caregiving, I mean providing unpaid care to a relative or friend who is aged 50 or older to help them take care of themselves.

> Caregiving may include help with personal needs or household chores. It might be taking care of a person's finances, arranging for outside services, or visiting regularly to see how they are doing. This person need not live with you.

To be included in this study, a caregiver had to be at least 18 years old and either currently providing informal care to a relative or friend aged 50 or older, or to have provided informal care to such a person at some point during the past 12 months. No stipulations were placed on the amount, frequency, or duration of care provided, or on where the care recipient resided.

The decision to use a broad definition of caregiving and caregiver was based on focus group discussions conducted with members of the target racial/ethnic groups prior to designing the survey instrument.

Intensity of Care: The Level of Care Index

A major purpose of this study was to understand how the level of demand presented by the caregiving situation (i.e., the difficulty of the tasks caregivers perform and the amount of time they devote to caregiving) impacts caregivers' lives and attitudes. To measure the intensity of caregiving, a Level of Care Index was developed which classifies caregivers into different levels of care according to the kinds and numbers of assistive activities they perform and the number of hours per week they devote to caring for their principal care recipient. (How the Level of Care Index was developed is discussed in detail in the Appendix at the end of this chapter.)

Each caregiver was classified into one of five levels, with Level 1 being the lowest in caregiving demand or intensity, and Level 5 being highest. Within each level, there is a range of activities and number of hours of care provided per week. Each successive level involves a higher degree of caregiving responsibility or demand. Level 1 caregivers, for example, provide no assistance with personal care activities such as dressing or bathing their care recipient, and typically provide care for a maximum of eight hours per week. Level 5 caregivers, in contrast, assist with at least two personal care activities and provide care for more than 40 hours per week. (See the Appendix for additional information.) Table 4.1 shows the distribution of caregivers in this survey by level of care provided.

Table 4.1. Caregivers by Level of Care

	Number of Caregivers	Percent of All Caregivers
Total	1,509	100.0
Level 1	389	25.8
Level 2	208	13.8
Level 3	287	19.0
Level 4	355	23.5
Level 5	185	12.3
Missing	85	5.6

Presentation of Findings

All findings presented in this report refer to caregiving and caregivers as defined. For ease of reporting, caregiving statistics are typically expressed in the present tense, whether or not the caregivers in question are currently providing care. Noteworthy findings, or key differences between subgroups, may be bulleted and/or italicized.

While some caregivers report that they care or cared for more than one person, the survey inquired only about relationships with and activities pertaining to the recipient for whom the caregiver provides the most care.

In addition, all percentages cited in this report refer to proportions of the entire U.S. population of informal caregivers, and not to the sample of caregivers included in this study. That is, the findings from this sample of caregivers have been adjusted or weighted to reflect accurately the distribution of U.S. telephone households with a caregiver, based on sampling techniques used by the contractor in combination with U.S. Census projections and estimates. (For a more complete discussion of weighting, see the Appendix.)

When percentages are cited and compared across subgroups, the differences are statistically significant at the .05 level or better, unless otherwise indicated. This means that no more than five times in 100 would the particular finding be expected to occur by chance, and that there is a 95 percent probability that the difference is a true difference between groups. When "no differences" are reported, it means that percentage differences found across comparison groups did not reach statistical significance at the .05 level and thus could have been due to chance.

Survey Findings:
Prevalence of Caregiving in the United States

- Just over 23% of all U.S. households with a telephone contain at least one caregiver,[5] of whom more than three-fourths (76%) are currently caring for a relative or friend who is at least 50 years old. The remaining 24% report having provided informal care to a relative or friend within the past 12 months, but are not currently doing so. Higher proportions of Level 1 and 2 caregivers are currently providing care than Level 4 and 5 caregivers.

- This translates into an estimated 22,411,200 caregiving households nationwide with English speaking caregivers,[6] of which there are approximately:

  - 18,290,000 White, non-Hispanic households

  - 2,380,000 Black, non-Hispanic households

  - 1,050,000 Hispanic households and

  - 400,000 Asian households.

  - The remaining caregiving households are of other races.

- The prevalence of informal caregiving is higher among Asian and Black households (31.7% and 29.4%, respectively) than among Hispanic households (26.8%) or White households (24%).

Demographic Profile of Caregivers

As shown in Table 4.2, the typical caregiver is a married woman in her mid-forties who works full-time, is a high school graduate, and has an annual household income of $35,000. Highlights of findings by race/ethnicity and other characteristics are presented below.

Age

- The average age of caregivers is 46.

- More than one in five caregivers is under age 35 (22%), close to four in 10 are 35 to 49 (39%), about one in four is 50 to 64 (24%), and 12 percent are 65 and older.

- Asian and Hispanic caregivers are significantly younger than Whites, with average ages of 39 and 40, respectively, compared with 47 for Whites. More than one-third of Asian and Hispanic caregivers are under 35, compared with just over one in five White caregivers.

- Level 5 caregivers are much more likely to be at least 65 years than any other caregivers: 30 percent, in contrast with only 10 percent of Level 1 caregivers, for example.

Gender

- More than seven in 10 caregivers (73%) are female and 27 percent are male.

- Asian caregivers are most evenly split among female and male caregivers: 52 percent of Asian caregivers are women (in contrast with 77% of Blacks, 74% of Whites, and 67% of Hispanics) and 48 percent are men.

Education and Income

- Thirty-five percent of caregivers are high school graduates, 23 percent have some college education, and 29 percent are college graduates or have post graduate education. Nine percent have less than a high school education.

- Asian caregivers in the sample are more highly educated than caregivers of other racial/ethnic groups, with 39 percent being college graduates and 21 percent having had graduate education. In contrast, only 15 percent of Blacks and 18 percent of

Hispanics are college graduates, and fewer than seven percent of either group have had graduate education. Sixteen percent of Black caregivers have less than a high school education, compared with only two percent of Asians.

- The median annual household income of caregivers is $35,000.

- Asian caregivers also report considerably higher annual household incomes than other groups (averaging more than $45,000, compared with just under $28,000 for Blacks, for example).The differences may reflect, in part, the fact that more recent Asian immigrants, whose incomes might be expected to be lower, were not included in the sample because they do not speak English.

Marital Status and Presence of Children under 18

- Close to two-thirds of caregivers nationwide are married (66%), 13 percent are single, 13 percent are separated or divorced, and eight percent are widowed.

- Black caregivers are the least likely to be married or living with a partner—just over half (51%) are, compared with two-thirds of Asians and Whites (68%), and 64 percent of Hispanics.

- While 41 percent of caregivers have one or more children under age 18 living in their households, more than half of all Black, Hispanic, and Asian caregivers report having one or more children under age 18 in their households, in contrast with 39 percent of White caregivers.

Employment Status

- Close to two in three caregivers (64%) are working, 52 percent full-time and 12 percent part-time; and 16 percent are retired. One in five (20%) say they are "not employed." Table 4.3 shows the percentages of working caregivers by age and other key characteristics.

- Of those not currently employed (36% of caregivers), about one in three (34%) said they had even been employed while taking care of their care recipient.

- Asian caregivers are more likely to be employed full- or part-time (77%) than Whites (65%), Blacks (66%), or Hispanics (65%), and also more likely to be employed full-time. This may

Table 4.2. Caregiver Profile (Base = Total Caregivers)

	Total	White	Black	Hispanic	Asian
Number interviewed (unweighted)	n=1,509	n= 623	n=306	n=307	n=264
Number in U.S. population (weighted)*	n=2,241	n=1,829	n=238	n=105	n= 40
Gender					
Female	72.5%	73.5%	76.8%	67.4%	52.3%
Male	27.5	26.5	23.2	32.6	47.7
Age of Caregiver					
Under 35	22.3%	20.5%	23.5%	37.1%	38.6%
35-49	39.4	39.0	44.4	37.5	43.6
50-64	26.0	26.8	22.5	21.2	14.4
65 or Older	12.4	13.6	9.5	4.2	3.4
Mean (years)	46.15	46.93	44.75	40.01	39.01
Marital Status					
Married or living with partner	65.7%	67.8%	50.9%	63.8%	64.4%
Single, never married	12.6	11.1	19.3	18.2	26.1
Separated or divorced	13.0	12.1	19.0	15.7	6.0
Widowed	8.0	8.3	9.8	2.0	3.0
Children under Age 18 in Household					
Yes	41.3%	38.8%	51.0%	58.3%	51.1%
No	57.8	60.2	48.4	41.7	48.1

Educational Attainment

Less than high school	9.0%	8.2%	16.3%	11.1%	2.3%
High school graduate	35.3	36.0	32.0	35.2	18.2
Some college	22.5	22.2	26.8	26.7	17.0
College graduate	20.1	20.4	15.4	18.2	39.0
Graduate School +	8.8	8.8	5.6	6.5	20.8
Technical school	3.5	3.5	3.3	2.3	1.9

Ever on Active Duty/U.S. Armed Forces

	11.5%	11.1%	11.1%	11.4%	7.2%

Current Employment

Employed full-time	51.8%	51.0%	55.6%	51.8%	63.3%
Employed part-time	12.3	12.7	10.5	13.4	14.0
Retired	15.9	17.0	13.7	6.8	4.2
Not employed	19.7	18.9	20.3	28.0	18.2

Household Income

Under $15,000	14.0%	11.7%	29.1%	21.1%	8.3%
$15K-24.9K	18.0	17.3	24.8	22.5	11.0
$25K-29.9K	9.3	9.5	9.8	7.8	8.0
$30K-39.9K	14.0	14.0	12.4	16.3	13.3
$40K-49.9K	10.3	10.4	7.8	11.1	14.0
$50K-74.9K	14.0	14.4	9.5	10.4	15.5
$75K or higher	10.9	12.1	3.0	6.2	19.7
Median	$35K	$35K	$22.5K		$27.5K
$45K					

Note: Column percentages may not total 100% because of refusals.
*Weighted numbers refer to numbers of caregiving households in the U.S. population. Each number must be multiplied by 10,000 to determine the U.S. population prevalence for that cell. For example, 2,241 means 22,410,000 (i.e., there are an estimated 22,410,000 caregiving households in the U.S.). All percentages are based on weighted data.

reflect the fact that, in general, their caregiving demands are lower than those of all other racial/ethnic groups.

- On the other hand, both White and Black caregivers are more likely to be retired than either Hispanics or Asians.

- Hispanic caregivers are more likely to report they are not working (28%) than either Asians (19%) or Whites (18%).

- Those providing Level 5 care are more likely to be retired (32%) than caregivers of any other level, which suggests that the persons they provide care for (including spouses) may themselves be older and require more care.

Military Status

- Eleven and a half percent of all caregivers and 38.9 percent of male caregivers have been on active duty in the U.S. Armed Forces. Fewer Asian caregivers (7.2%) than White (11.1%), Black (11.1%) or Hispanic caregivers (11.4%) had served in the military.

Table 4.3. Employment Status by Age and Other Characteristics (Percentages)

	Employed Full or Part-time
Total	64.2
18-34	77.2
35-49	75.8
50-64	60.3
65+	12.1
Asians	77.3
Women	60.5
HH income < $15,000	36.5
HH income > $50,000	77.8
R is primary caregiver	54.5
Care recipient has dementia	59.8
Level 1 caregivers	70.1
Level 5 caregivers	40.5

Characteristics of the Caregiving Situation

Number of Persons Cared For

- Close to seven in 10 caregivers (69%) provide care to just one person, 23 percent take care of two people, and eight percent care for three or more people.

- Asian and Black caregivers are more likely than White caregivers to be involved in caring for more than one person.

- Level 5 caregivers are more likely than Level 1, 2, and 4 caregivers to be taking care of only one person.

Duration of Caregiving

- The average duration of caregiving is 4.5 years.

- Close to two-thirds of caregivers (64%) have provided care to their primary care recipient for less than five years, while 21 percent have done so for five to nine years, and 10 percent for 10 years or more. There are no differences by caregiver level, except that Level 3, 4, and 5 caregivers are more likely to have been providing care for less than six months than are Level 1 caregivers.

Recipients of Care: To Whom Do Caregivers Provide Care?

Relationship between Caregiver and Care Recipient

- Overall, more than eight in 10 caregivers (85%) take care of a relative, and 15 percent take care of a friend or neighbor. Level 5 caregivers are more likely than other caregivers to be taking care of a relative and less likely to be taking care of a friend.

- Care recipients are typically female relatives: 31 percent of caregivers take care of their own mothers, nine percent care for their mother-in-law, and 12 percent take care of a grandmother. There are no differences by level of care.

- While only five percent of caregivers report taking care of a spouse,[7] 23 percent of Level 5 caregivers take care of a spouse (in contrast with less than one percent for Level 1 and Level 2 caregivers).

- Spousal caregivers are also much more common among caregivers aged 65+ (23%), when compared with all other age groups.[8]

- Of all racial/ethnic groups, Asian caregivers are the least likely to be caring for a spouse (only 1%) and the most likely to be assisting a father (18%).

- Hispanic caregivers are more likely to be caring for a grandparent (22%) than other caregivers (15%).

- Black caregivers are the most likely to be taking care of a relative other than an immediate family member or grandparent—14 percent, in contrast with nine percent of White, seven percent of Hispanic, and six percent of Asian caregivers.

Age of Care Recipient

- The average age of care recipients is 77years.

- About two in three care recipients (64%) are over age 75, and almost one in four (24%) is over age 85. There are no differences in the ages of care recipients by caregiver level.

- White caregivers, on average, care for persons who are older than those cared for by caregivers of other racial/ethnic groups: the mean age of care recipients of White caregivers is 77.6 years, compared with 75.2 for Blacks, 74.7 for Hispanics, and 74.4 for Asians.

- Asian caregivers provide care to persons least likely to be 85+ (only 15% are). The comparable figures for White and Black caregivers are 25 percent and 24 percent.

Health Status of Care Recipients

- Better than seven in 10 caregivers (71%) report that their care recipient's illness or condition is long-term or chronic in nature, and an additional 11 percent say the conditions/illnesses are both chronic and short-term. Twelve percent say their care recipient's illness or condition is short-term (expected to last up to three months), and six percent say they do not know. There are no differences by level of care.

Table 4.4 shows the main illnesses or problem of care recipients, as reported by their caregivers.

Table 4.4. Main Illness or Problem of Care Recipients

Illness	Percentage
"Aging"	15.5
Mobility problems	10.4
Dementia	9.7
Heart disease or condition	9.6
Cancer	8.6
Stroke	7.8
Arthritis	5.8
Diabetes	4.8
Lung disease	3.4
Blindness or vision loss	3.2
Mental or emotional illness	2.8
Broken bones	2.6
Neurological problems	2.2
High blood pressure	2.0

Presence of Dementia, Stroke, and Diabetes

- More than one in five caregivers (22.4%) say they take care of someone with Alzheimer's disease, confusion, dementia, or forgetfulness (hereafter referred to as dementia) as the primary or a secondary illness or condition. This finding translates into an estimated 5,020,000 caregiving households nationwide that provide care for someone with dementia.

- Black caregivers are more likely than any other group to report dementia in their care recipient (28%, in contrast with 22% of White, 20% of Hispanic, and only 3% of Asian caregivers). Asian caregivers also are less likely than other racial/ethnic groups to report dementia as the main illness or problem.

- Black caregivers also report a higher incidence of stroke (12%, in contrast with 7% for each other group.)

- Not surprisingly, higher percentages of Level 4 and 5 caregivers than Level 1 caregivers report that the main illness or problem of their care recipient is dementia. This is also the case for stroke.

- Higher proportions of Level 3, 4, and 5 caregivers report caring for someone with dementia as either the main or secondary problem. (See Figure 4.1.)

- Both Hispanic and Black caregivers are more likely than Whites to report diabetes as the care recipient's main illness (9.4% and 9.2% vs. 3.7%).

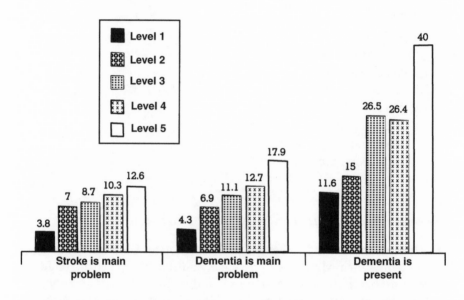

Figure 4.1. *Prevalence of Stroke and Dementia by Level of Care (percentages)*

Living Arrangements

Despite the frequency of chronic and long-term illnesses or conditions necessitating care, very few caregivers said their care recipient resides in a nursing home, assisted living facility, or group home. One-fifth of care recipients live in the same household as their caregiver, and this living arrangement was established in most cases (69%) because of the recipient's need for care. Slightly more than half of all care recipients live alone, either in their own home (37%) or in an apartment or retirement community (17%). The remaining 37 percent live with another family member or friend.

No matter where the care recipient lives, most caregivers and care recipients live in close proximity to each other. Not counting the 21 percent of care recipients who live with their caregiver, more than half of all care recipients (55%) live within a 20-minute commute of their caregiver, 69 percent live between 20 minutes and one hour away, and 94 percent live within two hours' commuting distance of their caregiver. Only six percent of care recipients live further than two hours away from their caregiver.

- While just over one in five care recipients (21%) live in the caregiver's home, 70 percent of those who receive Level 5 care live in the caregiver's home.

- Asian caregivers are more likely to live in the same household with their care recipient (36%) than Blacks (26%) or Whites (19%).

- Care recipients of Asian, Hispanic, and Black caregivers are more likely than those of White caregivers to live with another family member or friend if they do not live with the caregiver.

Intensity of Caregiving: Hours of Care Provided and Activities Performed

As discussed in the introduction to this report, and further elaborated on in the Appendix, a Level of Care Index was created to categorize caregivers according to the amount of time they devote to caregiving and the number and types of activities they assist with when caring for the person to whom they provide the most care. This section addresses these aspects of caregiving.

Estimated Hours Per Week of Care Provided

Caregivers in this survey provide anywhere from less than one hour of care per week to "constant care." Table 4.5 shows the mean number of hours of per week that caregivers estimate they provide, by level of care. Table 4.5 shows that the increases for Level 4 and 5 caregivers are dramatic.

- All Level 5 caregivers, by definition, provide "constant care" or 40 or more hours of care per week (an estimated 2,910,000 caregiver households nationwide), and 25 percent of Level 4 caregivers (or 1,200,000 caregiving households nationwide) also provide this amount of care. This means that a total of at least

4,110,000 caregiving households have a caregiver who provides at least 40 hours of care per week.

- On the other hand, close to all Level 1 (N=389) caregivers surveyed (99%), by definition, spend eight or fewer hours per week providing care.

- Almost half of all caregivers perform care for at least 8 hours per week, and 21% report spending between nine and 20 hours on caregiving per week.

- While the average caregiver provides care for 18 hours per week, close to one in five (18%) provides either "constant care" or at least 40 hours of care per week.

- Women spend significantly more time caregiving than men—an average of 18.8 hours per week, in contrast with 15.5 hours per week for men.

- While women constitute 73% of all caregivers, they are 79% of the constant/40-hour-per-week caregivers.

- Asian caregivers spend significantly less time providing care per week, on average, than other minority caregivers: 15.1 hours, in contrast with 20.6 hours for Blacks and 19.8 hours for Hispanics. (Whites average 17.5 hours of caregiving per week.)

Table 4.5. Mean Hours of Care Provided Per Week by Caregiver Level

Level	Number in Sample	Hours Per Week
All Caregivers	1,509	17.9
Level 1	389	3.6
Level 2	208	8.2
Level 3	287	9.1
Level 4	355	27.3
Level 5	185	56.5

Types of Assistance Caregivers Provide

1. Instrumental Activities of Daily Living (IADLs):[9] Managing Everyday Living

The majority of caregivers surveyed (98%) say they assist their care recipient with at least one IADL, and more than four in five (81%) assist with three or more IADLs.

- Almost eight in 10 caregivers (79%) say they help with transportation, 77 percent do grocery shopping, 74 percent do household chores, 60 percent prepare meals, and more than half manage finances (56%) and/or arrange or supervise the provision of outside services (54%).

- More than one in three caregivers (37%), or 8,370,000 caregiving households nationwide, give medications, pills, or injections to the person they care for. Black caregivers are more likely than either White or Asian caregivers to report that they give medications (51% vs. 35% and 38%); and Hispanic caregivers are more likely to give medications (45%) than Asian caregivers (38%).

- While men and women perform most ADLs in equal proportions, women are more likely than men to do housework (77% vs. 65%) and to prepare meals (65% vs. 47%).

- There are no differences in the incidence of assisting with IADLs by employment status (working compared with non-working caregivers).

- Income, however, does make a difference in the kinds of IADLs performed. For example, caregivers with household incomes under $15,000 are more likely than high-income caregivers (with household incomes of $50,000 or more) to provide assistance with housework (84% vs. 73%) and meal preparation (69% vs. 55%). Similarly, caregivers with household incomes over $50,000 are more likely than caregivers with household incomes under $15,000 to arrange for or supervise outside services (61% vs. 48%) and to manage finances (61% vs. 46%).

There are no differences by race/ethnicity in the extent to which caregivers provide help with IADLs, though there are differences by level of care, as shown in Table 4.6, which highlights differences between

Level 1 and Level 5 caregivers. Level 5 caregivers (and in most cases Level 4 caregivers, as well) are more likely than caregivers of any other level to provide assistance with each IADL.

Table 4.6. Performance of IADLS (percentages)

Instrumental Activity	Total	Level 1	Level 5
Transportation	79.3	72.0	89.6*
Grocery shopping	77.3	67.9	93.7*
Housework	73.6	53.2	96.0*
Preparing meals	60.0	28.9	94.6*
Managing finances	55.6	48.3	74.4*
Arranging/supervising outside services	53.9	42.9	74.6*
Giving medicine	37.3	0.0	86.6*
No ADLs	2.0	2.6	—*

*Differences between Level 5 and Level 1 caregivers are statistically significant at the .05 level.

2. Activities of Daily Living (ADLS):[10] Personal Care such as Bathing or Eating

More than half of all caregivers (51%) help with at least one ADL, and 29 percent help with at least three.

- Overall, women are more likely than men to assist with ADLs (54% vs. 45%), and higher proportions of women than men assist with dressing, bathing or showering, and with continence or diapers.

- Black caregivers are more likely to help with at least one ADL (60%) than Whites (50%) or Asians (44%); half of all White caregivers and 56 percent of Asian caregivers do not assist with any ADLs. Higher proportions of Blacks than Asians report assisting with each ADL, except for feeding.

- A higher percentage of Hispanic caregivers assist with at least one ADL (58%) than Asians (44%); and Hispanics are more likely than Whites to assist with dressing, bathing, toileting, and continence.

- Non-working caregivers are more likely to perform ADLs than employed caregivers (59% vs. 48%).

- While employed caregivers are as likely as those not employed to provide assistance with IADLs, a significantly smaller percentage provide assistance with any ADLs (48%, as compared with 59% of non-working caregivers).

While, by definition, Level 1 caregivers provide no help with ADLs, high proportions of Level 4 and 5 caregivers do, as shown in Table 4.7.

Table 4.7. Performance of ADLs (percentages)

Activity of Daily Living	Total	Level 4	Level 5
Getting in/out of chairs	36.8	56.7	77.8*
Dressing	31.4	56.2	79.9*
Bathing	26.6	47.4	77.5*
Toileting	26.2	47.8	63.2
Feeding	19.2	29.5	43.9
Continuence/diapers	13.6	20.2	44.6*
No ADLS	48.5	15.9	—*

*Differences between Level 5 and Level 4 are significant at the .05 level.

Receipt of Instruction in How to Perform Caregiving Activities

- Just over two in five caregivers (41%) report that someone taught them how to perform at least one of the activities they assist with, while 59 percent have received no instruction. There are no differences by level of care, gender, income, education, or employment status.

That fewer than half of all caregivers have received any instruction in providing care may reflect the fact that many activities they assist with, such as providing transportation or grocery shopping, require no particular skill to be performed satisfactorily.

- There are differences, however, by race/ethnicity. Asian caregivers are the least likely to have been taught how to perform any of the tasks they assist with—only 32% have received any training. This figure is significantly lower than for Black caregivers (46%).

Medication Management

More than seven in 10 caregivers say their care recipients take their own medications as directed—on time, in the right amount, and with no problem. Fewer than one in four caregivers (23%) report that their care recipient has trouble taking medicines, and six percent say their care recipient takes no medicines. There are no differences by race/ethnicity.

- Level 3, 4, and 5 caregivers are more likely than Level 1 caregivers to say their care recipient has trouble taking medications as directed (at least 30%, compared to 9% for Level 1 caregivers).

Of those who do help with medications, a very high percentage (96%) say they know how to administer them as prescribed (on time and in the right amount). Again, there are no differences by race/ethnicity or by level of care.

High proportions also report knowing what each medication is for (90%), the possible side effects of each medication (78%), and how medicines may react with each other (69%).

- Asians are less likely to know these things than caregivers of other racial/ethnic groups.

- Level 4 and 5 caregivers are more likely to be well-informed about these issues than Level 2 caregivers. (Level 1 caregivers do not administer medications.)

More than three in four caregivers who help with medications (77%) say they have asked someone about a medication that was prescribed. Asian caregivers who help with medications are less likely than either Whites or Hispanics to have consulted anyone about them (63% vs. 80% and 78%). There are no differences by level of care.

The person most frequently consulted is a doctor (61%), pharmacist (24%), or a nurse (9%). Four percent report having consulted a family member.

Caregiver Support: Who Also Helps Provide Care?

Almost three in four caregivers (73%) report that someone else also helps provide care to the care recipient. Typically the other helpers are the care recipient's daughter (34%), son (25%), spouse (9%), daughter-in-law (6%), grandson (6%), "the whole family" (5%), or son-in-law (5%). Sisters and nieces of the care recipient were each mentioned by four percent of caregivers. Thirteen percent of caregivers report that a friend or other unpaid non-relative also helps in providing care.

- Hispanic caregivers are more likely than Asians to report that a daughter of the care recipient also provides care (45% vs. 33%); and a higher proportion of Asians (11%) than any other racial/ethnic group report that daughters-in-law also provide care.

- Level 1 caregivers are more likely to say that a relative of the care recipient also helps provide care than are Level 5 caregivers (78% vs. 64%), and that person is less likely to be the care recipient's spouse for Level 5 caregivers than for Levels 2, 3, and 4 caregivers. (This latter finding reflects the fact that Level 5 caregivers are more likely to be caring for a spouse than lower level caregivers.)

Primary vs. Secondary Caregivers

Just over two in five caregivers (41%) say they provide most of the care or that no one else helps, while an equal percentage say someone else provides most of the care. This means that 41 percent of caregivers can be considered primary caregivers and an equal percentage can be considered secondary caregivers. Seventeen percent say the care is split equally between themselves and another person.

- A higher percentage of Black than Asian caregivers report that they themselves provide most of the care or that no one else helps (49% vs. 36%).

• While only 18 percent of caregivers report that no one else helps them with the caregiving, more than one in three Level 5 caregivers (34%) say no one else helps them (which amounts to 980,000 caregiving households), more than for caregivers of any other level.

Are Others Doing Their Fair Share of the Caregiving?

Just under half of all caregivers (49%) feel that other relatives are doing their "fair share" of the caregiving. One in five say their relatives are not doing their fair share, and just over three in 10 (31%) say no one else helps or they get help from a non-relative.

• Asian and Hispanic caregivers are more likely to feel that other relatives are doing their fair share of the caregiving (61% and 54%) than Blacks (43%), and Asians are also more likely to feel that way than Whites (49%).

• A higher proportion of Level 4 and 5 caregivers than Level 1 caregivers feel that other relatives are not doing their fair share (26% and 28% vs. 13%).

Perceptions of Family Conflict over Caregiving

Only five percent of all caregivers report that they experience a lot of family conflict over caregiving, just over one-fifth (21%) report some conflict, and 73 percent report no family conflict at all. There are no differences by race/ethnicity, but there are differences by level of care, by age, and by employment status.

• Level 1 caregivers are more likely to report no family conflict (80%) than either Level 4 or Level 5 caregivers (67% and 68%); and Level 3 caregivers are almost twice as likely as Level 1 caregivers to say they experience some family conflict (30% vs. 16%).

• Caregivers aged 18-34 are more likely than those over 65 to say they experience some family conflict over caregiving (27% vs. only 8%), and are less likely than caregivers aged 50-64 and 65+ to say there is no family conflict at all.

• Employed caregivers are more likely to report family conflict over caregiving (24%) than caregivers who are not working (16%).

Physical, Emotional, and Financial Strain and Stress of Caregiving

While relatively small percentages of all caregivers say their caregiving responsibilities have seriously interfered with their usual activities, caused them physical or mental health problems, been highly stressful physically or emotionally, or posed a serious financial hardship, there is considerable variation in the responses of caregivers by the level of care they provide, by race/ethnicity, and by other demographic variables.

Impact of Caregiving on Time for Family and Leisure Activities

More than four in 10 caregivers (43%) report that their caregiving responsibilities have caused them to have less time for other family members than before, and an equal proportion say that caregiving has necessitated giving up vacations, hobbies, or their own activities. More than half of all caregivers (55%) have experienced one or both of these.

- Not surprisingly, Level 3, 4, and 5 caregivers are more likely to report either of these situations than Level 1 or 2 caregivers. For example, two-thirds of Level 5 caregivers (68%) report having less time for family, in contrast with 22 percent of Level 1 caregivers and 35 percent of Level 2 caregivers; and almost three in four Level 5 caregivers (73%) have had to give up vacations, hobbies, or their own activities (as compared with 25% of Level 1 caregivers and 33% of Level 2 caregivers).

- Those caring for someone with dementia are more likely than other caregivers to have had less time for other family members or leisure activities (66%).

- Asian caregivers are less likely than caregivers of other racial/ethnic groups to say they have less time for other family members due to caregiving (only 31%, compared with 42%-44% of other caregivers). There are no other differences by racial/ethnic group.

- A higher percentage of caregivers with at least some college education report both less time for family and less time for leisure activities than those with a high school education or less.

Experience of Physical or Mental Health Problems

Fifteen percent of all caregivers report that they have suffered any physical or mental health problems as a result of caregiving, and 85 percent say they have not.

- Among Level 5 caregivers, however, more than three in 10 (31%) say they have experienced physical or mental health problems due to caregiving (compared with seven percent of Level 1 caregivers, 13 percent of Level 2 caregivers, and 12 percent of Level 3 caregivers.)

- A higher proportion of Black than Asian caregivers report having suffered physical or mental health problems as a result of caregiving (19% vs. 10%).

- Women are more likely than men to have experienced physical or mental health problems as a result of caregiving (17% vs. 9%), and non-working caregivers are more likely than working caregivers to have experienced such problems (19% vs. 12%).

- A higher proportion of caregivers aged 50-64 report having experienced physical or mental health problems (21%) than those aged 18-34 (9%) or 35-49 (13%).

Experience of Physical Strain

More than half of all caregivers (56%) report that their caregiving activities cause no physical strain at all (a rating of 1 on scale of 1 to 5, where 1 is low and 5 is high), and only six percent say that caregiving has been very much of a physical strain for them.

- Level 5 caregivers, however, experience more physical strain than caregivers of any other level. One in three (33%) rank their physical strain as a 4 or a 5 on the five-point scale.

- A higher proportion of Blacks (19%) report experiencing high levels of physical strain (a rating of 4 or 5) than either Whites or Asians (10% apiece).

- A higher percentage of women than men report experiencing physical strain (13% vs. 5%); and those with annual household incomes under $30,000 are more likely than those with incomes of at least $50,000 to experience high physical strain (17% vs. 6%).

Experience of Emotional Stress

One in four caregivers experience caregiving as emotionally stressful (a rating of 4 or 5 on a scale of 1 to 5), while more than half (55%) find it not very stressful (a rating of 1 or 2). In contrast, more than half of Level 5 caregivers (53%) find caregiving emotionally stressful.

• Of the racial/ethnic groups, Asians report the least amount of emotional stress.

• Women are more likely than men to experience their caregiving as stressful (30% vs. 13%), and a still higher percentage of those caring for a person with dementia say that caregiving is stressful (43%).

Experience of Financial Hardship

Only a small percentage of all caregivers (7%) report that caregiving is a financial hardship for them (a rating of 4 or 5 on a scale of 1 to 5), and more than three in four caregivers (76%) say that caregiving is not a financial hardship at all (a rating of 1).

• A higher percentage of Level 5 caregivers than caregivers of any other level say their caregiving responsibilities pose a financial hardship (21%).

• Whites are more likely than caregivers of any other racial/ethnic group to say that caregiving poses no financial hardship for them at all (78% vs. 70% of Hispanics, 66% of Asians, and 63% of Blacks).

• Black and Hispanic caregivers are more likely than Whites or Asians to say that caregiving is a financial hardship for them (a rating of 4 or 5); 13% and 11 %, compared with 6% of White and Asian caregivers.

• Not surprisingly, those with annual household incomes under $15,000 are more likely than those with higher incomes to say that caregiving poses a financial hardship (16% vs. only 1% for those with incomes of at least $50,000). Similarly, those who have not graduated from college are more likely to say that caregiving poses a financial hardship than those who have.

• Non-working caregivers are more likely to find caregiving a financial hardship (10%) than working caregivers (5%).

Estimated Out-of-Pocket Expenditures on Caregiving Other Than for a Spouse

For the 41 percent of caregivers who report that they know how much they spend of their own money on caregiving during a typical month, the average amount spent is $171, which totals approximately $1.5 billion per month spent out-of- pocket on caregiving nationwide.

Nine percent say they do not know how much they spend, and just under half of all caregivers (49%) say they spend no money of their own on caregiving during a typical month.

- Minority caregivers are more likely to have out-of-pocket expenditures for caregiving than Whites. Only 27 percent of Asians, 35 percent of Hispanics, and 37 percent of Blacks report no monthly personal expenditures on caregiving, in contrast with 53 percent of White caregivers.

- About twice as many Level 1 caregivers (67%) report no out-of-pocket expenditures for caregiving than Level 4 or Level 5 caregivers (31% and 34%).

- Excluding those who say they have no out-of-pocket expenses for caregiving, Level 5 caregivers spend considerably more than Level 1, 2, or 3 caregivers, averaging $357 per month, as compared with $95.42 for Level 1 caregivers, for example.

Caregiving Expenditures for Other Than a Spouse, as a Percentage of Monthly Income

More than three in four caregivers (77%) not involved in spousal caregiving report that they spend 10 percent or less of their own monthly income on caregiving, and fewer than one percent of all caregivers providing non-spousal care report that they spend more than 50 percent of their income on caregiving. Seventeen percent of all caregivers, and 26 percent of Level 5 caregivers, cannot estimate how much they spend per month.

- Of caregivers who can estimate how much they spend out-of-pocket on caregiving, Level 5 caregivers spend an average of 24 percent of their own monthly income on caregiving—a much higher percentage than for caregivers of any other level.

- Of those who spend any money out-of-pocket on caregiving, both Black and Asian caregivers report spending higher proportions of their income on caregiving (averaging 15% and 13%) than White caregivers (6%).

Dealing with Stress: Coping Mechanisms

Caregivers cope with the strains and stresses of caregiving principally through their personal resources or informal networks. The most common coping mechanisms are prayer (74%), talking with friends or relatives (66%), exercising (38%), and hobbies (36%). Relatively small percentages get help from counselors or other professionals (16%), use medications (7%), or resort to alcohol (3%).

* Prayer is the most common way of coping with the stresses and strains of caregiving—almost three in four caregivers (74%) use this method, but 88% of Black caregivers use prayer.

* Whites and Blacks are more likely than Hispanics or Asians to talk with friends and relatives to relieve stress.

* Asian caregivers are less likely to get help from a counselor or professional than either Whites or Blacks (6% vs. 17% and 14%).

Biggest Difficulty and Greatest Reward of Caregiving

Biggest Difficulty

One in five caregivers (20%) say the biggest difficulties they face in providing care are the demands on their time or not being able to do what they want; 15 percent say it is watching or worrying about their care recipient's deterioration; 10 percent say it is the care recipient's attitude (uncooperative, "demanding"); and four percent mention a problem with location, distance, or inconvenience. There were no differences by race/ethnicity.

More than one in four caregivers (26%) say they have no difficulty providing care, though this response was more frequent among Level 1 and 2 caregivers than among Level 4 and 5 caregivers.

* Perhaps not surprisingly, Level 3, 4, and 5 caregivers are more likely to say that watching or worrying about their care recipient's deterioration is their biggest concern (17-21%) than are Level 1 caregivers (just under 8%).

* Blacks are more likely than Whites to mention the physical demands of caregiving as their biggest difficulty (6% vs. 2%).

Biggest Reward

The biggest rewards of caregiving are knowing that the care recipient is well cared for, personal satisfaction in knowing one is doing a good deed, and the care recipient's appreciation or happiness. Each of these was mentioned by 16 percent of caregivers. Also mentioned are watching the care recipient's health improve (by 11%), family loyalty, "giving back," fulfilling family obligations (by 11%), and spending time together (by 10%). There are no differences by race/ethnicity.

- Level 2 caregivers are more likely to mention family loyalty or obligation as the biggest reward of caregiving (18%) than Level 4 or 5 caregivers (6%-7%).

Words Caregivers Use to Describe the Caregiving Experience

Positive Words

A majority of caregivers (57%) use positive words to describe the caregiving experience; and there are no differences in the overall positive comments by race/ethnicity or level of care.

Words used to describe the experience of caregiving by more than a handful of caregivers include "rewarded"/"rewarding" (mentioned by 19%); "happy," "helpful" (each by 7%); and "thankful"/"grateful," "enjoyable," and "love"/"loving" (each by 4%). Interestingly, Level 5 caregivers are more likely to report that they feel good, comfortable, content, or "OK" about caregiving than Level 1 or Level 2 caregivers (9% vs. 1%).

Negative Words

Just over one-third of caregivers (34%) use negative words to describe their experience as a caregiver. There are no differences by level of care provided or by racial/ethnic group.

The negative words caregivers most frequently use to summarize how they feel about caregiving are "stressful" (12%), "obligation"/"duty" (9%), "burdened" (3%), and "tired"/"exhausting" (3%). There are no differences by level of care.

- Hispanics are more likely than Whites to use the word "stressful" in describing their caregiving experiences (18% vs. 10%).

Eight percent of caregivers say they don't know how they feel about caregiving.

Utilization of Supportive Services Available in the Community

Almost three in four caregivers (74%) report having used one or more services or devices shown in Table 4.8. Not surprisingly, Level 3, 4, and 5 caregivers are more apt to have used wheelchairs or walkers, personal or nursing care services, home modification, and respite care (identified during the interviews as "temporary care services") than Level 1 or 2 caregivers. The number of such services and devices used also varies by level of care provided. For example, the average number of services used by Level 1 caregivers is 1.36, while for Level 5 caregivers it is 2.94.

- Caregivers who report that their care recipient has dementia are more likely to report the use of at least one of these services (83%) than caregivers overall (74%).

- Asian caregivers are the least likely of the racial/ethnic groups to report having used any of these services—only 62 percent, compared with 72-76% of caregivers of other racial/ethnic groups. This finding holds for wheelchairs and other devices, personal or nursing care services, and home-delivered meal services.

- White, Black, and Hispanic caregivers were more than twice as likely as Asian caregivers to have used personal or nursing care services (32% to 44% vs. only 15% of Asians), and Blacks were the most likely to have done so (44%).

It is not clear whether the lower rates of service utilization among Asian caregivers are a result of the overall lower level of care they provide, cultural factors, or something else.

- Both White and Hispanic caregivers were more likely to say they have made home modifications than Black caregivers (29% and 26% vs. 17%).

- Blacks and Hispanics are more likely to have used transportation services (more than 20% each) than Whites (only 14%), and Blacks are more likely than Whites to have used adult day care or senior centers (14% vs. 9%).

81

- Asians are the least likely to have used respite care services—only 8 percent have done so, compared with 15 percent of Whites, for example.

- Among Level 5 caregivers, use of respite care (by 23%), adult day care (by 16%), and support groups (by 15%) is modest, even though significantly higher than for caregivers providing lower levels of care. There were no differences by level of care in the extent to which meal services, help with housework, or transportation services are used.

- Female caregivers are more likely than male caregivers to have used a device such as a wheelchair or personal or nursing care services, and caregivers aged 65+ are more likely than caregivers of younger ages to have used a support group (14% vs. 4-8%).

- Not surprisingly, college graduates are more likely than caregivers of lower educational attainment to have used housework assistance or adult day care or a senior center to assist with care.

Sixteen percent of caregivers reported they had sought information on how to get financial assistance for the person(s) to whom they provide care. Use of financial information services is more common among Level 4 and 5 caregivers than among Level 1 and 2 caregivers, but does not differ by race/ethnicity (except that Hispanics are more likely to have used them than Asians) or other demographic variables.

Table 4.8. Utilization of Services (Base = Total Caregivers)

Service	Percentages
Acquiring a wheelchair, walker, or other device	46.7
Personal or nursing care services	37.8
Home modification	28.1
Home-delivered meal services	15.6
Assistance with housework	15.6
Financial information service	15.5
Transportation service	14.9
Respite care	14.1
Adult day care/senior center	9.5
Support group	6.6

More than one in four caregivers (27%) say they have used none of the services or devices. Not surprisingly, this is more typically the case among Levels 1 and 2 caregivers than among Levels 3, 4, and 5 caregivers, and also among Asian caregivers.

Service Providers

Almost half the caregivers who use any of these services or devices (49%) say they are or were provided by an individual or private commercial agency, paid for by the caregiver. Community or government agencies were a source of services or devices for 45% of the caregivers. Other sources include health care providers (used by 43% of caregivers using any services) and family, friends, and volunteers (used by 23%). Ten percent say the services are or were provided by a church or synagogue.

Level of Satisfaction with Providers of Assistive Services and Devices

As Table 4.9 shows, satisfaction with services and devices is relatively high, with more than four in five caregivers reporting that the devices/services they have used either fully or partially met their needs, except in the area of financial information services.

Caregivers who have used wheelchairs or other devices, home modifications, and transportation services are the most apt to say the service fully met their needs, and those who have used financial information services are least likely to say the services fully met their needs.

Table 4.9. Satisfaction with Services and Information (Base = Total Caregivers)

Service/Information	Met Need Fully	Met Need Partially
Wheelchair, walker, or other device	81.4	14.1
Home modification	77.9	17.6
Transportation Service	71.8	24.8
Home-delivered meal service	61.0	25.3
Housework	61.9	30.5
Personal care, nursing service	69.6	23.8
Adult day care/senior center	53.6	30.7
Respite care service	62.9	32.4
Support Group	53.4	37.8
Financial information service	33.5	40.7

Reasons for Non-Utilization of Assistive Services and Devices

For each of the 10 services inquired about, caregivers who said they did not use it were asked why. In the great majority of cases, the reason caregivers did not use a service is that they had no need for it, ranging from 61 percent for support groups to 96 percent for assistive devices.

Lack of Awareness of the Service

The second most frequent reason for not using a service was not being aware of it, mentioned by 18 percent of all caregivers, but by 30 percent of Level 5 caregivers (a higher percentage than for caregivers of any other level). This reason was cited by higher percentages of Blacks and Hispanics (27% and 29%) than Whites (17%), and by a higher percentage of primary caregivers (22%) than secondary or co-equal caregivers (16%).

"Too Proud" to Use It

An unusually high percentage of caregivers (15%) said they or their care recipient were too proud to use adult day care or a senior center—a much higher percentage than for any other service/device inquired about (two percent or fewer). There is probably also some confusion as to what adult day care is, because five percent of caregivers mentioned that they didn't use it because they didn't want an outsider coming in to their home. "Too proud" may also reflect resistance to services by the older person.

- This reason was more often cited by caregivers aged 50-64 (23%) than those aged 18-34 (12%), and by primary caregivers (25%) than secondary/co-equal caregivers (12%).

No Special Reason/Never Thought about It

Seventeen percent of caregivers who don't use a particular service said they had no special reason for not using it, or that they had never thought about it. Higher proportions of Level 4 and 5 caregivers mentioned this reason than Level 1 caregivers (23% vs. 12%), and so did higher percentages of Black and Hispanic caregivers (29% and 26%) than White caregivers (15%).

Too Busy

Ten percent of caregivers said they were too busy to use the service, with a higher percentage of Hispanic caregivers (21%) citing this reason than caregivers of any other race/ethnicity (10-11%). A higher percentage of primary caregivers than secondary caregivers also said that they were too busy.

Service Is Not Available

The perception or knowledge that a service is not available also contributes to its non-utilization. Interestingly, 17 percent of Level 5 caregivers and 13 percent of Level 4 caregivers mentioned this as a barrier, in contrast with only four percent of Level 1 caregivers. Those with incomes of less than $15,000 were more likely to cite this reason (15%) than those with incomes between $30,000 and $50,000 (only 4%).

Cost

Surprisingly, very few caregivers cited cost as a barrier to obtaining needed services. Factors influencing whether cost is mentioned include intensity of care, race/ethnicity, income, living arrangements, and primary vs. secondary/co-equal caregiver status.

- Although all percentages are small, higher percentages of Level 4 and Level 5 caregivers (9% and 11%, respectively) mention cost as a barrier to service utilization than Level 1 caregivers (1%), and a higher percentage of Hispanic caregivers (10%) cite this reason than Asians (2%).

- Not surprisingly, those with incomes under $15,000 were more likely to mention cost as a factor than those with incomes of at least $30,000. A higher proportion of caregivers whose care recipient lives with them cite cost as a reason for non-utilization of services (12%) than those whose care recipient lives up to an hour away (4%). Primary caregivers also are more apt to mention cost as a barrier than secondary/co-equal caregivers (8% vs. 4%).

Unmet Needs for Help, Information, or Support in Caregiver Role

Table 4.10 shows the kinds of assistance most frequently mentioned in response to a question concerning the kinds of help, information, or support caregivers would use, or would have used, in providing care.

While 38 percent said they didn't know what additional assistance they would use, or would have used, this figure escalates to 49 percent of Asian caregivers—higher than for all other racial/ethnic groups—and to 44 percent for those with a high school education or less (compared with about one-third of more highly educated groups).

Black caregivers were more likely than Whites or Asians to name at least one type of assistance they would use (51%, vs. 43% and 36%, respectively).

Those who have not used any services are more likely not to know what they would use, or would have used, than those who have (48% vs. 35%), and secondary/co-equal caregivers are less likely to know than primary caregivers (43% vs. 31%). This is also the case for higher percentages of Level 1 and 2 caregivers than for Level 5 caregivers.

While 19 percent of all caregivers said there was nothing they needed, those who had never used any services were more likely to say they didn't need any (25%) than those who had (16%).

Table 4.10. Kinds of Help, Information, or Support Caregivers Would Use/Would Have Used (Base = Total Caregivers*)

Help, Information, or Support	Percentages
Don't know	38.1
None/nothing/no help	18.5
Free time/time for self/a break	16.9
Help with housekeeping	9.8
Extra money/financial support	9.5
Central source of information	9.0
Information about paying for services such as nursing homes, adult day care	7.6
Someone to talk with/counseling/support group	6.0
Sitting services/someone to check up on care recipient	5.6
Help with ADLs/personal care	4.9
Help with shopping	4.3
Help with medications	3.2
Information about care recipient's condition	2.7

*Up to two responses per caregiver were coded.

Free Time/A Break from Caregiving

As expected, caregivers who provide the most intense and difficult kinds of care are the ones most likely to report needing more free time or a break from caregiving. There are no differences by race/ethnicity.

- While 17 percent of all caregivers say they could use more free time or a break from caregiving, Level 5 caregivers are more likely to say they need it (33%) than Level 1, 2, or 3 caregivers. Primary caregivers also are more likely to report needing a break than secondary/co-equal caregivers (21% vs. 14%).

- Caregivers taking care of someone with dementia also are more likely to mention needing more free time or a break from caregiving: 24%.

Caregivers who have used formal services are more likely to mention needing a break than those who have not (19% vs.10%).

Assistance with Housekeeping and Meal Preparation

Ten percent of caregivers say they could use help with housekeeping. Women are more likely to say this than men (11% vs. 7%). Both low- and high-income caregivers are more likely than middle-income caregivers to need help with housekeeping, as are primary caregivers compared with secondary/co-equal caregivers (13% vs. 8%), and those who have used formal services as compared with those who have not (12% vs. 5%).

Though the percentages are small, Black and Hispanic caregivers are more likely to report needing help with meal preparation than Whites (7% vs. 3%), as are spouse caregivers (9%) when compared to all caregivers (3%).

Needs for Financial Help

Very small numbers of caregivers mentioned needing money. Higher percentages of Blacks and Hispanics than Whites report needing extra money or financial support because of their caregiving responsibilities (14% vs. 9%).

Those caring for someone with dementia are also more likely to say they need extra money or financial support than the average caregiver (14% vs. 10%).

- Understanding how to pay for nursing homes, adult day care, or other services was more often mentioned by Hispanic caregivers (13%) than by Whites (7%), by caregivers with household incomes under $15,000 (16%) than by those with incomes above $15,000 (5% to 9%), by persons who have used formal services (9%) than by those who have not (3%).

- Not surprisingly, caregivers assisting persons with dementia were more likely than the typical caregiver to say they could use, or could have used, help in understanding how to pay for long-term care services such as nursing homes and adult day care (12% vs. 8%).

Central Source of Information

Having a central place to go to or to call to find out what help is available was mentioned by nine percent of caregivers as a need or service they would use, or could have used. Interestingly, this was mentioned more frequently by those with household incomes over $50,000 (15%) than by those with lower incomes (8%-10%), and more often by those with at least some college education (11-14%) than by those with a high school education or less (5%). It was also more frequently mentioned by those who had used services than those who had not.

Someone to Talk with, Counseling, Support Group

While only six percent of caregivers say they could use someone to talk with, counseling, or a support group, a higher percentage of Level 5 caregivers (25%) than all other groups say they could use this kind of assistance. Those caring for someone with dementia were also more likely than the average caregiver to say they could benefit from talking with someone (11%).

Women are more likely to say they could use this type of assistance than men (7% vs. 3%), and caregivers aged 50-64 and 65+ are more likely to say they need it than those aged 18-34 (9% and 10% vs. 2%). Those whose care recipients live with them are more likely to need someone to talk with than those who do not live with their care recipient (13% vs. 4%).

- Caregivers taking care of someone with dementia also are more likely to mention needing someone to talk with, counseling, or a support group (11%).

Impact of Caregiving on Work

Since the majority of caregivers are employed (64%), most of them full-time (52%), the impact of caregiving responsibilities on work life can be important.

While relatively few caregivers who ever worked while providing care to their care recipient (79% of caregivers) report having given up working entirely as a result of caregiving (6%), caregiving responsibilities do have a significant impact on caregivers' work life. For example, more than half the caregivers employed while caregiving for this care recipient (54%) have made changes at work to accommodate caregiving.

- Making changes in daily work schedule (going in late, leaving early, or taking time off during the day) are the changes most frequently reported: by 49% of caregivers who ever worked while caring for this care recipient.

- One-fifth of all caregivers ever employed while caring for this care recipient gave up work either temporarily or permanently: 11 percent took or have taken a leave of absence, four percent took early retirement, and six percent gave up working entirely.

- Seven percent report having changed from full-time to part-time work or taken a less demanding job.

- Relatively few report having lost their benefits (4%) or having turned down a promotion (3%) because of caregiving responsibilities.

- Hispanic and Asian caregivers are more likely to have had to take a leave of absence from work (18% and 22%) than Whites (10%).

As Table 4.11 shows, there is a correlation between the level of care provided and the likelihood of altering one's daily work schedule, taking a leave of absence, switching to part-time work, or giving up work entirely. For example, three in four Level 5 caregivers, in contrast with 41 percent of Level 1 caregivers, have made at least one of the work-related adjustments shown in Table 4.11.

- Thirty percent of Level 5 caregivers report having had to give up work entirely, and 26 percent say they took a leave of absence because of their caregiving responsibilities—much higher percentages than for Level 1, 2, or 3 caregivers.

Table 4.11. Work-Related Adjustments by Level of Care
(Base = Caregivers Ever Employed while Providing Care to This Care Recipient)

	Total	Level 1	Level 2	Level 3	Level 4	Level 5
Total unweighted +	(N=1,193)	(n=330)	(n=174)	(n=240)	(n=277)	(n=113)
Total weighted +	(N=1,716)	(n=530)	(n=245)	(n=331)	(n=363)	(n=166)
Made any changes listed below	**54.2**	**40.8**	**45.1**	**58.2***	**66.5***	**75.0***
Changed daily schedule: go in late, leave early, take time off during work	49.4	36.3	44.0	54.0*	61.5*	64.0*
Took leave of absence	10.9	5.5	5.9	9.1	17.8*	26.0*
Worked fewer hours, took less demanding job	7.3	2.0	3.8	6.5	11.7*	25.0*
Lost any job benefits	4.2	2.4	3.4	1.7	7.5	11.0*
Turned down a promotion	3.1	1.2	2.1	0.7	6.0	10.4*
Chose early retirement	3.6	1.2	0.3	3.0	5.1	14.8*
Gave up work entirely	6.4	1.3	0.2	4.4	10.2*	30.3*

+Unweighted numbers refer to numbers of caregivers in the sample, while weighted numbers refer to numbers of caregiving households in the U.S. population nationwide.
*Differences in percentages are significant at the .05 level.

Other factors associated with higher levels of care or more intense caregiving include caring for a person with dementia, living in the same household as the care recipient, helping with two or more ADLs, and being a primary caregiver. Table 4.12 shows the percentages of these types of caregivers who have made work-related adjustments as a result of caregiving.

Attitude of Employer toward Caregiver

More than four in five caregivers who have experienced any of these problems (81%) have found their employer's attitude toward the demands of caregiving to be either very understanding (63%) or somewhat understanding (18%). Seven percent said their employer was not very understanding, and 7% said their employer was not aware of their caregiving activities. There are no significant differences by level of care provided.

Summary and Conclusions

Family caregiving to persons aged 50 and older is widespread among the U.S. population. In close to one in four households there is at least one person aged 18 or older who presently provides care, or who has been a caregiver, to an older person at some point during the past 12 months. This person is typically a female and typically provided care to a female relative. About one in four caregivers is under 35 and more than one in three are age 50 or older, with the bulk of caregivers ranging in age from 35 to 49. The majority of caregivers have provided care to their primary care recipient for less than five years, while about one in five has done so for five to 10 years, and 10 percent have been providing care for at least 10 years.

Not only are family caregivers diverse in age and the length of time they have been providing care, they are also diverse with respect to the types of care and the number of hours of care they provide in a typical week, which range from very modest and non-taxing to heavy-duty, round-the-clock care involving assistance with multiple tasks and personal care. About half of all caregivers provide assistance with at least one personal care activity, and almost every caregiver provides assistance with some aspect of managing a household or coping with the demands of daily living. In general, caregivers and their care recipients live in close proximity to each other. About one in five lives in the same household with his or her care recipient(s)—typically the case with Level 5 caregivers—and of the remainder, almost

Table 4.12. Conditions Increasing the Likelihood of Work-Related Adjustments
(Base = Caregivers Ever Employed while Providing Care to This Care Recipient)

Work Adjustment	Alzheimer's or Confusion	Live in Same Household	Help with 2+ ADLs	Primary Caregiver
Total unweighted +	(n=239)	(n=270)	(n=426)	(n=460)
Total weighted +	(n=363)	(n=317)	(n=601)	(n=641)
Made any changes listed below	**62.7**	**64.9**	**68.2**	**65.7**
Changed daily schedule: go in late, leave early, take time off during work	57.5	57.3	62.1	61.5
Took leave of absence	9.9	15.1	18.5	15.8
Worked fewer hours, took less demanding job	13.7	14.0	14.0	9.6
Lost any job benefits	5.7	7.9	7.4	6.3
Turned down a promotion	5.8	7.4	5.3	4.5
Chose early retirement	6.9	10.2	6.2	6.6
Gave up work entirely	9.8	16.1	13.1	10.0

+Unweighted numbers refer to numbers of caregivers in the sample, while weighted numbers refer to numbers of caregiving households in the U.S. population nationwide.

seven in 10 caregivers live within an hour's commuting distance from their care recipient.

While a high percentage of caregivers use positive words to describe their feelings about caregiving, and relatively few say they experience family conflict over caregiving, the responsibilities involved in providing care do have an impact on family life, leisure time, work life, personal finances, and in some cases on physical and mental health. More than half of all caregivers report that their caregiving responsibilities cause them to have less time for other family members or have necessitated giving up vacations, hobbies, or their own activities. Not surprisingly, those whose caregiving activities are more intense and require a heavy investment of time are more likely to report these impacts.

Though relatively few caregivers who have ever worked while providing care to their care recipient(s) report that they have had to quit work entirely, more than half have made at least some work-related changes to accommodate the demands of caregiving. Most typically, these changes have involved modifying one's work schedule—going in late, leaving early, or taking time off during the day—though 11 percent report having had to take a leave of absence due to caregiving responsibilities. Level 5 caregivers, however, are much more likely than Level 1 or 2 caregivers to have made work-related changes of a more serious nature, more than 30 percent reporting that they gave up work entirely and 15 percent saying they took early retirement.

Among those caregivers who take care of someone other than a spouse and who report having out-of-pocket expenditures associated with caregiving, the average monthly outlay is $171. This estimate may be conservative, in that nine percent of all caregivers say they do not know how much they spend out-of-pocket on caregiving. Some caregivers experience considerable financial hardship due to caregiving responsibilities. For example, Level 5 caregivers, whose monthly outlay for caregiving averages $357, report out-of-pocket expenses constituting, on average, almost one-fourth of their monthly income. While a relatively small percentage of caregivers overall say that caregiving poses a financial hardship for them, Black and Hispanic caregivers are more likely than either Whites or Asians to say so, as are caregivers with annual household incomes under $15,000.

Again, while overall only a modest percentage of all caregivers report that they have suffered any physical or mental health problems as a result of caregiving, such problems are cited much more frequently by Level 5 caregivers than by persons providing lower levels of care, by women than by men, and by caregivers aged 50-64 than by younger caregivers. Additionally, more than half of Level 5 caregivers find caregiving emotionally stressful, in contrast with one in four caregivers overall. Women are more likely to experience emotional stress than men, and persons caring for someone with dementia are more likely to report that caregiving is emotionally stressful for them than those who are not.

Not surprisingly, utilization of supportive services available in the community, such as home-delivered meals, adult day care, or personal care/nursing services, is correlated with need, with Level 5 caregivers more likely to be using such services than Level 1 caregivers. Service utilization rates are lowest among Asian caregivers, for reasons that are unclear. Very few caregivers cited cost or "bureaucracy" as a barrier to service utilization. When asked what kinds of help, information, or support they would use, or would have used, a high percentage (38%) said they didn't know, and 19 percent said they didn't need any (additional) help. The most frequently cited need, however, was for free time, a "break" from caregiving, or time for oneself—particularly among Level 5 caregivers, those caring for someone with dementia, and primary caregivers.

This study suggests that family caregiving in the United States is prevalent and a normative experience that caregivers by and large accept as a necessary responsibility, and that they provide such care for the most part without many complaints or a perception that they lack access to services they might need. The findings also suggest, however, that the impact of caregiving on caregivers' lives varies considerably by the type and amount of care required and provided, by race/ethnicity, and also by other demographic factors such as age. More research is needed on the direct and indirect financial contributions of caregivers, and on how services provided are paid for. With the projected increase in the minority elderly population in the future, it will also be increasingly important to better understand the needs and experiences of minority caregivers. The present study has made a start in this direction.

Clearly, there is a segment of the caregiving population that provides very intense care that can involve extensive personal and financial sacrifice, as well as physical and/or emotional stress. Providing an average of more than 56 hours of care per week and assisting extensively with both IADLs and ADLs, Level 5 caregivers report spending more out-of-pocket on caregiving than caregivers of any other level, and close to one-third of them say they have experienced physical or mental health problems as a result of caregiving. These caregivers have also made more extensive work-related adjustments than caregivers providing less intense care. Three in four of them have made at least some change in their work life, 30 percent have had to give up work entirely, and 26 percent report having had to take a leave of absence due to caregiving responsibilities. Though a relatively small proportion of all caregivers, Level 5 caregivers would be appropriate candidates for intervention.

Appendix/Methodology

The Samples

Two samples were used to conduct the survey. The first was a fully-replicated, stratified, single-stage random-digit-dial (RDD) sample of U.S. telephone households generated in-house by ICR. The supplemental sample was extracted from ICR's EXCEL Omnibus Service, and included individuals who had previously identified themselves as Hispanic, Black, or Other Race. All respondents were known to be English speaking because they had been previously so identified by ICR. (Resources to conduct telephone interviews with non-English speaking Americans were not available.) The supplemental sample was used to over-sample by race for Black, Hispanic, and Asian caregivers. Because the EXCEL Omnibus Service uses a sampling model that is similar to the one in the RDD sampling model, the racial/ethnic oversamples extracted from that source are similarly representative of U.S. telephone households within these racial/ ethnic groups.

In total (both samples), 1,509 telephone interviews were conducted, all in English and averaging 20 minutes in length. The statistical margin of error for a sample of this size is plus or minus 2.52% at the 95% confidence level. This means that on a question answered by all 1,509 people, it is 95% certain that the total population would fall within 2.52 percentage points of the actual finding. The sampling error widens on questions answered by smaller groups of respondents.

The RDD sample yielded 754 interviews (consisting principally of interviews with Whites) that can be said to be accurate to within +/- 3.58% at the 95% confidence level. By race/ethnicity, the samples, and the 95% confidence interval for each, break out as is shown in Table 4.13.

Weighting of the Findings

To reflect the actual proportion of racial/ethnic groups in the U.S. population, all survey data were weighted using incidence levels derived from the RDD sample and U.S. Census projections. All findings reported are weighted so that they can be projected to U.S. telephone households with an informal caregiver, as defined for purposes of this survey.

Of an estimated 96,600,000 U.S. telephone households, the incidence of caregiver households was determined to be 23.2%, or 22,411,200 households. Frequencies shown in the tables in this report refer not to sampled caregivers, but to the U.S. population of caregivers, and must be multiplied by 10,000 to obtain accurate household projections nationwide. For example, the number 2,241 (the estimated number of U.S. caregiving households) is equivalent to 22.4 million households.

Weighted estimates of caregiver households by racial/ethnic group, together with their population percentage of all caregiver households, are shown in Table 4.14.

Table 4.13. Random-Digit-Dial Sample of U.S. Telephone Households

Racial/Ethnic Category	Sample Size n	95% Confidence Level
White (non-Hispanic)	623	+/-3.93%
Black (non-Hispanic)	306	+/-5.60%
Asian	264	+/-6.03%
Hispanic	307	+/-5.59%
Other	9	
Total	1,509	

Table 4.14. Weighted Estimates of Caregiver Households by Racial/Ethnic Group

Racial/Ethnic Category	Weighted n	Population Percentage
White (non-Hispanic)	18,287,539	81.6
Black (non-Hispanic)	2,375,587	10.6
Asian	403,402	1.8
Hispanic	1,053,326	4.7
Other	291,346	1.3

Factor Analysis

A factor analysis was conducted to determine which variables are most closely associated with the intensity, level of difficulty, or amount of wear and tear involved in informal caregiving.

Factor analysis is a statistical technique used to identify the underlying structure within a set of variables. It is used to reduce a large number of variables to a smaller set of factors that greatly simplify the description of the data and aid in its interpretation. Factor analytic techniques generate a smaller set of variables, called "factors," that represent the underlying dimensions of the original (larger) set of variables, based on the degree of association (or correlation) among them. Each factor is not a single, directly measurable entity, but rather a construct derived from the relationships among the original set of variables.

In this study, five questions were asked to assess different aspects of the amount of care, intensity of care, or degree of difficulty involved in informal caregiving, based on caregivers' reported experiences. These five questions concerned

1. the caregiver's estimate of the number of hours of care he/she provides per week;

2. the type of care he/she provides (the numbers of IADLs and ADLs he/she assists with);

3. the amount of physical strain experienced by the caregiver (a subjective measure);

4. the amount of emotional stress experienced by the caregiver (a subjective measure); and

5. the amount of financial hardship experienced by the caregiver (a subjective measure).

Only a single factor emerged from a factor analysis of these five items. It can be interpreted as a measure of intensity of care, which consists of the number of hours of care provided per week coupled with the type of care provided. (Physical strain, emotional stress, and financial hardship do not load on this factor.)

Level of Care Index

Based on the outcome of the factor analysis, a Level of Care Index consisting of five points was created. This enabled each caregiver to

Table 4.15. Coding of Assessment Questions

Variables	Response Categories
Hours of care per week	1 = 0 to 8 hours
	2 = 9 to 20 hours
	3 = 21 to 40 hours
	4 = 41 or more hours
Types of care provided	1 = 0 IADLs/0 ADLs
	2 = 1 IADL/0 ADLs
	3 = 2+ IADLs/0 ADLs
	4 = 1 ADL (with or without IADLs)
	5 = 2+ ADLs (with or without IADLs)
Physical Strain	1 Not at all a strain
	2
	3
	4
	5 Very much of a strain
Emotional Stress	1 Not at all stressful
	2
	3
	4
	5 Very stressful
Financial Hardship	1 No hardship at all
	2
	3
	4
	5 A great deal of hardship

be assigned for analytic purposes to one of the five levels, based on the intensity of caregiving provided.

The two variables on which the Index is based are "hours of care per week" (four levels, as shown above) and "types of care" (collapsed into four levels), as shown in Table 4.16.

Table 4.16. Level of Care Index

Variables	Response Categories
Hours of care per week	1 = 0 to 8 hours
	2 = 9 to 20 hours
	3 = 21 to 40 hours
	4 = 41 or more hours, or
	"constant care"
Types of care provided	1 = 0 IADLs/0 ADLs or 1 IADL/0 ADLs
	2 = 2+ IADLs/0 ADLs
	3 = 1 ADL (with or without IADLs)
	4 = 2+ ADLs (with or without IADLs)

Each caregiver's score on the two variables was summed, resulting in his/her assignment to one of seven levels (2, 3, 4, 5, 6, 7, or 8). Examination of the frequencies suggested that collapsing the seven levels into five, as shown in Table 4.17, would result in a useful and not very skewed distribution of caregivers across levels, with Level 1 being the least intense level of caregiving, and Level 5 being the most intense.

Table 4.17. Levels of Caregiving

	Combined Score	Resulting # of Caregivers (unweighted)	Percent of Sample
Level 1	2, 3	389	25.8%
Level 2	4	208	13.8%
Level 3	5	287	19.0%
Level 4	6, 7	355	23.5%
Level 5	8	185	12.3%
Missing		85	5.6%

References

A National Survey of Caregivers: Final Report. Conducted by Opinion Research Corporation for the American Association of Retired Persons and The Travelers Foundation. September 1988.

Caregiving Among American Indians: A Review of the Literature. Prepared by Ada-Helen Bayer, consultant to the Research Division/AARP. May, 1997.

Findings from an Excel Omnibus Survey of Caregivers Conducted May 19-28, 1995. Prepared for the Long-term Care Team/Health Advocacy Services/ Programs Division/AARP (August 28, 1995) by Jane Takeuchi of Evaluation Research Services/Research Division/AARP.

United States Census Bureau. May 1995. *Sixty-five Plus in the United States.* [http://www.census.gov/socdemo/www/agebrief.html]

Endnotes

1. These designations are adapted from OMB's "Directive No. 15," Race and Ethnic Standards for Federal Statistics and Administrative Reporting (as adopted on May 12, 1977). The term "White" refers to persons self-identified as White and having origins in any of the original peoples of Europe, North Africa, or the Middle East, but in this case exclusive of persons who designate themselves as of Hispanic origin. The term "Black" refers to persons who identify themselves as Black (having origins in any of the black racial groups of Africa), but in this case not of Hispanic origin. The term "Hispanic" refers to persons who identify themselves as of Mexican, Puerto Rican, Cuban, Central or South American, or other Spanish culture of origin, regardless of race. The term "Asian" refers to persons who identify themselves as having origins in any of the peoples of the Far East, Southeast Asia, the Indian subcontinent, or the Pacific Islands.

2. Funding for this survey was provided by a grant from Glaxo Wellcome, Inc., a research based company whose people are committed to fighting disease by bringing innovative medicines and services to patients, their families, and the health care providers who serve them.

3. Additional copies of this report and of any of its companion volumes may be obtained by writing the National Alliance for

Caregiving, 4720 Montgomery Lane, Suite 642, Bethesda, MD 20814-3425, or the AARP Fulfillment, 601 E Street, NW, Washington, DC 20049. Please use the order number when requesting reports.

4. Order a copy of the report on the Metlife Study of Employer Costs for Working Caregivers based on data from *Family Caregiving in the U.S.: Findings from a National Survey* from Metlife Mature Market Group, 57 Green Farms Road, Westport, CT 06880.

5. In a 1988 study of caregivers, 7.8 percent of U.S. households were identified as having a caregiver when a more restrictive definition of caregiving was used than in the present study. In the 1988 study, to be defined as a caregiver, a person must have been helping with at least two Instrumental Activities of Daily Living (IADLs) or one Activity of Daily Living (ADL). See *A National Survey of Caregivers: Final Report,* (D13203) conducted by Opinion Research Corporation of Washington, DC, for the American Association of Retired Persons of Washington, DC, and The Travelers Foundation of Hartford, CT. September 1988.

6. The 1988 report estimated that there were seven million U.S. caregiving households at that time, based on the definition of a caregiver used for that study. Applying the same definition of a caregiver as used in the 1988 study to the current study (i.e., the caregiver must be providing assistance with at least two Instrumental Activities of Daily Living or one Activity of Daily Living), the number of caregivers providing this level of care as of 1996 is 21,290,000, or triple the number in 1988.

7. A 1995 survey of caregivers aged 18 and older that used a very similar definition of caregiving found almost the same low percentage of caregivers taking care of a spouse (4%). (See *Findings from an Excel Omnibus Survey of Caregivers* Conducted May 19-28, 1995, prepared for AARP's Long-term Care Team/Health Advocacy Services/Programs Division by Jane Takeuchi, Evaluation Research Services/Research Division/ AARP, August 28, 1995.)

8. This finding is consistent with the 1995 survey, in which 14 percent of caregivers aged 65+ were caring for a spouse.

9. Instrumental Activities of Daily Living (IADLs) are activities performed to manage one's daily life or maintain a household and live independently, such as preparing meals, grocery shopping, driving or using transportation systems, doing light housework, taking medications, managing finances and paying bills, and using the telephone.

10. Activities of Daily Living (ADLs) are activities involving personal care, such as eating, toileting, getting in and out of bed and chairs, bathing, dressing and grooming, and managing continence or changing adult diapers/briefs.

Chapter 5

Balancing Caregiving with Work and the Costs Involved

Introduction

Family caregiving for persons aged 50 and over is widespread in the United States and is on the increase. Nearly 25% of all households have at least one adult who has provided care for an elderly person at some point during the past 12 months. Over the next 10 years, the total number of employed caregivers in the United States is expected to increase to between 11 and 15.6 million working Americans— roughly one in ten employed workers.[1] This landmark study is the first ever to examine the long-term costs these caregivers face when they disrupt their work to accommodate the needs of their older loved ones.

Background

In 1997, to understand the challenges faced by family caregivers, the National Alliance for Caregiving (NAC) and AARP conducted a national survey of 1509 individuals aged 18 and over who provide unpaid care to a relative or friend aged 50 or older.[2] It measured the prevalence and intensity of caregiving in the United States. The study found that—in addition to their caregiving responsibilities—64% of these caregivers are employed, creating a "juggling" act between work and caregiving obligations. The same year, MetLife sponsored a study of the cost to business of caregiving in lost productivity. This study

Reprinted with permission, "The MetLife Juggling Act Study, November 1999," © National Alliance for Caregiving.

used data from the national caregiver survey to estimate the loss to U.S. employers of between $11.4 to $29 billion per year.[3]

New Information

In early 1999, the MetLife Mature Market Institute sponsored a pilot study following up on a subset of the 1997 respondents to determine the total financial and personal costs of caregiving to workers. This study was produced by the National Alliance for Caregiving and the National Center on Women and Aging at Brandeis University. In the past, studies have measured the costs of eldercare by approximating the value of the services that would have been required if a family member did not provide them. This study offers a more complete accounting of the losses faced by caregivers by measuring the long-term effects from wage reductions, lost retirement benefits, compromised opportunities for training/promotion, lost "plum" assignments, and stress-related health problems.

Methodology

The follow-up research is based on 55 in-depth interviews with caregivers who have made some type of work adjustment—either formal or informal—as a result of caregiving responsibilities. This is not a representative sample of the U.S. population. Rather, these respondents were recruited from the 81% of 1997 NAC/AARP survey respondents who volunteered to participate in future research studies and who met the following criteria:

- Age 45 or older in 1996

- Made some type of work adjustment (formal or informal) due to their caregiving responsibilities

- Reported providing at least eight hours of caregiving per week and at least two caregiving tasks.

In more specific terms, the starting point was the original nationally representative sample of 1509.

- Of the 1509, 1216 agreed to do future studies

- Of the 1216, 525 were 45 years of age or older

- Of the 525, 223 reported experiencing a type of work disruption due to caregiving

- Of the 223, 202 had been providing care for 6 months or longer
- Of the 202, 157 provided at least eight hours of caregiving per week and at least two caregiving tasks.

This study provides an in-depth look at the costs that 55 of these 157 individuals face in caring for their elderly loved ones. While this is not a representative sample, it is a detailed, "real life" study into the working and caregiving experiences of these 55 people.

Key Research Findings

The MetLife research reveals that working caregivers can incur significant losses in career development, salary, and retirement income, and substantial out-of-pocket expenses as a result of their caregiving obligations. The primary research findings, segmented into eight key themes, follow.

The "Juggling Act": Underestimating the Obligation

"Initially, I didn't think I'd have to modify anything [at work], but as time wore on I did."

Caregivers often underestimate the time required for caregiving and the impact of their obligation on their work. Most of the caregivers surveyed started out providing a small amount of care, gradually taking on more and more responsibility. Respondents expecting care to last six months or less actually spent more than a year providing care. Similarly, a majority of those anticipating one or two years of caregiving actually spent four or more years providing care. Caregivers also underestimated the number of hours that would be required, per week, during these years. Among the respondents, the average length of caregiving was about eight years, with roughly one-third providing care for ten years or more.

Work Schedules: Burning the Candle at Both Ends

"Well, at the time I had a full-time job. I had two children in college...it was necessary for me to work. I kind of hoped we'd get through it."

"When I was full-time, I had to interrupt my job too much with phone calls and leaving work. With part-time, I am 'here' when working, and then I have more free time to help my father when I am off." [4]

"I needed to take care of Mom. I reduced my hours so much that management had to give my accounts to someone else."

Work schedules were often compromised to meet the obligations of these caregivers. Almost all of the respondents made informal adjustments to their work schedules.

Altogether, 84% of the respondents made at least one formal adjustment to their work schedule.

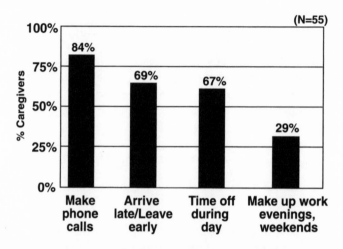

Figure 5.1. *Informal Adjustments to Work Schedule Due to Caregiving*

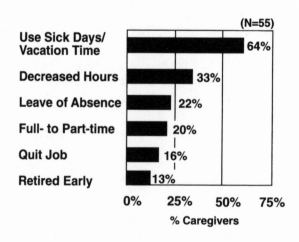

Figure 5.2. *Formal Adjustments to Work Schedule Due to Caregiving*

Career Tracks: Standing Still at Best

"I needed to take a few courses, and the school was willing to reimburse me for some of those. And I wasn't able to take them because I didn't have the luxury of going to night school because of taking care of Mother. So, I... didn't get the teaching certificate... a change of jobs was out."

"When people in higher authorities, when they realize that you're a caregiver, they start looking for somebody else that doesn't have those responsibilities—somebody younger, or somebody single...who may not have children or have other responsibilities. So, it impacts you."

Responsibilities at home can mean missing out on promotions and training at work. Almost three in 10 of the caregivers surveyed said that caregiving limited their skills training, while two in 10 reported turning down the opportunity to work on a special project and almost as many steered clear of work-related travel. Overall, a total of 40% of the survey respondents reported that caregiving affected their ability to advance in the job in one or more of the following ways:

- 29% passed up a job promotion, training, or assignment
- 25% passed up an opportunity for job transfer or relocation
- 22% were not able to acquire new job skills
- 13% were not able to keep up with changes in necessary job skills.

Wage and Retirement Loss: Significant Impact

Loss in Wages: Paychecks Pared

"I had to go on part-time right away because of surgery my father had."

Income can be cut severely as a result of caregiving obligations. Nearly two-thirds of the respondents reported that caregiving had a direct impact on their earnings—and 30 of those reporting such a loss were able to provide enough information to quantify the monetary impact. Among those providing monetary information, the total loss in wage wealth was substantial, with an average total loss of $566,443.

Wage wealth is the present value of life-time wages calculated as of the date of retirement.

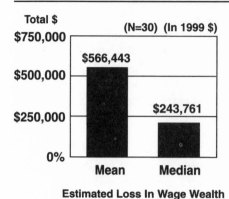

Figure 5.3. Estimation of Caregiving's Impact on Total Wage Wealth

Retirement Income: Less to Count On

"I think I would have been able to make more headway and more money if I'd had a full-time job, could keep a full-time job."

As well as current income, caregivers' retirement savings suffer. As a result of their caregiving, the respondents estimated Social Security benefits decreased an average of $2,160 annually. Over their retirement years, their lost Social Security wealth averages $25,494.

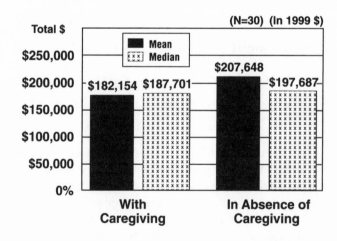

Figure 5.4. Estimation of Caregiving's Impact on Total Social Security Wealth

Among those respondents eligible for pensions and able to provide information about them, estimated average annual pension benefits fell by $5,339 annually as a result of caregiving, or $67,202 in pension wealth, on average, over their retirement years.[7]

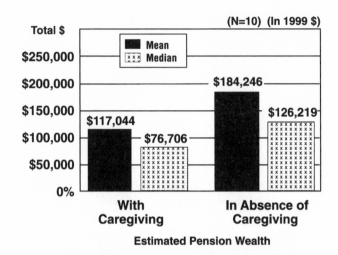

Figure 5.5. *Estimation of Caregiving's Impact on Total Pension Wealth*

Total Wealth Lost: Substantial Loss

The average loss in total wealth experienced by these caregivers as a result of caregiving is estimated by aggregating lost wages ($566,443), Social Security ($25,494), and lost pension benefits ($67,202).[4] Their loss was substantial, averaging $659,139 over the lifetime.

Economic Adjustments: Caregiving Expenses and Reduced Discretionary Income

Out-of-Pocket Expenses

Almost all respondents reported that they paid one or more expenses in order to help the care recipient. Food, transportation, and medications were their three most common expenses. The highest average amount expended by caregivers per month went for assistance with rent or mortgage ($364), with expenses for home care professionals ($322) following closely behind. On average, caregivers helped with these expenses for two to six years, and spent a total of $19,525 in out-of-pocket expenses.

Reductions in Savings and Spending

Roughly one-quarter of the caregivers surveyed were able to estimate reductions in money they would otherwise be putting into savings, investments, and/or home improvements due to the costs of caregiving.

	Somewhat	A lot	Average Total Amount
Savings/Investments	16%	11%	$25,028
Home Improvements	16%	9%	$7,626
Vacations	9%	9%	$2,043
Buying a Car	13%	7%	$8,660
IRA	4%	11%	$3,610
College Costs	6%	9%	$20,133

Figure 5.6. *Estimated Limitations on Spending/Savings Due to Expenses of Caregiving*

Health: Whiplash

"I had migraine headaches and depression and needed to take sick time."

Caregiving responsibilities often take a toll on the health of the caregiver—and on employee productivity due to increases in absenteeism, early retirement and turnover, and decreases in on-the-job effectiveness. Almost three-quarters of the caregivers surveyed said that caregiving had an impact on their health, with more than two in 10 reporting significant health problems.

Of those who reported an impact of their caregiving responsibilities on their health, nearly half cited additional visits to a health care provider as a result. Of those requiring such visits, half reported more than eight additional visits per year, representing another out-of-pocket expense for caregivers and increased absenteeism for employers.[8]

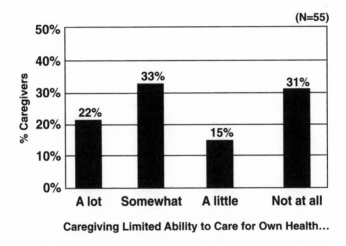

Figure 5.7. Perceived Impact on Caregiver's Own Health

Worker Productivity: Stretched Thin

"Because of the stress, I wasn't as effective on the job. My ability to focus on work was affected."

It seems inevitable that the pressures of caregiving for an elderly relative or friend will sometimes have an impact on the employee's performance at work. While almost half of the respondents reporting health problems did not believe that their work was influenced by their health status, one-quarter felt their ability to work was somewhat affected, and more than one in 10 said that it was greatly affected.

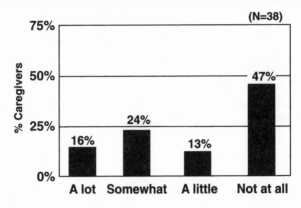

Figure 5.8. *Caregiving-Associated Health Issues and Impact on Work*

Employer Costs and Workplace Support

"I would go to my friend who was a co-worker for 20 years, and who also goes to the same church I do. She gave me emotional support."

"A program to take time off in emergencies would have helped."

"I would talk with my closest friends at work when I was a little down... the company didn't have any policies that would assist me on that."

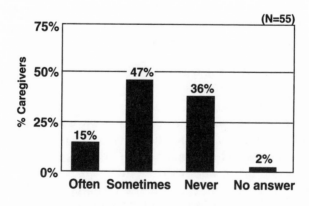

Figure 5.9. *Frequency of Seeking Support at Work*

As noted earlier, the decline in caregivers' productivity at work translates into significant economic losses for employers.

Sixty-two percent of caregivers surveyed in the current study reported asking someone at work—supervisors, coworkers, or management—for support or help around their caregiving responsibilities. However, the support was primarily informal. Few companies have employer-sponsored programs or eldercare services which formally support caregivers and minimize productivity losses.

Conclusions

The MetLife Juggling Act study confirms that employed caregivers shoulder enormous burdens in providing informal care for elderly friends and relatives. Initially, most caregivers underestimate the time that caregiving requires; they start out providing small amounts of care and gradually take on more and more responsibility. Among the caregivers surveyed, the average amount of time spent caring for an elder is eight years, with roughly one-third of the respondents providing care for ten or more years. Key costs incurred over that time period include:

Lost Wealth—Employees often suffer significant drops in income as a result of a caregiving obligation. Nearly two-thirds of the caregivers surveyed reported that their eldercare responsibilities had a direct impact on earnings. Among those able to quantify the monetary impact, the loss in average total wage wealth over the lifetime equaled $566,443. Losses in lifetime wealth from Social Security averaged $25,494, and, for those eligible, losses in lifetime wealth from pensions averaged $67,202. The total lost wealth was significant, averaging $659,139.

The Caregiver "Glass Ceiling"—Almost three in 10 of the caregivers surveyed said that caregiving limited their opportunities for skill building, while two in 10 reported turning down the opportunity to work on special projects, and almost as many steered clear of work-related travel. Overall, nearly 40% of the respondents reported that caregiving affected their ability to advance on the job.

Employer Costs and Lost Productivity—Employers find that caregiving takes a toll on worker productivity and boosts employee turnover, absenteeism and early retirement. One-quarter of the survey respondents with health problems reported that their ability to work was somewhat affected by health problems related to caregiving. And, more than one in 10 said that their work was greatly affected. As noted, a prior MetLife study has estimated that U.S. businesses lose $11.4 to $29 billion per year due to caregiving.

Despite the losses both employers and employees incur, only 23% of companies with 100 or more employees have programs in place to support caregivers.[5] While about 60% of caregivers surveyed reported seeking support at work, the arrangements that were made were informal and not incorporated into company policy.

Today, as the nation struggles with Social Security and Medicare reform, and the increasing need for long-term care, more Americans will bear the costs associated with caregiving. And, with the age of eligibility for Medicare and Social Security benefits expected to rise, the cost to caregivers is likely to rise as well.

Clearly, current and future caregivers need to plan carefully for their—and their loved ones'—long-term care needs. To help caregivers meet this challenge, employers, communities, and public and private sector organizations need to work together to develop and fund affordable policies and services for working caregivers, such as:

- Flexible benefits such as flextime, telecommuting, job-sharing, and compressed work weeks

- Community-based programs such as respite, adult day care, and caregiver support groups

- Information, referral, and educational programs

- Employee and/or employer funded long-term care insurance

- A more favorable tax environment for caregivers and their employers.

As we enter the new millennium, Americans need a greater awareness of the realities of caregiving and new models to support working caregivers. In addition, continued research and discussion are needed on employer-, employee-, and community-sponsored partnerships that will address the multifaceted challenges that working caregivers bear.

About the Respondents

Demographic Profile

The group of 55 caregivers who completed the in-depth telephone interviews is demographically diverse. These respondents were selected and recruited from the final sample of the 1997 NAC/AARP survey—a nationwide sample of 1509 caregivers, including an over-sampling of African-American, Hispanic, and Asian-American caregivers. The characteristics of this Juggling Act sample are similar to the unweighted sample of the 1997 study.

Three-quarters of the 1999 caregivers surveyed are female, six in 10 are married and almost three in 10 are divorced or widowed. Roughly four in 10 have a high school education or less, while just as many have a college degree. Just over one-fifth of the caregivers reported living alone.

Employment Profile

All but five percent of the respondents were employed at the start of their caregiving experience. The remaining caregivers became employed later during caregiving, saying that they started to work because they needed the income or that they wanted to get out of the house for a few hours during the day.

Three-quarters of the participants worked for only one employer during their caregiving experience, while one quarter worked for two employers or more. Roughly one-quarter of the respondents worked in retail sales, one-fifth in education, and one-fifth in health care, with the remaining working in other occupations including manufacturing, government, and social services.

Nearly two-thirds of the respondents reported a lengthy tenure—11 years or more with their employer.

Survey Methodology

The MetLife Juggling Act Study builds on the information gathered in the 1997 National Alliance for Caregiving (NAC) and AARP national survey, *Family Caregiving in the U.S.* A total of 55 caregivers completed an in-depth telephone interview which focused on balancing work with caregiving, and the decisions and consequences that are involved in that enterprise. Recruitment and interviewing were conducted by the National Center on Women and Aging at Brandeis University. Interviews took between 30 minutes and two hours to complete.

Researchers used data on wages to determine the potential impact of caregiving on wages, Social Security and pension benefits. For 30 cases with a measurable impact on wages, the researchers calculated actual lifetime wages and estimated what workers' earnings and benefits would have been in the absence of caregiving. The differences were then converted to losses in wage, Social Security, and pension wealth. The survey instrument and a full report of the in-depth analysis are available upon request.

Footnotes

1. Wagner, D.L., (June, 1997). *Comparative Analysis of Caregiver Data for Caregivers to the Elderly 1987 and 1997.* National Alliance for Caregiving.

2. National Alliance for Caregiving/AARP (June, 1997). *Family Caregiving in the U.S.: Findings from a National Survey.*

3. Metropolitan Life Insurance Company (June, 1997). *The MetLife Study of Employer Costs for Working Caregivers.*

4. For respondents who were unable to provide sufficient data for pension loss, missing values have been replaced with the mean.

5. Families and Work Institute (1998). *Business Work-Life Study.*

Chapter 6

Work and Elder Care: Facts for Caregivers and Their Employers

An Aging Population, Women Workers, and Elder Care

Today people are living longer and the elderly population is growing.

- In 1995, life expectancy at birth was 75.8 years, compared to only about 35 years when the U.S. was founded.

- In January 1997, 32.3 million (12 percent) of the 261.6 million civilian noninstitutional population in the United States was 65 years of age or older, and the Census Bureau projects that by the year 2050 as many as 1 in 5 Americans could be elderly.

- Between 1990 and 1995, the elderly population 75 years and over was one of two age groups whose rate of population increase outstripped that of other segments. The "oldest old"—those aged 85 and older—are the most rapidly growing elderly age group.

Most elderly are not in nursing homes, and the number of nursing home residents 85 years of age and over (per 1,000 population) actually decreased 10 percent between 1985 and 1995. Elderly women are much more likely than elderly men to live alone. Eight in 10 noninstitutionalized elderly who lived alone in 1993 were women.[1]

"Work and Elder Care," Fact Sheet No. 98-1, U.S. Department of Labor Women's Bureau, May 1998.

An estimated 7.3 million elderly persons—nearly one-quarter of the Nation's elderly population—required assistance with activities of daily living (ADLs) or instrumental activities of daily living (IADLs) in 1994. ADLs include seven personal care activities: eating; toileting; dressing; bathing; walking; getting in and out of bed or chair; and getting outside.

IADLs include six home management activities: preparing meals; shopping for personal items; managing money; using the telephone; doing heavy housework; and doing light housework. In 1994 only about 1.6 million of the elderly requiring assistance with ADLs or IADLs were residing in nursing homes.[2]

Caregivers to the Elderly

Women are the traditional caregivers to the elderly, and because many also participate in the paid labor force, many must face the challenge of meeting both work and family obligations.

In 1997, 59.8 percent of women 16 years of age and over were in the civilian labor force, i.e., working or looking for work. Only 13 percent of all families fit the traditional model of husband as wage-earner and wife as homemaker. In 61 percent of married couple families, both husband and wife work outside the home.

Today a significant proportion of American households are providing care for an elderly relative or friend and many more expect to do so in the future. Women are more likely than men to be caregivers and to receive care, although an increasing number of men have parental responsibility. Many caregivers are caring for both children and elders. Caregiving impacts on work, causing caregivers to come in late, work fewer hours, and even give up work or retire early.

An estimated 22.4 million U.S. households—nearly one in four—are currently providing informal care to a relative or friend age 50 or older or provided such care at some point during the last twelve months, according to a 1996 survey conducted by the National Alliance for Caregiving and the American Association of Retired Persons.[3]

Examples of caregiving included help with personal needs or household chores, taking care of a person's finances, arranging for outside services, or visiting regularly to see how the person cared for is doing. (The person being cared for was not necessarily living with the caretaker).

The typical caregiver is a 46-year-old woman who is employed and also spends around 18 hours per week caring for her mother who lives nearby (although 4.1 of the 22.4 million households spend at least 40 hours per week and another 1.6 million spend 20-40 hours per week).

The average duration of caregiving is 4.5 years. The typical care recipient is a 77-year-old woman who lives alone and has a chronic illness. The study also found that:

- Seventy-two percent of caregivers are women. Asian caregivers are most evenly split among female and male caregivers (52 percent of Asian, 77% of Black, 74% of White, and 67% of Hispanic caregivers are women).

- Sixty-four percent of caregivers are working full- or part-time.

- Forty-one percent of caregivers are caring for children under 18 at the same time as elderly relatives or friends.

- Half of employed caregivers reported taking time off, coming in later, or working fewer hours, six percent gave up work entirely due to caregiving, and 3.6 percent took early retirement.

- When asked what kind of help or information caregivers could use most, survey respondents requested "free time, time for myself" most frequently, and 38 percent said that they didn't know what help or information they could use.

An earlier study found that of the seven percent of workers who cared for an elderly parent, grandparent, in-law, relative, friend, or spouse, 50 years or older, 56 percent were women and 44 percent were men. It also found that 72 percent of the elders cared for were female; the average age of the elders was 74; 92 percent of elders cared for were family members; and 19 percent of elders lived with their caregivers, 46 percent lived 20 minutes or less from the caregiver, and 18 percent lived over one hour away.

Elders received, on average, eight hours of direct personal care such as bathing, dressing, and feeding, and an additional 3.7 hours of indirect care such as phone calls and shopping. Women provided more direct care than men (14.2 hours vs. 7.5 hours per week), and female caregivers spent an average of 19.9 hours in direct and indirect care compared to the 11.8 hours spent by male caregivers.[4]

A 1986 study of 143 employed and 141 not employed caregivers found that, among employed caregivers:[5]

- most (72%) said working made caring for their relative easier;

- caregivers who fared the best continued to work more than 40 hours a week and could afford substantial in-home help, adult day care, or nursing home care for their relatives;

- an employed caregiver who had to work to make ends meet had a very stressful predicament;

- more than half those employed half-time or more reported missing time at work due to caregiving responsibilities (an average of 9.3 hours);

- over half employed 20 hours or fewer said caregiving caused them to reduce their hours;

- one-fifth (22%) of the not-employed had quit their jobs to provide care full-time;

- and caregivers who quit or reduced their hours drastically had the highest level of stress, had relatives with the most severe behavioral problems, and when they quit, their annual income loss was about $20,400 each.

More than half of Americans (54 percent) say it is likely that they will be responsible for the care of an elderly parent or relative in the next ten years, according to a 1998 national public opinion poll conducted for the National Partnership for Women & Families. Four in ten Hispanic women (40 percent) say it is very likely.[6]

Types of Elder Care Assistance

Geriatric Care Managers[7]

Professional geriatric care managers (GCM) are professionals in the field of human services (registered nurses, licensed clinical social workers, gerontologists, psychologists) trained and experienced in assessment, coordination, and monitoring of services for older adults and their families.

Services may include in-home assessment, arrangements for home care, monitoring/coordination of services, counseling, consultation, placement, information and referral, crisis intervention, and financial management/entitlements.[8]

Homemakers and Home Health Aides.

A "homemaker" or "personal care worker" is supervised by an agency or the caretaker and provides personal care, meal planning and household management, and medication reminders. A home health aide, certified nurse assistant, or nurses aide is supervised by an agency's registered nurse and provides personal care, help with transfers, walking, and exercise; household services that are essential to health care; and assistance with medications.[9]

Companions / Friendly Visitors

A "companion" or "live-in" is supervised by an agency or the caretaker and may provide personal care, light housework, exercise, companionship, and medication reminders.[10]

One way in which the Federal government helps provide companion services is through the Senior Companions program. Under the Senior Companions program, a program of the Senior Corps of the Federal Corporation for Public Service, people age 60 and older provide assistance and friendship to elderly individuals who are homebound and, generally, living alone. They can do such things as take care of simple chores, provide transportation to medical appointments, and provide respite care to relieve live-in caretakers for short periods of time.

Senior companions usually serve two to four clients, providing 20 hours of weekly service. The National Senior Service Corps hotline can be reached at 1-800-424-8867.

Telephone Reassurance Systems

Telephone reassurance systems may be available through such organizations as area agencies on aging, the American Red Cross, or police departments. For example, the Fairfax (VA) Area Agency on Aging provides a free telephone reassurance service whereby a volunteer is matched with an elderly (age 60 or above), homebound, or socially isolated individual. The volunteer calls the elderly person weekly.

Through volunteers, the Harlem, Manhattan, and Queens chapters of the American Red Cross in Greater New York provide companionship, reassurance, and a link with community services to isolated homebound seniors through weekly telephone calls (the Telephone Reassurance Club).

The Senior Call Back Program of the Falls Church, VA Police Department is a computer-run program which, once a day, Monday through Friday, dials up seniors who live or are left alone and who ask to participate. If the senior doesn't answer, he/she will be called twice more, and if he/she still doesn't answer the third call, the police will follow up to make sure the senior is all right.

121

Respite Care

Respite care refers to time off for caregivers, and may be provided in the home, e.g., through home health agencies, or in the community, e.g, by hospitals, nursing homes, churches, or board and care facilities. Some respite care programs are offered free by voluntary organizations and some are subsidized by public funds.

Temple University's Center for Intergenerational Learning has a program—Time Out—in which college students provide respite to families caring for frail elders. Employers can help by covering some of the costs associated with hiring a caregiver so that employees can obtain respite from their caregiving responsibilities.

Daily Money Managers

Daily money managers can organize and keep track of financial and medical insurance papers, assist with writing checks, and/or maintain bank accounts.[11]

Home-Delivered Meals

One source of home-delivered meals is Meals on Wheels. Meals on Wheels is a non-profit, volunteer-based service that delivers nutritious meals to people who are elderly or disabled, homebound, and unable to prepare their own meals. The typical recipient is a woman over 75 years of age living alone.

Programs are organized by local communities, churches, charitable organizations, and concerned citizens. Meals-on-Wheels Greater San Diego has a program called "ElderCare" which offers a network of services, including information and referral, needs assessment, counseling and problem solving, daily money management, and WorkSaver. Through WorkSaver, businesses can refer their employees to Meals-on-Wheels Greater San Diego for solutions to working while trying to care for an elderly relative locally or elsewhere.

Chore and Home Repair

An example of a delivery mechanism for chore and home repair is Minnesota Chore Corps, which serves the seven county metro area of Minneapolis/St. Paul and was created by the Minnesota Department of Human Services. Originally designed for seniors and their families, Minnesota Chore Corps matches callers with businesses that can meet their needs. Seniors need and are searching for products and services that can help them remain independent for as long as possible. Such products and services include housing developments; pet-walking services; transportation services; legal services; shopping assistance; house cleaning; nutritious, home-delivered meals; self-defense classes; minor/major home repair services; financial planning; customized banking services; companionship; in-home personal care; and weekly in-home services such as doing laundry and taking out the trash.

Participating businesses are screened for appropriate liability insurance, bonding, licensing, and references. Chore Corps businesses charge reasonable rates and may offer senior Chore Corps discounts.

- **Legal assistance or resources** through such organizations as the National Academy of Elder Law Attorneys, Inc. and the American Bar Association's Commission on Legal Problems of the Elderly. Materials produced by the latter, such as the fact sheets packet on law and aging, could be made available at the worksite.[12] The packet addresses legal resources for older persons and includes a fact sheet written for older persons and their families.

- **Family and Medical Leave**. Under the Federal Family and Medical Leave Act (FMLA), a covered employer must grant an eligible employee up to 12 work weeks of unpaid leave in a 12 month period to care for an immediate family member (spouse, child, or parent—but not a parent "in-law") with a serious health condition.[13] The law permits an employee to elect, or the employer to require, the employee to use accrued paid leave, such as vacation or sick leave, for some or all of the FMLA leave period. Employees may also be eligible for family and medical leave to care for an elderly relative through voluntary policies offered by their employer or negotiated by a labor organization. For example, in 1995 American Federation of State, County, and Municipal Employees (AFSCME), Local 1635, negotiated a contract which allows employees to use paid accrued sick leave, personal leave, and vacation credits to care for a sick child or family member.

Federal employees have a variety of options for obtaining and taking leave related to caregiving responsibilities. In addition to FMLA, the Federal Employees' Family Friendly Leave Act permits employees to use up to 13 days of sick leave without pay each year for routine family medical purposes. Moreover, employees can use up to 24 hours of leave without pay for elderly relatives' health or care needs. There are also leave transfer and leave bank programs.

- **Assistance with financing care** may be available from both public and private sources, e.g., Medicare, Medicaid, private health insurance, and employers.

A major public source of financing is the health insurance commonly known as Medicare, which provides health insurance protection to the aged, disabled, and those suffering from end-stage kidney disease. There are two parts to the Medicare program. **Medicare hospital insurance** (Part A) helps pay for inpatient hospital care, inpatient care in a skilled nursing facility, home health care and hospice care. **Medicare medical insurance** (Part B) helps pay for physician services, outpatient hospital services, outpatient physical therapy, and other medical services, supplies and equipment not covered by Medicare Part A. Medicare does not cover long-term or custodial care. Part A pays the full cost of medically necessary home health care and 80 percent of the approved cost for durable medical equipment supplied under the home health benefit. With regard to home health services, Part B generally pays 80 percent of the Medicare approved amounts for home health services to those beneficiaries who do not have Part A.[14] Some respite care may be covered by Medicare, Medicaid, private health insurance, or programs under the jurisdiction of State agencies.[15]

The Federal Medicaid law authorizes Federal matching funds to assist the states in providing health care for certain low-income persons. The states have considerable flexibility in structuring their programs and there are substantial variations from state to state. Medicaid provides health and long-term care coverage to approximately 37 million Americans and their families. It covers several million senior citizens for long-term care benefits that provide financial protection for beneficiaries, spouses, and the adult children of those requiring nursing home care. Home and community-based services waivers enable states to use home care as an alternative to costly nursing home care. Case management services are among the most frequently covered optional services that States may elect to provide.[16]

An example of financial assistance in the private sector is the child and elder care fund Hotel and Restaurant Employees, Local 2, negotiated with the San Francisco Hotels Multi Employer Group in 1994. Currently, the hotels contribute 15 cents for eligible members for every hour worked. It reimburses members for care for a disabled spouse, disabled domestic partner, parent, current parent-in-law, or grandparent living in the Bay Area (up to $150/month). Services that are reimbursable must be related to the health or well-being of the older/disabled adult.

Ways Employers/Labor Organizations Are Helping/Can Help Employees with Elder Care

MetLife has estimated that the aggregate cost of caregiving in lost productivity to U.S. business is $11.4 billion per year, based on data from findings from a national survey on caregiving. They consider this calculation to be very conservative. The total costs would exceed $29 billion per year if caregivers providing care at lesser levels of caregiving (Levels I and II), those working part-time, and long-distance caregivers were included in the calculation.[17]

In 1994, 33 percent of full-time employees in small private establishments were eligible for elder care benefits in the form of paid leave, paid leave of absence policies, employer-sponsored adult day care centers, and employer-subsidized day care for the elderly. Elder care resource and referral services were not included. Although smaller establishments typically provide fewer benefits than larger establishments, full-time employees in medium and large private establishments were slightly less likely to be eligible for elder care benefits (31 percent).[18]

A survey of work and family benefit plans for salaried employees of 1,050 major U.S. employers (Fortune 100 and 500 companies) by Hewitt Associates found that in 1996, nearly one-third of the employers offered elder care programs, an increase of 17 percent over the number offering elder care assistance in 1991.

The most common approach to elder care assistance was resource and referral programs, offered by 79 percent of the employers with elder care programs. Long-term care insurance was offered by 25 percent of the employers with elder care programs, up from five percent in 1991.[19] According to another study, a 1997 study of wage and salary workers in the U.S., only one in four employees have access to elder care resource and referral services through his or her employer.[20]

In the 1992 National Study of the Changing Workforce, the Families and Work Institute pointed out that primary reliance on workplace programs results in an unequal distribution of benefits in society. Higher-income workers and better-educated workers have far more access to health insurance and pension plans, flexible time and leave programs, and dependent care assistance than their less advantaged counterparts.

Supervisors' attitudes and behavior are also important in influencing usage when work/life benefits are offered. In a survey by Intracorp many respondents report that a benefit may exist on paper, but managers send mixed signals if employees try to use the benefit. The survey also found that employees' comfort level in using work/life benefits ties directly to managerial encouragement and supportiveness of the work environment.[21]

That said, the following are some of the ways in which employers and labor organizations are helping and can help their employees with elder care.

Needs Survey

Employers can determine their employees' need for and interest in assistance with elder care by conducting a needs survey.[22] For example, in 1990 the Social Security Administration and the American Federation of Government Employees conducted a joint needs assessment survey. SSA has 14,000 employees at its Headquarters in Baltimore, two-thirds of whom are women. Over 2,000 responded that they needed support with their caregiving responsibilities. Whirlpool Corporation of Benton Harbor, Michigan, also did a dependent care needs assessment by location.

Elder Care Resource and Referral

Resource and referral services for elder care helps familiarize employees with the array of services for the elderly, including medical, custodial, legal, and counseling services. Employers also provide needed information about elder care through seminars, support groups, handbooks, hotlines, and employee assistance programs. For example, through the Metropolitan Employers Dependent Care Association (MEDCA) in Colorado, administered by The Work Options Group, participating small- to mid-sized employers offered a broad range of "dependent care" programs to their employees.

Among the services MEDCA provides are a national adult care consultation and referral service. Through a toll-free number, the Care Connection offers a free phone consultation with a professional care counselor to assist with such things as identifying adult day care needs, personalized resources and referrals to anywhere in Colorado where the caller's relative lives, general resources for those with relatives outside the state, and educational materials and helpful tips.

Coopers & Lybrand, a big six accounting firm with 19,000 employees nationwide, offers its employees and their families Life Balance Partners, which is provided by Ceridian Performance Partners. This is a nationwide resource, referral, and consulting service designed to assist employees with childcare, parenting, elder care, and work/life balance needs. Employees call a toll-free number to speak with a consultant who will research their concerns and provide comprehensive educational and consultation assistance.

In 1995, Bausch & Lomb introduced LifeWorks, a broad spectrum program to assist employees in several areas, including elder care resource and referral. At Bausch & Lomb, elder care resource and referral is among the most frequently used services provided by the LifeWorks program.

Based upon specific requests at corporate headquarters, Whirlpool Corporation introduced an elder care referral service provided by Senior Services of Kalamazoo, MI. Resource information can also be provided by means of handbooks, guides, or guidebooks. For example, in 1989, ELC Associates of Cupertino, California prepared for Region IX of the U.S. Department of Labor an elder care resource guidebook, which provides basic information and lists community resources in Northern and Southern California areas. The University of California, Berkeley, has prepared *A Guide for Balancing Work and Family*, which has a section on Elder/Adult Dependent Care, with information on setting up a care plan, home care and day care, housing options, nursing homes, financial and legal concerns, death and dying, and selected community resources.

Seminars

Seminars may be used to provide basic information, to help assess needs,[23] or to supplement another kind of service. Formats may include presentations by experts or brown bag lunches and may consist of single workshops or a series, usually on-site. Blue Cross and Blue Shield of Massachusetts began offering brown bag luncheon seminars on life topics in 1995.

Support Groups

Support groups are sponsored by hospitals, nursing homes, social service agencies, and health associations.[24] AARP Online sponsors a caregiver support chat group on America Online.

Employee Assistance Programs

In one study, among respondents using employee assistance programs, the heaviest users were employees with both elder care and child care responsibilities.[25] Employee Assistance Programs could serve in a variety of roles to coordinate and assist in the development and procurement of elder care services.[26]

Caregiver Fairs

Caregiver fairs are another vehicle for providing caregivers with information on resources. For example, the Social Security Administration holds a senior services exhibition every two years. It prepares a publication listing the participating organizations, which it passes out in advance of the exhibition.

Exhibitors include organizations dealing with Social Security and Medicare, adult day care services, chore service/companions care, financial services and long-term care insurance, home health services, hospice care services, legal services, long distance caregiving information, transportation services, and more.

Some companies participating in the American Business Collaboration for Quality Dependent Care, such as Citibank and GE Capital Services, offer on-site caregiver fairs. They are usually four hours long and held in a strategic location such as a cafeteria or lobby and include creative promotional activities, elder care service vendors who run exhibits, and 6-8 mini-tip sessions in conjunction with the fair to address a variety of elder care issues.

Counseling

The University of California, Berkeley has a pilot program under which an on-site counselor, a licensed clinical social worker, provides assessment and counseling to faculty and staff on elder care and adult dependent care issues.

Long-Term Care Insurance

This type of insurance helps employees pay for long-term care for themselves or dependent children, spouses, or parents. It is designed to fill gaps in Medicaid and Medicare coverage. Long-term care insurance may cover home care, assisted living facilities, or hospice care, and some policies pay for family caregiving.

Long-term care insurance was one of eight work/life benefits getting the most frequent use in a study of acceptance and use of work/life benefits in U.S. companies with 500 or more employees nationwide;[27] however, in 1994, only one percent of full-time employees in small private establishments and six percent of full-employees in medium and large private establishments were eligible for long-term care insurance.[28]

The greatest increase in long-term care insurance has occurred in employer-sponsored group long-term care insurance, a 60 percent increase in the last two years. Almost one-third of the States have passed laws providing for tax deductions for long-term care.[29]

Visiting Nurse Services

Companies can provide reimbursement or direct subsidies to employees for visiting nurse costs, thereby making it easier for employees to go to work when medical needs arise among elderly dependents.

Adult Day Care, including Intergenerational Day Care

Employers can support local, adult day care centers with financial or in-kind contributions. Although there is no legislation authorizing Federal agencies to use space for adult day care centers, Easter Seals and the Employee Activities Association (EEA) located at the Social Security Administration (SSA) and the Health Care Financing Administration (HCFA) in Baltimore, Maryland, are sponsoring Break-a-Way, a conveniently located, affordable senior adult day program for elderly relatives of employees.

The EEA is a non-profit employees group that provides services (e.g., fitness centers and child care centers) to employees at SSA and HCFA. The center is a public-private partnership, with the Baltimore County Department of Aging coordinating the provision of meals and donating furniture, and the University of Maryland medical system, Kernan Hospital, providing medical oversight, including comprehensive geriatric medical care.

The center opened in 1997 and serves up to 50 people a day. Although it is designed to serve elderly adults, younger adults with disabilities may also enroll. The center is open from 7:00 A.M. to 6:00 P.M., but there are options for extended care before and after the daily program or for four-hour blocks during the normal daytime hours. There is transportation from home and back for persons who live within a 3-mile radius of the center.

Emergency Care

The purpose of emergency care is to assure that care will be available when regular arrangements are not, or when other circumstances dictate a short-term need. In 1995 the Bay Area Emergency Care Consortium, a consortium of seven San Francisco Bay area businesses, primarily law firms, began a program, at no cost to employees, for emergency in-home child and elder care. The program is administered by Caregivers on Call. The service, which is either fully or partially subsidized, is available 24 hours per day, seven days per week, year-round, when employees' usual child or elder care arrangements fall through or are not available at a time when the employee must go to work or fulfill a work assignment.

Flexible Spending or Dependent Care Accounts

In Dependent Care Assistance Programs (DCAPs), the popular name for salary reduction plans, the employer and employee agree to reduce the employee's income by a certain amount to be placed in a dependent care assistance fund for the employee. Through such an agreement, the employee is not taxed on the amount set aside for dependent care assistance. This program is more likely to benefit higher income workers because low income workers may not be able to afford to have their income reduced. Employee benefit surveys suggest that only a small percentage of employees use such accounts, although some companies subsidize employee contributions to the accounts.[30]

Flexible Schedules and Leaves of Absence

Blue Cross and Blue Shield of New Jersey has a policy allowing alternative work scheduling. The arrangements—telecommuting, compressed work weeks, job sharing, part-time employment, flextime, and biweekly work arrangements—vary by division based on operational needs.

Case Management

Some employers make in-home assessment available to their employees. For example, under one of the components of the City of Scottsdale, Arizona's, comprehensive elder care program, a Certified Independent Social Worker can go to the elder relative's home, conduct an interview, make an assessment, and provide the employee with recommendations and resources.

This helps the employee determine if their relative can continue to live alone, what services are necessary to do so, and the availability and cost of these services. Follow-up service and coordination is provided as necessary to ensure families' satisfaction with the care plan. The service is available to all city employees, at no cost to the employee, whether their elder relative lives in the Scottsdale area or elsewhere.

Transportation

Transportation is one of the instrumental activities of daily living that caregivers help elderly relatives and friends with the most. Almost eight in 10 family caregivers (79 percent) say they help with transportation.[31] The American Business Collaboration for Quality Dependent Care (ABC), a national coalition led by 22 member companies, is helping to create a national model on escorted transportation for the elderly dependents of employees.

ABC resources are being used to develop national guidelines and expand existing programs by finding transportation providers and recruiting and training those who drive and escort older adults. Once the program is established in a community, elderly dependents of employees of ABC companies can call on these transportation providers whenever they require transportation. Usually there is a nominal fee. Because considerable caregiver time can be spent transporting elderly relatives to medical appointments and for other needs during business hours, the provision of escorted transportation can help lower absenteeism, reduce workday disruptions and stress, and improve productivity.[32]

Elder care assistance for employees doesn't have to be costly. Low-cost and no-cost ways for employers to provide employees with eldercare information include: community resource directories, brochures on eldercare, and posters or tabletop displays available from area agencies on aging; "lunch and learn" presentations; including a segment on caregiving in pre-retirement planning programs; articles in company newsletters; and dependent care booklets containing information on such employee benefit policies as leaves of absence, sick leave, flexible work schedules, telecommuting, and flexible spending accounts.[33]

Labor organizations can obtain additional ideas for helping employees they represent who have elder care needs from the fact sheet Bargaining for Elder Care prepared by the Labor Project for Working Families and the Working Women's Department of the AFL-CIO.

Resources

Elder Care Locator
Toll-Free: 800-677-1116

Elder Care Locator is a public service of the Administration on Aging, U.S. Department of Health and Human Services, administered by the National Association of Area Agencies on Aging, and the National Association of State Units on Aging. It helps caregivers locate services for older adults in their own communities.

Administration on Aging
U.S. Department of Health and Human Services
330 Independence Avenue, SW
Washington, DC 20201
Tel: 202-619-0724
Fax: 202-260-1012
TDD: 202-401-7575
Website: http://www.aoa.gov
E-mail: aoainfo@aoa.gov

National Association of State Units on Aging (NASUA)
1225 I Street, NW, Suite 725
Washington, DC, 20005
Tel: 202-898-2578
Fax: 202-898-2583
Website: http://www.nasua.org
E-mail: staff@nasua.org

NASUA is a national, non-profit, public interest organization which provides information, technical assistance, and professional development support to its members—the 57 State and territorial government agencies on aging. The organizational units of NASUA include home and community based services, elder rights, aging program management and administration, and communications and development. NASUA operates a National Resource Center on Long-Term Care and the National Information and Referral Support Center, both funded by the Administration on Aging, as well as AGE-NET, an electronic bulletin board. It also collaborates with other organizations on the Eldercare Locator, the National Resource Center on Elder Abuse, and the National Long Term Care Ombudsman Resource Center Programs.

National Association of Area Agencies on Aging, Inc.
927 15th Street, N.W., 6th Floor
Washington, DC 20005
Tel: 202-296-8130
Fax: 202-296-8134
Website: http://www.n4a.org

Represents a majority of the more than 660 area agencies on aging. Its mission is to assist older Americans, allowing them to stay in their own homes and communities with maximum self-dignity and independence for as long as possible. Publishes the *National Directory for Eldercare Information and Referral*.

The Medicare Hotline
Health Care Financing Administration
U.S. Department of Health and Human Services
Toll-Free: 800-638-6833
TTY: 877-486-2048
Website: http://www.medicare.gov

American Association of Retired Persons
601 E Street, N.W.
Washington, DC 20049
Toll-Free: 800-424-3410
Website: http://www.aarp.org
E-mail: member@aarp.org

"Survival Tips for New Caregivers" (video) and "Before You Buy: A Guide to Long-Term Care Insurance."

National Alliance for Caregiving
4720 Montgomery Lane
Bethesda, MD 20814
Tel: 301-718-8444

The NAC is a non-profit joint venture of several national aging organizations that have allied themselves to focus attention on the issue of family caregiving of the elderly through research, program development, and public awareness activities. NAC has published the brochure *Linkages, Resources for People Caring for Older Relatives*, and has sent to libraries across the country information on caregiving books and videos, helping caregivers find local community services, Internet resources, and resource organizations.

Children of Aging Parents (CAPS)
1609 Woodbourne Road, Suite 302A
Levittown, PA 19057
Toll-Free: 800-227-7294
Tel: 215-945-6900
Website: http://www.caps4caregivers.org

CAPS is a non-profit, charitable organization with a national mission to assist the caregivers of the elderly with reliable information, referrals, and support.

Worklife Enrichment & Studies Team
Center for Employee Services
Social Security Administration
G122A West High Rise Building
6401 Security Boulevard
Baltimore, MD 21235
Tel: 410-965-0479

Family Caregiver Alliance
690 Market Street, Suite 600
San Francisco, CA 94104
Toll-Free in California: 800-445-8106
Tel: 415-434-3388
Fax: 415-434-3508
Website: http://www.caregiver.org
E-mail: info@caregiver.org

Family Caregiver Alliance was the first community organization in the country created to assist families and caregivers of adults suffering from Alzheimer's Disease and other brain disorders that are acquired in adult years. It operates 11 nonprofit Caregiver Resource Centers in California, modeled after the Family Caregiver Alliance (FCA), which provide a range of service options for family caregivers, including working caregivers, in addition to information and referral, family support services such as counseling and respite care, community education, and technical assistance.

Bay Area Emergency Care Consortium
Managing Director or Director
Caregivers on Call: 800-225-1200

Human Resources Representative
Bausch & Lomb
One Bausch-Lomb Place
Rochester, NY 14604
Tel: 716-338-6000
Fax: 716-338-6007
Website: http://www.bausch.com

Local 2/Hospitality Industry Child and Elder Care Plan
209 Golden Gate Avenue
San Francisco, CA 94102
Tel: 415-864-8770, Ext. 720

Human Resources Manager
Whirlpool Corporation
2000 N. M-63
Benton Harbor, MI 49022-2692
Tel: 616-923-5000
Website: http://www.whirlpoolcorp.com

Director of Work/Life Initiatives
Pricewaterhouse Coopers
400 Renaissance Center
Detroit, MI 48243
Tel: 313-394-6000
Website: http://www.pwcglobal.com

Vice-President, AFSCME Local 1635
2680 Ridge Road, West Suite 203
Rochester, NY 14626
Tel: 716-227-3210

Consultant/Human Resources
Blue Cross and Blue Shield of New Jersey
P.O. Box 820
Newark, NJ 07101
Toll-Free: 800-355-2583
Website: http://www.bcbsnj.com
E-mail: comments@horizon-bcbsnj.com

The Work Options Group
1017 South Boulder Road
Suite F
Louisville, CO 80027
Toll-Free: 888-610-CARE
Tel: 303-604-6545
E-mail: workopts@indra.com

Manager, CARE Services
Tang Center, Room 3100
2222 Bancroft Way
University of California
Berkeley, CA 94720-4300
Tel: 510-643-7754
Fax: 510-642-7411
E-mail: careserv@uhs.berkeley.edu

Easter Seals
230 W. Monroe St.
Suite 1800
Chicago, IL 60606
Toll-Free: 800-221-6827
Tel: 312-726-6200
Fax: 312-726-1494
TTY: 312-726-4258
Website: http://www.easter-seals.org

National Academy of Elder Law Attorneys, Inc.
1604 North Country Club Road
Tucson, AZ 85716
Tel: 520-881-4005
Fax: 520-325-7925
Website: http://www.naela.com

Publishes "Questions and Answers When Looking for an Elder Law Attorney."

Worklife Coordinator, City of Scottsdale
7575 E. Main
Suite 205
Scottsdale, AZ 85251
Tel: 408-312-5000

Working Women's Department, AFL-CIO
815 16th Street, N.W.,
Washington, DC 20006
Tel: 202-637-5064
Fax: 202-637-5058
Website: http://www.aflcio.org
E-mail: feedback@aflcio.org

Center for Intergenerational Learning
1601 North Broad Street, Room 206
Philadelphia, PA 19122
Tel: 215-204-6970
Fax: 215-204-6733
Website: http://www.temple.edu/cil

National Meals on Wheels Association of America
1414 Prince Street, Suite 202
Alexandria, VA 22314
Toll-Free: 800-999-6262
Tel: 703-548-5558
Fax: 703-548-8024
Website: http://www.mealsonwheelsassn.org

American Business Collaboration for Quality Dependent Care
200 Talcott Avenue West
Watertown, MA 02472
Toll-Free: 800-447-0543
Website: http://www.abcdependentcare.com

Endnotes

1. *Health United States 1996-97 and Injury Chartbook*, DHHS Publication No. (PHS) 97-1232, U.S. Department of Health and Human Services, Centers for Disease Control.

2. *Long-Term Care for the Elderly*, CRS Issue Brief, Congressional Research Service, Updated December 1, 1997; Chapter I (Health Status) in *Chartbook on Health Data on Older Americans,* Centers for Disease Control and Prevention, National Center for Health Statistics, (year). And Prevention, National Center for Health Statistics, July 1997; U.S. Population Estimates by

Age, Sex, Race, and Hispanic Origin: 1990 to 1996, U.S. Bureau of the Census, Population Division, Population Projections Branch; *Sixty-Five Plus in the United States*, Statistical Brief, U.S. Census Bureau, May 1995.

3. *Family Caregiving in the U.S.,* National Alliance for Caregiving and American Association of Retired Persons, June 1997.

4. *The National Study of the Changing Workforce*, Families and Work Institute, 1993.

5. "Overworked, Underestimated, the Employed Caregiver Doing Double Duty," a research summary from *Family Survival Project*, a Resource Center for families of brain-damaged adults. Contains a section on "What Can Employers Do?" See Resources.

6. Family Matters: A National Survey of Women and Men, National Partnership for Women & Families, February 1998.

7. "Doing What's Best for Mom and Dad without Doing Yourself In," *Guide to Retirement Living,* Summer/Fall 1997, Free from Douglas Publishing, Inc., Steve Gurney, Publisher, Box 7512, McLean, VA 22106-7512, 800-394-9990.

8. "When an older person needs assistance... call a Professional Geriatric Care Manager," the Mid Atlantic Chapter of National Association of Professional Geriatric Care Managers, 703-897-8212.

9. "Elderaction: Action Ideas for Older Persons and Their Families," Administration on Aging, U.S. Department of Health and Human Services, http://www.aoa.dhhs.gov/aoa/eldractn/caregive.html.

10. Ibid.

11. "Daily Money Management," *The Guide to Retirement Living*, Summer/Fall 1997.

12. "ABA Resources Guide the Elderly through Important Legal Steps," *FOCUS on Federal Employee Health and Assistance Programs*, U.S. Office of Personnel Management, Volume 8, Number 3, May/June 1997.

13. *Compliance Guide to the Family and Medical Leave Act*, WH Publication 1421, December 1996, U.S. Department of Labor, Employment Standards Administration, Wage and Hour Division.

14. *The Social Security Handbook*, SSA Publication No. 65-008, 13th Edition, August 1997, Social Security Administration.

15. *Finding Your Way Through the Home Care Maze: A Practical Guide for the Home Care Consumer*, developed by the Fairfax Area Agency on Aging in cooperation with the Fairfax Home Care Task Force, produced by the Home Care Development Program, April 1997 Edition.

16. *Medicaid*, HCFA Fact Sheet, March 1997, Health Care Financing Administration, U.S. Department of Health and Human Services; Testimony of Donna E. Shalala, U.S. Secretary of Health and Human Services before the U.S. House of Representatives Commerce Committee, June 11, 1996.

17. *The MetLife Study of Employer Costs for Working Caregivers*, MetLife Mature Market Group, Westport, CT, (203) 221-6580, June 1997.

18. *Employee Benefits Survey*: A BLS Reader, Bulletin 2459, U.S. Department of Labor, Bureau of Labor Statistics, February 1995; *Employee Benefits in Small Private Establishments*, 1994, Bulletin 2475, U.S. Department of Labor, Bureau of Labor Statistics, April 1996; *Employee Benefits in Medium and Large Private Establishments*, 1993, Bulletin 2456, U.S. Department of Labor, Bureau of Labor Statistics, November 1994.

19. *Work and Family Benefits Provided by Major U.S. Employers in 1996*, Hewitt Associates.

20. *The National Study of the Changing Workforce*, Families & Work Institute, 1998.

21. *Too Seldom is Heard an Encouraging Word, A Study of Work / Life Programs and Corporate Culture's Impact on Utilization*, Intracorp, Philadelphia, PA, 1998.

22. "Eldercare Belongs in EAP," *Employee Assistance Quarterly*, Vol. 7(4) 1992.

23. "Eldercare: An Emerging Employee Assistance Issue," *Employee Assistance Quarterly*, Vol. 8(3) 1993.

24. *Age Lines, Support Groups Aid Caregivers*, National ELDER CARE Institute on Long Term Care and Alzheimer's Disease at the Suncoast Gerontology Center, University of Florida.

25. *Too Seldom is Heard an Encouraging Word*, Intracorp, Philadelphia, PA, 1-800-345-1075.

26. "Eldercare Belongs in EAP," *Employee Assistance Quarterly*, Vol. 7(4) 1992.

27. *Too Seldom is Heard an Encouraging Word, a Study of Work/Life Programs and Corporate Culture's Impact on Utilization*, Intracorp, Philadelphia, PA, 1998.

28. Op. Cit. *Employee Benefits in Small Private Establishments*, 1994, and *Employee Benefits in Medium and Large Private Establishments*, 1993.

29. Presentation by Barbara Stucki, American Council of Life Insurance, at Round Table on Long-Term Care for the Baby Boom Generation, Challenges and Options, sponsored by The Robert Bosch Research Foundation Scholars Program in Comparative Public Policy & Comparative Institutions at American Institute for Contemporary German Studies, December 16, 1997, Washington, DC.

30. "Odd Jobs," *The Washington Post*, February 27, 1994; "Making dependent-care spending plans user-friendly," *Glamour,* July 1993.

31. *Family Caregiving in the U.S.*, op. cit.

32. "Elder care transit driving down stress," *Business Insurance*, June 23, 1997.

33. *Low-Cost and No-Cost Eldercare Programs*, the Eldercare Connection, a joint project of the National Association of Area Agencies on Aging and the Employee Assistance Professionals Association under AoA Grant # 90-AM0616.

Chapter 7

The Extent and Impact of Dementia Care

Caregiving is a family issue, as evident by the much cited fact that the bulk of care for chronically ill or disabled older people is provided by family and friends (e.g., Schulz & O'Brien, 1994). This is especially true when considering care for persons with dementia. With the aging of the population, the number of people with Alzheimer's disease and related disorders is expected to increase from nearly two million Americans age 65 and over afflicted with the disease in 1995 to nearly three million people by the year 2015 (General Accounting Office, 1998). The personal, social, and financial impacts of dementia caregiving have been well documented (Schulz, O'Brien, Bookwala, & Fleissner, 1995), with a recent study providing more precise estimates on the costs of both family and institutional care at different stages of illness (Leon, Cheung, & Neumann, in press).

Given the characteristic cognitive, behavioral, and affective losses associated with the progression of the disease, caring for someone with dementia is assumed to be more difficult and burdensome than caring for loved ones with other chronic conditions and disabilities (Light, Niederehe, & Lebowitz, 1994). However, this assertion has never really been adequately examined in a large representative population of caregiving including both dementia and nondementia caregivers.

Excerpts from "The Extent and Impact of Dementia Care: Unique Challenges Experienced by Family Caregivers," by Marcia G. Ory, Ph.D., Jennifer L. Yee, Ph.D., Sharon L. Tennstedt, Ph.D., and Richard Schulz, Ph.D., National Institute on Aging (NIA), April 1999.

Recent innovations—such as the development of new cognitive enhancing drugs or the emergence of new residential care facilities— are likely to affect the course and care of people with dementia. Similarly with a rapidly expanding population of older adults, smaller family sizes, and more women in the paid labor force, there are concerns regarding the availability and willingness of future generations of family caregivers (Hooyman & Gonyea, 1995; Kaye & Applegate, 1990; Marks, 1996). However, functional deficits are still likely to occur, particularly at the later stages of the disease, and there is no reason to believe that, for the foreseeable future, families will not remain primary caregivers throughout most of the course of illness.

Health Effects of Dementia Caregiving

The extent to which caregiving affects the physical and mental health of the caregiver is an important policy question and has been addressed by numerous studies carried out in the past decade. Research on caregiving remains a priority because of the need to strengthen family members' abilities to provide care without jeopardizing caregivers' own health or well-being or relinquishing their caregiver responsibilities prematurely (Schulz & Quittner, 1998).

Researchers have assessed psychiatric morbidity attributable to caregiving by using a standardized self-report measures such as the CES-D [Center for Epidemiologic Study—Depression Study] (Radloff, 1977) or Beck Depression Inventory (Beck, Ward, Mendelson, Mock, & Erbaugh, 1961), structured diagnostic interviews, such as the Diagnostic Interview Schedule (DIS) or the Hamilton Depression Rating Scale (HDRS, Hamilton, 1967), as well as indicators of psychotropic drug use (see Schulz et al.,1995). On the whole, studies using self-report inventories show a consistent pattern of increased depression and anxiety symptomatology among dementia caregivers when compared to age and gender based norms (e.g., Collins & Jones, 1997; Haley et al., 1995; Irwin et al, 1997; King & Brassington, 1997; Majerovitz, 1995; MaloneBeach & Zarit, 1995; Rose-Rego, Strauss, & Smyth, 1998; Schulz et al., 1997). Studies that include clinical diagnoses as an outcome report elevated rates of major depression among dementia caregivers when compared to age-matched controls, and in some studies, elevated rates of generalized anxiety (Irwin et al., 1997; Redinbaugh, MacCullum, & Kiecolt-Glaser, 1995; Vitaliano, Russo, Scanlon, & Greeno, 1996; Vitaliano, Scanlon, Krenz, Schwartz, & Marcovina, 1996; Schulz et al., 1995). The use of psychotropic drugs as an indicator of psychiatric morbidity has been examined in only a few studies and the results have varied widely, making it difficult to reach conclusions about the effects of caregiving on the use of these medications (Schulz et al., 1995).

Studies of physical health outcomes among caregivers have used a broad range of measurements, which can be classified into four major types of outcomes: self-rated global health; the presence of chronic conditions, illnesses, physical symptoms, and disabilities; health-related behaviors, medication use, and health service utilization; and physiological indices (Bookwala, Yee, & Schulz, 1998). In contrast to the consistent findings for psychiatric health effects among ADRD [Alzheimer's Disease and Related Disorders] caregivers, findings based on physical health outcomes are less conclusive.

A common assessment of physical health status that has been employed in caregiving studies is a single question that asks respondents to rate their current overall health on a scale from poor to excellent. In general, most studies have found that caregivers perceive their health to be somewhat poorer than noncaregivers or community samples (Beach, Schulz, Yee, & Jackson, 1998; Mui, 1995; Pruchno, Peters, & Burant, 1995; Rose-Rego et al., 1998; Schulz et al., 1997).

Contrary to the findings for self-rated global health, findings concerning the other types of physical health measures are more equivocal. With respect to self-reported physical illness and disability, common measures employed by researchers include symptom checklists such as the Cornell Medical Health Index or the Physical Health Section of the OARS [Older Americans Resources and Services] (Duke University, 1978), and asking respondents to report if they have experienced various illnesses or diseases. A few recently published studies suggest that caregiving may be related to the presence of illness, physical symptoms, and disabilities (Bass, Noelker, & Rechlin, 1996; Canning, Dew, & Davidson, 1996; Cochrane, Goering, & Rogers, 1997; Fuller-Jonap & Haley, 1995; Jutras & Lovie, 1995). For example, Fuller-Jonap and Haley (1995) reported that caregiving husbands reported more respiratory problems than a comparison group. Jutras and Lovie (1995) noted that more caregivers than noncaregivers reported having diabetes and back problems than those that did not reside with a disabled elder. In addition, Cochrane et al.(1997) reported that caregivers mentioned having more physical health problems in the previous year, and more "limited activity days" and "days that required extreme effort" compared to noncaregiving controls. However, in contrast to these studies, other studies have failed to find an association between caregiving and self-reported illness or disability (Brodaty & Hadzi-Pavlovic, 1991; Irwin et al., 1997; Pruchno et al., 1995; Shaw et al., 1997).

With regard to health-related behaviors, some studies have found that caregivers report less physical activity, sleep, and rest than noncaregivers (Burton, Newsom, Schulz, Hirsch, & German, 1997; Fuller-Jonap & Haley, 1995; Glaser & Kiecolt-Glaser, 1997; Kiecolt-Glaser, Glaser, Gravenstein, Malarkey, & Sheridan, 1996; Schulz et al., 1997). However, inconsistent evidence was found with regard to differences in other health-related behaviors, such as alcohol consumption, smoking, weight change, finding time to see the doctor, and missing doctor's appointments. In terms of medication use, Schulz et al. found increased medication use among caregivers and Burton et al. reported that caregivers were more likely to forget to take their medications. A few studies examined utilization of health services, such as hospitalizations and physician visits as physical health indicators. However, a consistent association has not been found between caregiving and health care utilization (Schulz et al., 1995).

An important emerging area of caregiving health outcomes research focuses on changes in sub-clinical disease such as immune functioning, hypertension, pulmonary function, blood chemistries, and cardiac arrhythmias as indicators of health status. However, evidence supporting the association between caregiving and such physiological indices is mixed. In two recent studies, Kiecolt-Glaser and her colleagues reported that compared to matched controls, caregivers showed poorer immune response after exposure to an influenza virus vaccine and to infection by a latent herpes simplex virus (Glaser & Kiecolt-Glaser, 1997; Kiecolt-Glaser et al., 1996). Similarly, Pariante and associates (1997) found that caregivers had lower levels of T cells, a higher percentage of T supressor/cytotoxic cells, and a lower T helper:suppressor ratio compared to matched controls. With regard to cardiovascular risk factors and functioning, Vitaliano and associates (1996) found that men caregivers had higher lipids than age-and sex-matched control and women caregivers reported less aerobic activity than their noncaregiving counterparts. In addition, Moritz, Kasl, and Ostfeld (1992) showed increased systolic blood pressure among male ADRD caregivers. Although some studies found caregiving to be related to physiological indices of health, others found no association (e.g., Irwin et al., 1997; Schulz et al., 1997).

If we ask the question, what factors predict negative health effects among caregivers, two distinct patterns emerge. One pattern of findings indicates that predictors generally known to be risk factors for negative health outcomes in all populations emerge in these studies as well. Thus, physical and psychiatric morbidity is associated with being female, low financial adequacy, high levels of stress, and personality variables, such as high levels of neuroticism, and low levels of mastery (e.g., Bookwala & Schulz, 1998; Burton et al., 1997; Draper, Poulos, Poulos, & Ehrlich, 1995; Dura, Stukenberg, & Kiecolt-Glaser., 1991; Hooker, Monahan, Frazier, & Shifren, 1998; Morrisey, Becker, & Rupert, 1990; Mui, 1995). Similarly, the relation between depression, anxiety, social support, and physical health morbidity have been frequently reported in the literature and are characteristic of the caregiving literature as well (e.g., Li, Seltzer, & Greenberg, 1997; Redinbaugh et al., 1995). The second pattern concerns those associations that are unique to the caregiving context. For dementia caregivers, two factors are important in predicting negative health effects in addition to those already listed above. Patient problem behaviors are consistently linked to both psychiatric and physical morbidity of the caregiver and patient cognitive impairment is consistently related to physical morbidity of the caregiver (Li et al., 1997; Majerovitz, 1995; Moritz et al., 1992; Schulz et al., 1995).

Evaluating links between caregiving stress and health outcomes will ultimately require us to specify complex, multivariate models that are tested prospectively. Minimally, such models will include objective measures of stressors, assessments of how those stressors are perceived by caregivers, and a repertoire of health outcomes that includes categorical clinical disease, sub-clinical disease markers, health care utilization data, and self-reported health. In developing and testing such models, it is important to keep in mind that we must identify not only patterns of relations among variables but also that the observed morbidity effects exceed some absolute standard for classifying an individual as ill or at risk of illness. This can be achieved by selecting health measures with well-established age and gender norms.

In articulating such stress-health models, it may be fruitful to focus on outcomes that reflect the exacerbation of existing health conditions. The demands of caregiving may not precipitate an illness event per se, but rather may aggravate existing vulnerabilities. Thus, attempts should be made to assess whether illness results from existing conditions being exacerbated or represents new conditions unrelated to prior medical history or risk factors. Illness effects will most likely be found among individuals with elevated risk factors who are exposed to higher levels of stress (Vitaliano, Schulz, Kiecolt-Glaser, & Grant, 1997).

Finally, to the extent that illness effects are observed in future studies of caregiving, it will be important to determine the mechanisms that account for those effects. It must be remembered that mechanisms accounting for symptom reporting, health care utilization, and disease processes may differ from each other.

Implications for Policy and Practice

Contrary to the continued concerns of public policy makers, families do not relinquish their caregiving role unnecessarily. Data from a longitudinal study by Tennstedt and colleagues (1993b) support the conclusion that services are used as intended—to support and sustain the informal caregiving arrangement or to fill gaps in needed care. While home and community-based services are used by many, informal care typically predominates in these mixed care arrangements (Tennstedt, Sullivan, McKinlay, & D'Agostino, 1990; Tennstedt et al. 1993b, 1996).

In the case of dementia care, use of formal services is not only appropriate but also clinically indicated as severity increases. From a practice perspective, it is important to determine the optimal mix of formal services and informal care in order to ensure the well being of both care recipient and caregiver. Transition to a special care environment is another important juncture in this regard. Assistance with appropriate timing and with negotiating a role for continued involvement of the caregiver(s) will facilitate what might be interpreted as another in a series of losses by a caregiver who sees this transition as loss of an important role.

From a policy perspective, the issue of eligibility criteria for services is important. For both publicly and privately (i.e., third party payer) funded services, eligibility typically is based on functional disability in the performance of specified ADLs. The Advisory Panel on Alzheimer's Disease (1989) has advocated for the expansion of eligibility criteria to provide services in situations where the degree of cognitive impairment interferes with the person's ability to complete either IADLs or ADLs without substantial supervision. The cost analyses performed by Paveza and associates (1998) "suggest that changes in cognitive impairment are independent factors affecting cost regardless of the magnitude of ADL/IADL impairment" (p. 79). Similar findings from the National Long-Term Care Channeling Demonstration Project were reported by Liu, McBride, & Coughlin (1990). These findings support the notion of applying a cognitive weighting factor to the degree of ADL/IADL impairment in establishing eligibility for services.

Finally, we should not lose sight of the fact that caregiving is imbedded in the family experience, history, and values. How caregivers respond to the presenting needs for care, how they perceive the personal impact of that care, and how they interface with the formal service system will by shaped by their personal situation. As we have argued for recognition of the heterogeneity of older adults, as researchers, practitioners, and policy makers we must recognize the heterogeneity of their caregivers.

Table 7.1. Demographic Characteristics of Dementia and Nondementia Caregivers

Demographic Variable	Dementia	Nondementia
Mean Age	46.26	42.99
Mean Age of Care Recipient	78.39	75.65
Percent Female	72.5	68.1
Race (percent)		
White	42.8	41.0
Black	26.9	18.4
Asian	10.3	19.4
Hispanic	19.4	20.5
Relationship to Recipient (percent)		
Spouse/Partner	7.2	3.1
Parent/Parent-In-Law	48.9	52.8
Sibling/Sibling-In-Law	3.1	2.9
Child	0.0	0.2
Grandparent/Grandparent-In-Law	16.9	18.0
Aunt/Uncle	0.6	0.9
Other Relative	14.4	16.0
Non Relative/Friend	0.0	0.0
Median Income Category	$30,000 but less than $40,000	$30,000 but less than $40,000
Median Highest Education Level	Some College	Some College
Marital Status (percent)		
Married/Living with Partner	62.3	63.8
Single, Never Married	14.2	17.4
Divorced/Separated	16.5	12.5
Widowed	7.0	6.3
Children Present (percent)		
Employment Status		
Full or Part-time (percent	61.6	68.3
Retired	16.6	10.8
Not Employed	20.9	21.9

Table 7.2. Caregiver Involvement

Characteristic	Dementia	Nondementia
Duration of Care (Years)	5.10	5.07
Hours of Care (Weekly)	17.6	12.45

Table 7.3. Total Task Performance for Dementia and Nondementia Caregivers

Types of tasks performed	Dementia	Nondementia
IADL's*	4.78	4.37
ADL's**	2.29	1.36
Total	7.07	5.73

*IADL's include: giving medicines, pills, injections; managing finances; grocery shopping; housework; preparing meals; transportation; arranging services.

**ADL's include: getting in or out of beds or chairs, getting dressed; getting to and from the toilet; bathing and showering; continence or dealing with diapers; feeding.

Table 7.4. The Effects of Physical, Emotional, Financial, and Role Stress on Dementia and Nondementia Caregivers

Item	Dementia	Nondementia
Give up vacations, hobbies, or your own activities (percent)	55.0	40.9
Less time for other family members (percent)	52.0	38.1
Other relatives doing their fair share of caregiving (percent)	59.4	74.1
Extent of family conflict over caregiving (mean out of a one to three range)	1.55	1.34
Emotional strain of caregiving (mean out of a one to five range)	2.99	2.22
Physical strain of caregiving (mean out of a one to five range)	2.40	1.80
Did you suffer mental or physical problems as a result of caregiving (percent)	22.3	12.6
Financial hardship of caregiving (mean out of a one to five range)	1.87	1.50
Own money spent per month (mean)	104.00	106.22

Table 7.5. Percentages of Dementia and Nondementia Caregivers Reporting the Feeling That Best Describes Caregiving

Feeling Category	Dementia	Nondementia
Anger	5.1	1.5
Sadness/Fear	2.5	1.5
Burden	15.2	10.6
Obligation	11.0	12.9
Love	17.4	18.4
Happiness	48.9	54.5

References

Bass, D. M., Noelker, L. S., & Rechlin, L. R. (1996). The moderating influence of service use on negative caregiving consequences. *Journal of Gerontology: Social Sciences, 51B,* S121-S131.

Beach, S. R., Schulz, R., Yee, J. L., & Jackson, S. (1998). Negative (and positive)health effects of caring for a disabled spouse: Longitudinal findings from the Caregiver Health Effects Study. Manuscript submitted for publication to *Psychology and Aging.*

Beck, A. T., Ward, C. H., Mendelson, M., Mock, J., & Erbaugh, J. (1961). An inventory for measuring depression. *Archives of General Psychiatry,* 4, 561-571.

Bookwala, J., & Schulz, R. (1998). The role of neuroticism and mastery in spouse caregivers' assessment and response to a contextual stressor. *Journal of Gerontology: Psychological Sciences,* 53B, P155-P164.

Bookwala, J., Yee, J. L., & Schulz, R. (1998). Caregiving and Detrimental Mental and Physical Health Outcomes. Manuscript in preparation.

Brodaty, H., & Hadzi-Pavlovic, D. (1991). Psychosocial effects on carers of living with persons with dementia. *Australian and New Zealand Journal of Psychiatry,* 24, 351-361.

Burton, L. C., Newsom, J. T., Schulz, R., Hirsch, C. H., & German, P. S.(1997). Preventative health behaviors among spousal caregivers. *Preventative Medicine,* 26, 162-169.

Canning, R. D., Dew, M. A. & Davidson, S. (1996). Psychological distress among caregivers to heart transplant recipients. *Social Science and Medicine,* 42, 599-608.

Cochrane, J. J., Goering,P. N., & Rogers, J. M. (1997). The mental health of informal caregivers in Ontario: An epidemiological survey. *American Journal of Public Health,* 87, 2002-2007.

Collins, C., & Jones, R. (1997). Emotional distress and morbidity in dementia carers: A matched comparison of husbands and wives. *International Journal of Geriatric Psychiatry,* 12, 1168-1173.

Draper, B. M., Poulos, R. G., Poulos, C. J., & Ehrlich, F. (1995). Risk factors for stress in elderly caregivers. *International Journal of Geriatric Psychiatry*, 11, 227-231.

Dura, J. R., Stukenberg, K. W., & Kiecolt-Glaser, J. K. (1991). Anxiety and depressive disorders in adult children caring for demented parents. *Psychology and Aging*, 6, 467-473.

Fuller-Jonap, F. & Haley, W. E. (1995). Mental and Physical health of male caregivers of a spouse with Alzheimer's disease. *Journal of Aging and Health*, 7, 99-118.

General Accounting Office (1998). Alzheimer's disease: Estimates of prevalence in the United States (GAO/HEHS - 98-16). Washington, DC: United States General Accounting Office, Health, Education, and Human Services Division.

Glaser, R., & Kiecolt-Glaser, J. K. (1997). Chronic stress modulates the virus-specific immune response to latent herpes simplex type 1. *Annals of Behavioral Medicine*, 19, 78-82.

Hamilton, M. (1967). Development of a rating scale for primary depressive illness. *British Journal of Social and Clinical Psychology*, 6, 278-296.

Hooker, K., Monahan, D. J., Frazier, L. D., & Shifren, K.(1998). Personality counts for a lot: Predictors of mental and physical health of spouse caregivers in two disease groups. *Journal of Gerontology: Psychological Sciences*, 53B, P73-P85.

Hooyman, N. R., & Gonyea, J. (1995). *Feminist perspectives on family care: Policies for gender justice.* Thousand Oaks, CA: Sage.

Jutras, S., & Lavoie, J. P. (1995). Living with an impaired elderly person: The informal caregiver's physical and mental health. *Journal of Aging and Health*, 7, 46-73.

Kiecolt-Glaser, J. K., Glaser, R., Gravenstein, S., Malarkey, W. B., & Sheridan, J.(1996). Chronic stress alters the immune response to influenza virus vaccine in older adults. *Proceedings of the National Academy of Sciences*, USA, 93, 3043-3047.

King, A. C., & Brassington, G. (1997). Enhancing physical and psychological functioning in older family caregivers: The role of regular physical activity. *Annuals of Behavioral Medicine*, 19, 91-100.

Leon, J., Cheng, C.K., Neumann, P. J. (in press). Health service utilization costs and potential savings for mild, moderate, and severely impaired Alzheimer's disease patients, *Health Affairs*.

Li, L. W., Seltzer, M. M., & Greenberg. J. S. (1997). Social support and depressive symptoms: Differential patterns in wife and daughter caregivers. *Journal of Gerontology: Social Sciences*, 52B, S200-S211.

Light, E., Niederehe, G., & Lebowitz, B. D. (1994). *Stress effects on family caregivers of Alzheimer's patients: Research and interventions*. New York: Springer.

Liu, K., McBride, T.D., & Coughlin, T.A. (1990). Costs of community care for disabled elderly persons. *The policy Implications Inquiry*, 27, 61-72.

Majerovitz, S. D. (1995). Role of family adaptability in the psychological adjustment of spouse caregivers to patients with dementia. *Psychology of Aging*, 10, 447-457.

Malone Beach, E. E. & Zarit, S. H. (1995). Dimensions of social support and social conflict as predictors of caregiver depression. *International Psychogeriatrics*, 7, 25-38.

Morrissey, E., Becker, J., & Rupert, M. P. (1990). Coping resources and depression in the caregiving spouses of Alzheimer patients. *British Journal of Medical Psychology*, 63, 161-171.

Mui, A. (1995). Perceived health and functional status among spouse caregivers of frail older persons. *Journal of Aging and Health*, 7, 283-300.

Pruchno, R. A., Peters, N. D., & Burant, C. J. (1995). Mental health of coresident family caregivers: Examination of a two-factor model. *Journal of Gerontology: Psychological Sciences*, 50B, P247-P256.

Radloff, L. S. (1977). The CES-D scale: A self-report depression scale for research in the general population. *Applied Psychological Measurement*, 1, 385-401.

Redinbaugh, E. M., MacCullum, R. C., & Kiecolt-Glaser, J. K. (1995). Recurrent syndromal depression in caregivers. *Psychology in Aging*, 10, 358-368.

Rose-Rego, S. K., Strauss, M. E., & Smyth, K. A. (1998). Differences in the perceived well-being of wives and husbands caring for persons with Alzheimer's disease. *The Gerontologist, 38,* 224-230.

Schulz, R., & O'Brien, A. T. (1994). Alzheimer's disease caregiving: An overview. *Seminars in Speech and Language, 15,* 185-193.

Schulz, R., O'Brien, A. T., Bookwala, J., & Fleissner, K. (1995). Psychiatric and physical morbidity effects of dementia caregiving: Prevalence, correlates, and causes. *The Gerontologist, 35,* 771-791.

Schulz, R., & Quittner, A. L. (1998). Caregiving through the lifespan: An overview and future directions. *Health Psychology, 17,* 107-111.

Tennstedt, S.L., Sullivan, L., McKinlay, J.B., & D'Agostino, R. (1990). How important is functional status as a predictor of service use by older people? *Journal of Aging and Health, 2,* 439-461.

Vitaliano, P. P., Russo, J., Scanlon, J. M., & Greeno, K. (1996). Weight changes in caregivers of Alzheimer's care recipients: Psychobehavioral predictors. *Psychology and Aging, 11,* 155-163.

Vitaliano, P. P., Scanolon, J. M., Krenz, C., Schwartz, R. S., & Marcovina, S. M.(1996). Psychological distress, caregiving, and metabolic variables. *Journal of Gerontology: Psychological Sciences, 51B,* P290-P299.

Vitaliano, P. P., Schulz, R., Kiecolt-Glaser, J. K., & Grant, I. (1997). Research on physiological and physical concomitants of caregiving: Where do we go from here? *Annals of Behavioral Medicine, 19,* 117-123.

Chapter 8

Grandparents Raising Grandchildren

Many older Americans approaching or in retirement suddenly find themselves caring for and raising their grandchildren. A grandparent stepping in to raise grandchildren or other relatives is not a new development. What is new is the growth in this phenomenon. According to the U.S. Census Bureau, in 1997 3.9 million children were living in homes maintained by their grandparents, up 76 percent from 2.2 million in 1970. In a majority of the cases, grandparents are the primary caregivers. Researchers report that at some point more than one in ten grandparents raise a grandchild for at least six months. Typically, grandparents are caregivers for periods that are far longer. Grandparents who are caregivers tend to be women. The majority of grandparents raising their grandchildren are younger than age 65. Based on 1996 Census data, 48 percent of grandparent caregivers are between age 50 and 64; 33 percent are younger than age 50; and 19 percent are age 65 plus.

Why the Increase?

There are many reasons why grandparents step in to care for their grandchildren, including:

- Death of parents
- Incarceration of parents

"Grandparents Raising Grandchildren," Fact Sheet, Administration on Aging (AoA).

- Unemployment of parents
- Substance abuse by parents
- Teen pregnancy
- Family violence
- HIV/AIDS

Grandparent Caregivers Face Challenges

Grandparent caregivers face a myriad of challenges in nearly all aspects of their lives when they assume the role of parent. They are prone to psychological and emotional strain as well as feelings of helplessness and isolation. Many grandparents raising grandchildren face financial difficulties, too. In fact, researchers have reported that grandparent caregivers are 60% more likely to live in poverty than are grandparents not raising grandchildren. Grandparent caregivers often neglect their own physical and emotional health because they give priority to the needs of their grandchildren. Often the grandchildren in their care have unmet physical, emotional, and developmental needs that require special assistance.

Grandparents raising grandchildren encounter problems that can require them to seek legal authority in order to make decisions on behalf of their grandchildren. Grandparents may need legal authority to get their grandchildren medical care, enrollment in school, and to enable them to receive immunizations and vaccinations, public assistance, and supportive services. Grandparents can find themselves in need of respite services, affordable housing, and access to medical care.

Resources

State and Area Agencies on Aging across the country have instituted programs and services to assist grandparent caregivers. Many have published information guides and have established resource centers to assist grandparent caregivers to identify and access available services. Other important interventions offered around the country include respite services and support groups.

To learn about grandparent caregiver resources in your community, contact the local Area Agency on Aging, listed in the government section of your telephone directory, usually under aging, elderly, or senior services. An Area Agency on Aging can also be located by contacting the Eldercare Locator at 800-677-1116.

Many national organizations provide information and assist grandparent caregivers deal with the challenges of raising their grandchildren. An extensive list of resources and valuable links is available on the Administration on Aging website at http://www.aoa.gov.

Grandparent Information Center
AARP
601 E. Street, N.W.,
Washington, DC 20049
Toll-Free: 800-424-3410
Website: http://www.aarp.org
E-mail: gic@aarp.org

AARP Grandparent Information Center provides a needed link between grandparents and the resources that can help them care for their grandchildren. The Center is a national clearinghouse for information about programs, support groups, research activities, and resources for grandparent-headed families. A number of publications, a quarterly newsletter, and referrals to national and local resources are available from the Center.

The Brookdale Foundation
126 East 56th Street, 10th Floor
New York, NY 10022
Website: http://www.ewol.com/brookdale
E-mail: bkdlfdn@aol.com

The Brookdale Foundation began a grandparents raising grandchildren initiative in 1991. A current effort is the Relatives as Parents Program (RAPP), a program designed to establish community-based services for grandparent caregiving. There are currently 43 state and local programs operating around the country.

Child Welfare League of America (CWLA)
440 First St. N.W.
Washington, DC 20001
Tel: 202-638-2952
Fax: 202-638-4004
Website: http://www.cwla.org

Child Welfare League of America began advancing a national initiative in kinship care in 1993. CWLA can provide information on grandparent caregiving and is currently developing a training curriculum for kinship care service workers.

Creative Grandparenting, Inc.
100 W. 10ᵗʰ Street, Suite 1007
Wilmington, DE 19801
Tel: 302-656-2122
Fax: 302-656-2123

Creative Grandparenting, Inc. is a non-profit organization aimed at educating, enabling, and empowering grandparents. A newsletter and other publications are available.

The Foundation for Grandparenting
108 Farnham Rd.
Ojai, CA 93023
Website: http://www.grandparenting.org
E-mail: gpfound@grandparenting.org

The Foundation for Grandparenting is a not-for-profit, tax-exempt corporation dedicated to the betterment of society through intergenerational involvement. The Foundation sponsors a week-long Grandparent-Grandchild Summer Camp.

Generations United
122 C St. NW, Suite 820
Washington, DC 20001
Tel: 202-638-1263
Fax: 202-638-7555
Website http://www.gu.org

Generations United (GU) is a national coalition dedicated to intergenerational policies, programs, and issues. GU can provide general information on grandparent caregiving.

GrandsPlace
154 Cottage Rd.
Enfield, CT 06082
Tel: 860-763-5789
Website: http://www.grandsplace.com
E-mail: Kathy@grandsplace.com

GrandsPlace is an internet website devoted to grandparents raising grandchildren. Site provides useful links to a wide array of resources.

The National Foster Parent Association
P.O. Box 81
Alpha, OH 45301
Toll-Free: 800-557-5238
Fax: 937-431-9377
Website: http://www.nfpainc.org

The National Foster Parent Association has a booklet entitled, "Grandparents Raising Grandchildren: A Guide to Finding Help and Hope," which discusses the needs of grandchildren, the problems of the parents, and the legal and social issues confronting the grandparents. The booklet provides sources to turn to for help and support. It is available for $3.00 which covers postage and handling.

National Coalition of Grandparents
137 Larkin Street
Madison, WI 53705
Tel: 608-238-8751

National Coalition of Grandparents is a national coalition of grandparent caregivers working for legislation and other policy changes in support of relative caregivers.

National Committee to Preserve Social Security and Medicare
10 G St., NE, Suite 600
Washington, DC 20002
Toll-Free: 800-966-1935
Fax: 202-216-0447

National Committee to Preserve Social Security and Medicare has two publications designed to assist grandparent caregivers. "Grandparents as Parents" and "Grandparents' Guide to Navigating the Legal System" provide excellent information for grandparent caregivers.

R.O.C.K.I.N.G., Inc
P.O. Box 96
Niles, MI 49102
Tel: 616-683-9038

Raising Our Children's Kids: An Intergenerational Network of Grandparenting, Inc. (R.O.C.K.I.N.G.) is a national organization that helps relative caregivers access support groups and other resources in their area.

Consumer Information Center
Tel: 719-948-4000
Website: www.cpsc.gov/whatsnew.html

The U.S. Consumer Product Safety Commission (CPSC) and Pampers Parenting Institute offer a booklet entitled, "A Grandparents' Guide to Family Nurturing and Safety" (item number 606E). The booklet encourages grandparents to develop caring relationships with the grandchildren in a healthy and safe environment. Cost: Free. The electronic version is on CPSC's website.

Administration on Aging
U.S. Department of Health and Human Services
303 Independence Avenue, SW
Washington, DC 20201
Tel: 202-619-0724
Fax: 202-401-7620
Website: http://www.aoa.gov
E-mail: aoainfo@aoa.gov

Eldercare Locator
Toll-Free: 800-677-1116, Monday-Friday

Part Two

Caregiving Responsibilities and Concerns

Chapter 9

Addressing Declining Abilities

As an illness like Alzheimer's disease progresses, the impaired person becomes less able to do many things safely. The world seems confusing, even frightening. The person becomes less and less able to recall what things are and how they work, what is dangerous and what is safe. He or she loses both adult judgment and the physical skills to perform adult tasks. These abilities are not lost all at once. Different ones decline below safe levels at different times. As a result, judging when an impaired person's activities pose a danger to self or others becomes a hard task for the caregiver. Some things that may become dangerous come to mind at once. These are complex tasks using equipment which could be dangerous. Tasks like driving, cooking on a stove, working with power tools, and using guns or sharp tools are among these. Some activities such as smoking seem simple enough but require great caution. The person may dispose of matches safely, for instance, but forget a burning cigarette. The danger of other tasks may be less easy to see. Watering the lawn can be a problem if the person might wander off, for instance. Taking a shower, using a hair dryer, even climbing stairs can be dangerous if a person's skills and judgment have declined past a certain point.

These changes can frustrate and make the impaired person feel useless and unhappy. An activity may mean a great deal. A lot of the

Reprinted with permission "Dealing with a Patient's Declining Abilities," by Beverly Evans, MPH, OTR and Chief, Occupational Therapy Section of the Department of Veterans Affairs Medical Center, Minneapolis, Minnesota, © Kenneth Hepburn, Ph.D.

person's self-esteem may be wrapped up in being able to perform that task. Perhaps it had to do with something important about the person's role in the family. Fixing meals for the family or being the driver, for instance, may seem like his or her special job.

These losses can lead the impaired person to angry outbursts and difficult behavior. Even safe tasks then become problems. For instance, setting the table could be a problem if the person is no longer able to remember all the needed steps and becomes angry and upset.

As caregiver, you will often be called on to deal with problems caused by the impaired person's waning skills and judgment. As the disease goes on, you need actively to manage the daily life of the impaired person. This will involve taking over more and more. You will first take over the harder tasks themselves. Then you will take over deciding what the impaired person should and should not do. This is a big job in itself. You will also need to look carefully at your home. Does the home make life easier or harder for the impaired person (and for you)? You may well have to change your home as time goes by to work better for the impaired person and for you. Chapter 12 of this book,"Creating a Safe and Workable Environment," deals further with controlling the impaired person's surroundings and watching over activities.

The first step in dealing with the impaired person's growing needs involves overcoming any fear you may feel about the problem. Admitting that the impaired person is losing skills may heighten the sense of loss you feel already. You may feel swamped with new burdens. You may prefer to look the other way a little longer. Try not to wait so long that a crisis occurs. Begin as soon as you can to regularly assess the impaired person's skills and the home setting.

In bringing up these issues, the subject of finding help when you need it comes up, too. You can't be alert and on-the-job all day every day. You will need a network of care to cope with the increasing need for supervising the impaired person.

Your goal becomes seeing to the safety and reasonable happiness of the impaired person while also making sure that your caregiving tasks don't overwhelm you. What do you need to do? The answer to this question involves three steps: observation, judgment, and response.

Observation

You can't spend your day following the person in your care to see if he or she can still function well. This would be a grim chore for you and would likely upset the person. Instead you will need to become sensitive to early clues and then follow them up with care. Often some small event will occur that will alert you to the need to observe an activity more closely. Perhaps the person has left the electric coffee-pot plugged in after taking the last cup of coffee. Or perhaps he or she failed to observe a traffic light change and had to slam on the brakes to avoid running a red light. You may find that the oven has been left on, the phone is off the hook, or cigarettes have been left to burn down in the ashtray.

When you pick up a clue or have a hunch, then observe more carefully. You may want to seek help from an expert. Occupational therapists or visiting nurses are trained in what to look for and can suggest what activities might pose problems. Here are some questions to help you:

1. Is the person able to concentrate long enough to do an activity safely?

    • When cooking, for instance, does he or she become too distracted by the radio to tend to the food properly or to turn off the stove?

2. Does the person have enough judgment and good sense to perform the task safely?

    • Does he or she know when food is fit to eat or not?
    • Does he or she properly dispose of matches?

3. Can the person perform all the coordinated actions needed to do a certain task?

    • Can these still be done in a time you think is safe?
    • For instance, is the person able to stop the car quickly when needed?

4. Is the person apt to become frustrated or angry too easily? Does the person become flustered and lose control often?

Judgment

If you are the primary caregiver for an impaired person, keep in mind that you have the authority to judge when an activity is no longer safe. Once you have observed carefully, your job is to decide whether or not any activity might be dangerous enough to harm the impaired person or anyone else. If yes, you will need to respond promptly. If no, leave well enough alone for the time being. You want to avoid giving yourself extra work sooner than needed. You also want to guard against becoming too protective. But do watch carefully.

Driving

One activity deserves mention as a special case. Impaired persons should not drive. Driving is one of the most complex activities most people do. Accidents cause an enormous number of deaths and injuries every year. Most experts who write about caring for persons with dementia stress the importance of stopping the patient from driving very early in the disease. You may want to seek help in deciding that a certain activity has to be stopped or curtailed. Once again your health care team members can be of great help. They can assess the person's skills. Your family can also help observe the impaired person and help you decide about setting limits. Support groups are another source of help and of ideas. Members can offer each other useful tips about many types of problems. Contact the Alzheimer's Disease and Related Disorders Association toll free at 1-800-621-0379 to learn more about a support group near you.

Response

Once you have decided an activity is no longer safe, you need to restrict that activity. There are a number of ways you might go about doing this tactfully.

- Don't bring up the subject. Learn to choose your words with care, and don't invite trouble. Don't suggest, for instance, that you fix dinner together if the impaired person becomes upset during the bustle of preparing meals. Try to get in the habit of not even mentioning what needs to be done, if the impaired person will not be involved.

- Be prepared to offer a diversion when the need arises. Keep a written list of simple, repetitive activities the person enjoys doing. Then you will be ready with a good substitute activity on short notice.

- Learn any advance signals the impaired person may give, and try to divert the person's attention when you notice these warnings. When the person seems about to begin a problem activity, you should suggest without delay one of the activities from your list. Preventing problem activities.

- Develop other techniques for preventing certain problem activities. If diversion does not work, you will need to develop other techniques to prevent the impaired person from attempting the problem activity. You may find it helpful to equip your home with devices that prevent the impaired person from beginning activities you determine unsafe. These need not be fancy or costly. At the simplest level, what you want is something that will slightly distract the person until the impulse to try a certain activity has passed and been forgotten. Latches in odd positions (up high or down low) can stop an impaired person at a door or window. You may hide the car keys, or your garage mechanic can show you several simple things to do to keep a car from starting. Your gas or electric company can help you find ways to make the stove and furnace safe. Many inexpensive products designed to "childproof" the home will also work with an impaired person.

A special problem arises if you decide that a certain activity is unsafe, but the person is still alert enough to outsmart your preventive measures. For instance, a person who may still be able to figure out how to get the car started may not have the skills to drive safely. In a case like this, the person still must be kept from the activity.

How you do this will vary from person to person and will depend on how much the impaired person is still able to understand. You may be able to explain, very simply, that the activity is no longer safe and that the person must not do it. You may have to deny access (take away keys, lock a room). Or you may have to enlist outside help. The authority of other family members, a doctor or nurse, a police officer, or a member of the clergy can be helpful in convincing a person that he or she is no longer allowed to perform certain activities. For instance, showing a written statement from the doctor may help persuade the impaired person that an activity such as driving or hunting is no longer allowed.

Dealing with Your Own Feelings

Caring for a person with declining powers presents you with many hard problems. You may need to change your home to fit the person's needs. You will surely have to increase the amount of time you spend watching over the person. You will also have to deal with your own feelings. You may grieve to see the impaired person's declining powers. You may feel that you are losing the person to the illness.

Another major source of trouble comes up when the impaired person can no longer do tasks that you have always relied on him or her to do. These may include driving, cooking, cleaning, yard work, home finances, home repairs, or clothes mending. Then the loss will mean that you may have to take over these jobs yourself. At the very least you will have to find someone else to do them or decide you can live without them. If you decide to do the jobs yourself, you may have to learn how to do them first. You may begin to feel swamped.

All in all, you may find that you do not want to look too closely at how well the impaired person is doing. Deep down, you may not be fully ready to accept the illness and what it means.

Such feelings are normal. Don't keep these feelings inside. Talk to your doctor, a counselor, family member, or friend about how you feel. Sharing your feelings with members of a support group can be very helpful too.

Give yourself time to adjust, and make sure you get away from your caregiving role once in a while. Even a few hours to yourself can refresh you.

Chapter 10

Activities of Daily Living

Activities of daily living include tasks such as bathing, grooming, dressing, preparing food, eating, and caring for the home. Walking and general mobility—getting from place to place—are also important aspects of a person's life. Individuals with declining abilities may have difficulty caring for themselves. People with Parkinson's disease often have tremors, rigidity, and slowness of movement, all of which may interfere with their ability to care for themselves.

This chapter contains suggested techniques and useful aids which can help people to remain independent and assist with activities of daily living. The adaptive devices mentioned can be purchased at a surgical supply store or through the catalogues listed in the reference section. There are many things that can be done to increase independence and safety in self-care and mobility. For further information, consult your physician, occupational therapist, or physical therapist.

The Bedroom

The bedroom should be kept free of clutter and be large enough to allow free access to the bed, bureau, closet, and hallway doors. Scatter rugs increase the risk of falling and should be avoided. If they are used, they must be taped or tacked to the floor even if they have non-skid rubber pads beneath them. Casters should be removed from

"Be Independent," reprinted with permission of the American Parkinson Disease Association, Inc., © 1999.

furniture, since objects that roll provide unstable handholds. Shoes and other small objects should be kept off the floor, especially at night.

Special equipment and aids can be used in the bedroom to help maintain independence and safety while increasing comfort.

Bedroom Equipment

1. Bed pulls can be attached to the frame at the end of the bed. They are useful to assist in rising to a seated position or turning in bed, and can be either purchased or made at home. To make: Braid three pieces of tightly woven fabric, such as sheeting, together in a length that reaches from the base of the bed to your hand when you are lying down. Sew a large

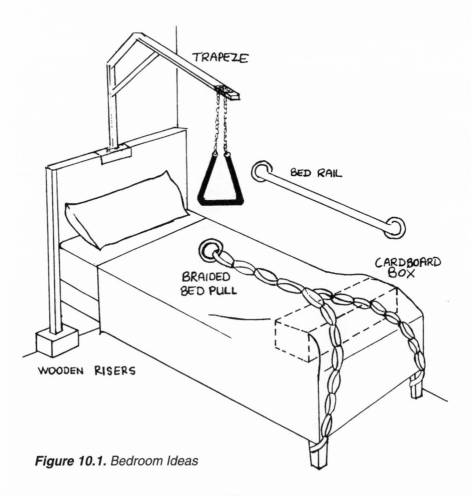

Figure 10.1. Bedroom Ideas

wooden curtain ring to the end to serve as a grasp. Then sew a small binder clip near the ring so that the bed pull can be clamped to the bedding and remain within your reach. Bed pulls can also be attached to the sides of the bed to assist in turning.

2.   A trapeze installed over the head of the bed can help individuals to change position. It may be purchased at a surgical supply store and can be mounted to most standard beds.

3.   A sturdy cardboard box can be placed under the covers at the foot of the bed. This "bed cradle" keeps feet and lower legs free of the sheets while turning.

4.   A urinal may be kept within reach on a bed table, or a commode may be placed at the bedside for nighttime use. The urinal or commode helps reduce walks to the bathroom.

5.   Disposable incontinence garments are designed to address the problem of accidental urination and may be especially helpful at night.

6.   A chair with armrests and a firm seat should be part of the bedroom furniture. Dressing can be accomplished while sitting in the chair, thus eliminating the risk of falling. Try to avoid sitting in a low chair. A firm pillow, secured to the chair, makes it easier to rise from a low surface.

7.   The bed should be no lower than knee height for ease in getting in and out. If the bed is too high, a carpenter can cut two or three inches off the legs. If the bed is too low, use a thicker mattress or mattress padding.

8.   A railing can be installed on a bedroom wall ten inches higher than the level of the bed, and the bed placed against the wall under the railing. The railing becomes an assist for rising from and turning in bed. Commercially made bedrails are available and can be mounted on most beds. Satin sheets are smooth and can also facilitate turning.

9.   For difficulty in sitting up in bed, place a foam wedge cushion under the mattress at the head of the bed, or place wooden risers under the legs at the head of the bed.

10.   Nightlights should be installed in a wall socket near the bedroom door, in the hallway leading to the bathroom, and in the

bathroom. They are indispensable in helping you avoid accidents.

11. A communication device such as a bell or intercom system may be needed to ensure safety at night, especially if you have decreased voice volume.

The Bathroom

Safety is essential in the bathroom. It is the most dangerous room in your house. The tile floor is slippery and the surfaces of the shower or tub are extremely slick, especially when wet. The average bathroom is often small and furnished with porcelain fixtures that jut out from the walls and restrict walking space. A call for help may go unheard, especially if the water is running or the door is closed.

It is important that the bathroom be made as safe as possible. Adequate equipment and awareness of danger increases the ease and safety of bathing and grooming. Bathing is easier if you are organized and keep everything that you need arranged safely within or near the tub.

Bathroom Safety

1. Non-skid decals or strips, attached to a tub or shower floor, or the use of a rubber mat, help to eliminate falls. Small bathroom rugs are easy to trip over, and should not be used. Use a large rug that covers most of the floor, wall-to-wall carpeting, or bare flooring. Do not wax the floor.

2. Grab bars or tub rails placed in strategic locations provide balance and support for getting in and out of the tub or shower. Never use towel racks or wall soap holders as grab bars. They are not designed for this and may break away under pressure.

3. Tub seats or shower chairs make bathing easier and safer. A flexible shower hose or a hand-held shower massage allows for safer bathing while seated. A shower nozzle with a turn-off knob is more convenient than a free-flow nozzle.

4. A raised toilet seat makes sitting on and rising from the toilet easier. Arm rails attached to the toilet, or a grab bar installed on the wall adjacent to the toilet, provide convenient hand holds.

5. If you have difficulty holding objects, do not use glass tumblers. Paper or plastic cups are safer.

6. A nightlight should always be installed in a bathroom wall socket.

7. The hot water heater in your house should be turned down to prevent accidental scalding.

Grooming

1. Soap on a rope keeps soap conveniently within reach while showering or taking a tub bath.

2. A suction nailbrush makes grooming easier and safer. It can be secured to the tub, reducing the risk of injury from falling.

3. A long-handled sponge reaches the lower legs, feet, and back. It helps eliminate bending and is necessary if you have a problem with balance. A curved bath sponge can be useful for washing your back.

4. Wash mitts are terry cloth gloves that eliminate the need for holding onto a washcloth.

5. An electric razor should be used for safety, particularly if you have hand tremor. A variety of electric razor holders, which make grasp easier, are commercially available.

6. Round-headed faucets require a twisting motion to operate. This is difficult for people with impaired strength or coordination. They can be replaced with a lever-type handle or a single arm control faucet. The round-headed faucet can be improved by adding tap-turner adaptations.

7. Adding a commercially made built-up handle, a bicycle handle or a wrist cuff makes your tooth brush, hairbrush or comb handles larger and easier to grip. Extension handles may be helpful if your shoulder or arm movement is limited.

Dressing

The fine hand coordination and strength needed for dressing is sometimes impaired. Pain and stiffness in the limbs can also complicate putting on and taking off clothing, particularly underwear, socks,

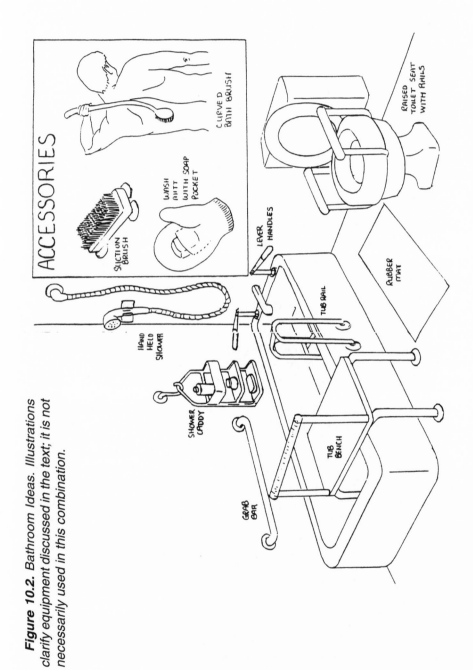

***Figure 10.2.** Bathroom Ideas. Illustrations clarify equipment discussed in the text; it is not necessarily used in this combination.*

and slacks. There are many simple and useful aids that can help people remain independent.

Try to choose clothing that is easy to manage. Loose fitting, stretchy clothes with simple fastenings are easier to put on and take off. For some people, pullover tops may be more convenient. They eliminate the need for buttoning. Front-closing garments are easier to manage than zipper and button-back garments.

Knee-length stockings can be worn instead of panty hose only if they have wide elasticized tops to prevent constriction of circulation. **Never** wear stockings rolled down and secured with a rubber band or garter. This impairs circulation.

Clothing should be placed, in order of wear, on a chair near the individual. Take time and, if possible, do not allow anyone to rush the care recipient. Try to maintain their independence.

Dressing Devices

1. Velcro closures are excellent substitutes for buttons and zippers. Sew tabs of velcro over the buttonhole and on the underside of the button. Press the velcro strips together to fasten your shirt.

2. A button hook or button aid slips through the buttonhole and pulls the button back through it. The handles of these tools are more easily grasped than a small button when fine hand coordination is impaired.

3. Large, easily grasped zipper pulls or rings make opening and closing trouser flys, jackets, and coats less difficult.

4. Small cuff buttons can be difficult to manipulate. Use elastic thread to sew buttons onto cuffs. Keep them buttoned all the time and slide your hand through. You can also join the cuff with a velcro closure.

5. A dressing stick or reacher is useful for pulling pants and undergarments up over your legs. It allows you to remain seated while dressing and reduces the risk of falling. Reachers are also useful for picking up objects that have dropped to the floor.

6. Elastic shoelaces need to be tied only once, thus converting laced shoes to slip-on shoes. Standard tie shoes can be closed with Velcro strips. A shoemaker can stitch them on.

7. A front-closing bra is easier to put on and take off. You can adapt a back-closing bra by sewing up the rear closure, cutting the front open and attaching velcro strips.

8. A long-handled shoehorn and a sock donner reduce bending and straining when putting on socks and shoes.

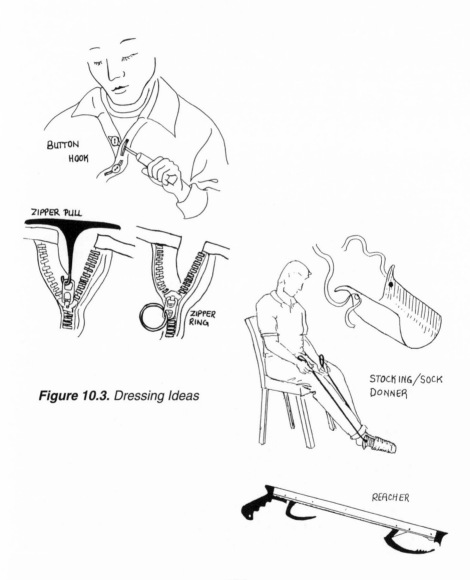

Figure 10.3. Dressing Ideas

The Kitchen

Decreased strength, range of motion, and coordination problems can limit your ability to perform kitchen activities such as: meal preparation, food storage, eating, cleaning, and clearing up after meals. Many ingenious aids have been devised to improve safety and efficiency in the kitchen.

The kitchen should be kept well organized with dishes, utensils, and foods stored near to where they are used and within easy reach. Coffee and tea for instance, should be stored as close as possible to the tea kettle. Store utensils you rarely use behind those used everyday. If there is wall space, install a pegboard at an accessible height and hang utensils there.

Pace yourself during kitchen activities and plan before you start to avoid unnecessary energy-consuming steps. If you have impaired balance, slowness of movement, or decreased hand coordination, meal preparation is safer and easier if done while seated.

Kitchen Equipment

1. A Lazy Susan, placed in the center of the kitchen table or on a counter, holds numerous frequently used items and eliminates the need to gather each one before meals. The Lazy Susan can also be used as a shelf organizer to reduce the need to reach for objects at the back of the shelf.

2. Reachers can be used in the kitchen to pick up light objects that fall to the floor. Heavy objects should be placed in counter-height cabinets.

3. A rubber pad or wet dishcloth can be placed under bowls and pans to stabilize them while you are preparing food.

4. Electric can openers are useful and convenient, especially if fine hand coordination is impaired.

5. A jar opener eases the problem of opening jars.

6. A cutting board with a raised edge prevents diced vegetables and small pieces of meat from scattering off the board. A nail hammered into the board skewers food while dicing or cutting. The nail also helps when buttering bread or toast. Suction cups can be attached to the bottom of your cutting board to prevent it from sliding.

7. A microwave, used instead of a stove, reduces the risk of injury from burns.

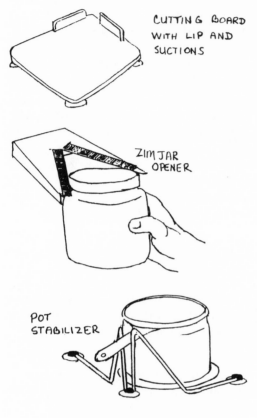

CUTTING BOARD WITH LIP AND SUCTIONS

ZIM JAR OPENER

POT STABILIZER

Figure 10.4. Kitchen Ideas

8. A long-handled dustpan enables you to collect floor sweepings without bending to the floor. A sponge mop should be kept accessible as spills should be wiped up immediately to reduce the chance of falling.

9. Your strength and hand function should affect your choice of pots and pans. If you have limited strength, use aluminum pots and pans and lightweight dishes. Make sure that the shape and size of the handles are suited to your grasp strength. A long pot handle allows for two-handed lifting.

10. A pot stabilizer keeps the handle steady when you stir.

11. Kitchen scissors can help you to open plastic packages and boxes that are difficult to rip.

Mealtime

There are many attractive and durable commercially available mealtime aids. They have been designed to enable people to continue to eat with as much independence as possible.

If a special or adapted piece of silverware is used at home, take it along when dining in a restaurant. If a person has difficulty cutting food, ask the waiter to have the food cut in the kitchen before it is presented. This prevents someone from having to reach across the table to assist. Take time while eating and try not to rush.

Mealtime Equipment

1. Attachable plate guards provide a rim on one side of the plate. Food, especially small vegetables, can be pushed against the guard, where they fall onto the fork. Plate guards also prevent spills. Scoop dishes contoured with raised edges serve the same purpose.

2. Silverware with built up plastic handles is more easily grasped. Tubular foam padding can be attached to the utensil to widen the grip.

Soup spoons can be used instead of forks when eating small pieces of food. Sporks are a combination spoon and fork. This one utensil can spear as well as hold food. A rocking knife may be used instead of a straight knife if you have problems with coordination. Weighted utensils may help to decrease hand tremors, thus allowing the utensil to reach your mouth more easily.

3. If you have a tremor, flexible plastic straws help you to drink.

4. A mug with a large handle for easy grasp should be used if your tremor is severe. An insulated mug with a lid reduces the risk of burns from spills when drinking hot liquids.

5. A rubber pad or a moist paper towel can be placed under plates, cups, and serving dishes to keep them from sliding.

Walking

The ability to get from one place to another inside or outside the home is very important. There are a number of assistive devices that can help a person with decreased balance, coordination, or mobility to walk safely.

Canes can be used to compensate for minor balance problems. They come in a variety of shapes and sizes and increase an individual's base of support.

The standard J-Handle cane offers some stability as well as a sense of security. An ortho-cane or a quad cane may also be used. Each offers an increasing degree of support and balance.

If more assistance than a cane is needed, a walker can be prescribed. A walker that folds is good if you need to store or transport it in limited space—for example, in a car. Wheels can be added if you have difficulty coordinating the advancement of the walker or are unable to lift it off the floor. A braking mechanism which locks with

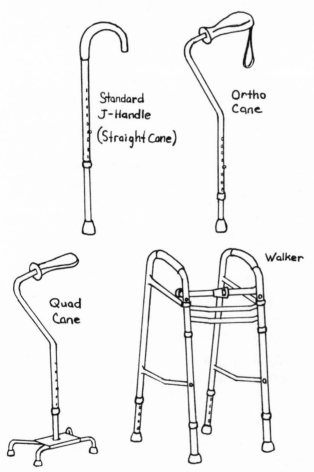

Figure 10.5. *Walking Ideas*

downward pressure can be attached to the front or back wheels. It is important to note, however, that although the rolling walker is easier to advance, it can be unsafe on rugs and other uneven surfaces.

If you are unable to walk, or can walk only short distances in your home, a wheelchair provides more functional mobility.

In order to best suit your individual needs, a physical therapist should be consulted so that the appropriate ambulatory device or wheelchair is provided.

Negotiating Stairs

Stairs often become a major barrier to a person who has limited strength, balance, and mobility. The following guidelines make stair climbing easier.

If there is a handrail available, use it as long as it is well secured. Hold onto the handrailing with one hand and an assistive device, if needed, in the other hand. Both hands can also be placed on the handrail to sidestep up and down the stairs one at a time.

If you are unable to go up or down the stairs safely in a step-over-step manner, negotiate the stairs one step at a time. Place one foot on the step; place the second foot on that same step before you move on to the next.

If someone is assisting you, that person should stay by your side. The assisting person should stagger their feet so that their lead foot is one step down from yours. This maintains good balance.

If you cannot safely climb stairs, you can be carried up and down in a wheelchair. A lift may be installed, but it is expensive.

Specific instructions for walking up and down the stairs or being assisted in a wheelchair can best be given by a physical therapist.

Getting In or Out of a Car

There are ways to make getting in or out of a car easier. First, the car must be parked far enough away from the curb so that you can step onto the level ground before you go into or get out of the car. To get into a car turn so that you back in for the last steps. Your buttocks should lead. Then sit down and swing your legs in.

To exit the car, swing both legs out together and stand up. Sit in the front or back seat, whichever gives you more room. Use pillows to make it easier to get up from a low car. Specific techniques should be taught by and practiced with a physical therapist or occupational therapist.

Miscellaneous Tips

If you have a problem with shuffling, small steps, and stopping while walking, arrange the furniture so as to avoid congested areas. Keep hallways free of obstacles. Plan a route through the house so that there is always a safe handhold available in case you lose your balance.

Railings can be installed on the walls to provide support. Your family should consult with you before they rearrange the furniture so that you do not lose familiarity with your surroundings.

Avoid low couches and chairs as it is often extremely difficult to rise from them without help. A straight-back chair with armrests and a firm seat is easier to get up from. A firm cushion can be used to acquire the height that is suitable for you. Pneumatic lifter seats can assist someone who has severe difficulty rising from a chair.

Handrails should be installed on all staircases, especially those outside.

Use a carpet sweeper instead of a vacuum. It is lighter and easier to manipulate.

The "Fone Holder" is a long, flexible shaft that attaches to most tables and can be positioned to hold the telephone receiver so a person can use the handset without having to move or even touch it. Another device adapts huge push buttons to the small touch-tone buttons of a standard phone to make dialing easier.

Handwriting can be a serious problem for persons with Parkinson's disease. Various pens, pencils, and writing devices are available to stabilize your grip. A weighted pen may help reduce tremors and improve writing.

A door knob turner fits over the door handle and converts the round knob into a lever. This makes it easier to open.

A Word to the Family

In order to preserve independence in activities of daily living, people should do all that they can for themselves. Because of tremor, rigidity, and slowness of movement, each activity may take more time than it used to.

It is tempting to do or to complete tasks for people. It saves time and, perhaps, frustration. However, this may lead to dependence, because it decreases people's motivation to help themselves.

The physical ability of persons with Parkinson's disease varies throughout the day in response to anti-Parkinson's medication. Tremor, rigidity, and slowness of movement may be more pronounced in the morning than in the afternoon. People's ability to dress or to eat may be impaired at one time and not another.

To decrease misunderstanding and further frustration, families should be aware that their relatives are not malingering but that it is the variability of the disease that causes fluctuation in independence. People may require help some of the time, but not all of the time.

It is vitally important for the families of people with Parkinson's disease to help them remain as independent as possible.

Resources for Independent Living

Listed are some companies that feature products, equipment, and clothing designed to make self-care skills easier.

Adaptability
P.O. Box 513
Colchester, CT 06415
Toll-Free: 800-243-9232

After Therapy Catalog
North Coast Medical
18305 Sutter Blvd.
Morgan Hill, CA 95037-2845
Toll-Free: 800-821-9319

American Walker
4683 Schneider Dr.
Oregon, WI 53575
Tel: 608-835-9255

Bell Atlantic Center for Customers with Disabilities
280 Locke Drive, 4th Floor
Marlboro, MA 01752
Toll-Free: 800-974-6006
Fax: 508-624-7645
Website: http://www.bellatlantic.com
E-mail: baccd@bellatlantic.com

Bruce Medical Supply
411 Waverly Oaks Rd.
Suite 154
Waltham, MA 02454
Toll-Free: 800-225-8446
Fax: 781-894-9519
Website: http://www.brucemedical.com

Comfort House
189-V Frelinghuysen Avenue
Newark, NJ 07114-1595
Toll-Free: 800-359-7701
Website: http://www.comforthouse.com

Dr. Leonard's Health Care Catalog
100 Nixon Lane
Edison, NJ 08818
Toll-Free: 800-785-0880
Fax: 732-572-2118
Website: http://www.drleonards.com

Dressing Tips and Clothing Res. for Making Life Easier

The Best 25 Catalogues Resources for Making Life Easier
933 Chapel Hill Road
Madison, WI 53711
Website: http://
www.makinglifeeasier.com
E-mail:
help@makinglifeeasier.com

Metro Medical Equipment

12985 Wayne Road
Livonia, MI 48150
Toll-Free: 800-877-7285
Fax: 734-522-9380

Durable Medical Equipment (over 3500) Plate Guards, Aids for Daily Living

Yes I Can
35325 Date Palm Dr., Suite 131
Cathedral City, CA 92234
Toll-Free: 800-366-4226
Tel: 760-321-1717

Fashion Ease

1541 60th Street
Brooklyn, NY 11219
Toll-Free: 800-221-8929
Tel: 718-871-8188
Fax: 718-436-2067
Websitet: http://
www.fashionease.com

Independent Living Aids Inc.

200 Robbins Lane
Jericho, NY 11753-2341
Toll-Free: 800-537-2118
Fax: 516-937-3906
Website: http://
www.independentliving.com

J C Penny's Special Needs Catalog

P.O. Box 2021
Milwaukee, WI 53201

Patients Transfer Systems

Beatrice M. Brantman, Inc.
207 E. Westminster
Lake Forest, IL 60045
Toll-Free: 800-232-7987
Fax: 847-615-8894

Personal Pager

The Greatest of Ease Company
2443 Fillmore Street, #345
San Francisco, CA 94115
Tel: 415-441-6649

Sammons Preston

P.O. Box 5071
Bolingbrook, IL 60440-5071
Toll-Free: 800-323-5547
Fax: 800-547-4333
Website: http://
www.SammonsPreston.com

Sears Health Care Catalog

Sears Roebuck and Company
P.O. Box 804203
Chicago, IL 60680-4203
Toll-Free: 800-326-1750

The Speedo Aquatic Exercise System

7911 Haskell Avenue
Van Nuys, CA 91409
Toll-Free: 800-547-8770

The Do Able Renewable Home

Consumer Affairs Program
Dept.
American Association of Retired
Persons (AARP)
Toll-Free: 800-424-3410

Voice Amplifiers

Rand Voice Amplifier

Park Surgical Company, Inc.
5001 New Utrecht Avenue
Brooklyn, NY 11219
Toll-Free: 800-633-7878
Tel: 718-436-9200
Fax: 718-854-2431
Website: http://
www.parksurgical.com

Luminaud Inc.

8688 Tyler Blvd.
Mentor, OH 44060-4348
Toll-Free: 800-255-3408
Fax: 440-255-2250
Website: http://
www.luminaud.com

Anchor Audio, Inc.

3415 Lomita Blvd.
Torrance, CA 90505
Toll-Free: 800-262-4671
Tel: 310-784-2300
Fax: 310-784-0066
Website: http://
www.anchoraudio.com

Walkers

Noble Motion Inc.

P.O. Box 5366
Pittsburgh, PA 15206
Toll-Free: 800-234-9255
Fax: 412-363-7189
Website: http://
www.wheels4walking.com

Chapter 11

Health Care Issues

Contents

Section 11.1

Nutrition

"Growing Older, Eating Better," by Paula Kurtzweil, *FDA Consumer*, March 1996, revised December 1996, Publication No. (FDA) 97-2301, and excerpts from "The Elderly Nutrition Program," Fact Sheet, Administration on Aging, 1999.

Growing Older, Eating Better

When Bernadette Harkins, 89, of Rockville, Maryland, could no longer feed herself properly, she moved to an assisted-living residence. Today, she can enjoy three meals a day served to her and about 30 other people in their home-like communal dining room.

When Harry, 85, of Moscow, Pennsylvania, could no longer feed himself properly, he moved in with his daughter and her family. With her guidance, he ate six times a day, snacking on high-calorie, high-protein foods, and maintaining a near-normal weight.

Harry, who asked that his last name not be used, and Harkins typify many of today's older generation. Living alone in most cases, they often are unable to meet their dietary needs and are forced to make compromises.

Harry didn't know how to cook. He developed cancer, which made it even more important that he eat a well-balanced diet. Harkins knew how to cook but didn't take time to prepare adequate meals for herself. "I would snack is what I'd do," she said. "I would think about getting a meal and then just have a cup of tea and toast. I knew I wasn't doing the right thing as far as nutrition was concerned."

Their eating problems stemmed from loneliness and lack of desire or skill to cook. Other older people may eat poorly for other reasons, ranging from financial difficulties to physical problems. The solutions can be just as varied, from finding alternative living arrangements to accepting home-delivered meals to using the food label recently revised by the Food and Drug Administration and the U.S. Department of Agriculture. Physical activity also is important in maintaining a healthy lifestyle.

Why the Concern?

Nutrition remains important throughout life. Many chronic diseases that develop late in life, such as osteoporosis, can be influenced by earlier poor habits. Insufficient exercise and calcium intake, especially during adolescence and early adulthood, can significantly increase the risk of osteoporosis, a disease that causes bones to become brittle and crack or break.

Good nutrition in the later years still can help lessen the effects of diseases prevalent among older Americans or improve the quality of life in people who have such diseases. They include osteoporosis, obesity, high blood pressure, heart disease, certain cancers, gastrointestinal problems, and chronic malnutrition.

Studies show that a good diet in later years helps both in reducing the risk of these diseases and in managing the diseases' signs and symptoms. This contributes to a higher quality of life, enabling older people to maintain their independence by continuing to perform basic daily activities, such as bathing, dressing, and eating. Poor nutrition, on the other hand, can prolong recovery from illnesses, increase the costs and incidence of institutionalization, and lead to a poorer quality of life.

The Single Life

Whether it happens at age 65 or 85, older people eventually face one or more problems that interfere with their ability to eat well. Social isolation is a common one. Older people who find themselves single after many years of living with another person may find it difficult to be alone, especially at mealtimes. They may become depressed and lose interest in preparing or eating regular meals, or they may eat only sparingly.

In a study published in the July 1993 *Journals of Gerontology*, researchers found that newly widowed people, most of whom were women, were less likely to say they enjoy mealtimes, less likely to report good appetites, and less likely to report good eating behaviors than their married counterparts. Nearly 85 percent of widowed subjects reported a weight change during the two years following their spouse's death, as compared with 30 percent of married subjects. The widowed group was more likely to report an average weight loss of 7.6 pounds (17 kilograms). According to the study, most of the women said they had enjoyed cooking and eating when they were married, but, as widows, they found those activities "a chore," especially since there was no one to appreciate their cooking efforts.

For many widowed men who may have left the cooking to their wives, the problem may extend even further: They may not know how to cook and prepare foods. Instead, they may snack or eat out a lot, both of which may lead people to eat too much fat and cholesterol and not get enough vitamins and minerals.

Special Diets

At the same time, many older people, because of chronic medical problems, may require special diets: for example, a low-fat, low-cholesterol diet for heart disease, a low-sodium diet for high blood pressure, or a low-calorie diet for weight reduction. Special diets often require extra effort, but older people may instead settle for foods that are quick and easy to prepare, such as frozen dinners, canned foods, lunch meats, and others that may provide too many calories, or contain too much fat and sodium for their needs.

On the other hand, Mona Sutnick, Ed.D., a registered dietitian in private practice in Philadelphia, pointed out that some people may go overboard on their special diets, overly restricting foods that may be more beneficial than detrimental to their health. "My advice for a 60-year-old person might be 'watch your fat' but for an 80-year-old who's underweight, I'd say, 'eat the fat, get the calories,'" Sutnick said.

Physical Problems

Some older people may overly restrict foods important to good health because of chewing difficulties and gastrointestinal disturbances, such as constipation, diarrhea, and heartburn. Because missing teeth and poorly fitting dentures make it hard to chew, older people may forego fresh fruits and vegetables, which are important sources of vitamins, minerals, and fiber. Or they may avoid dairy products, believing they cause gas or constipation. By doing so, they miss out on important sources of calcium, protein, and some vitamins.

Adverse reactions from medications can cause older people to avoid certain foods. Some medications alter the sense of taste, which can adversely affect appetite. This adds to the problem of naturally diminishing senses of taste and smell, common as people age.

Other medical problems, such as arthritis, stroke, or Alzheimer's disease, can interfere with good nutrition. It may be difficult, if not impossible, for example, for people with arthritis or who have had a stroke to cook, shop, or even lift a fork to eat. Dementia associated with Alzheimer's and other diseases may cause them to eat poorly or forget to eat altogether.

Money Matters

Lack of money is a particular problem among older Americans who may have no income other than Social Security. According to 1994 U.S. Census Bureau data, nearly 12 percent of people 65 and over are below the average poverty level for their age group. In 1994, the poverty level for a person 65 and over was $7,108 a year.

According to the 1994 data, the mean annual income for people 65 and over was $16,709, almost $10,000 less than what they earned on average between ages 55 and 64. Lack of money may lead older people to scrimp on important food purchases—for example, perishable items like fresh fruits, vegetables, and meat—because of higher costs and fear of waste. They may avoid cooking or baking foods like meats, stews, and casseroles because recipes for these foods usually yield large quantities. Financial problems also may cause older people to delay medical and dental treatments that could correct problems that interfere with good nutrition.

Food Programs

Many older people may find help under the Older Americans Act, which provides nutrition and other services that target older people who are in greatest social and economic need, with particular attention on low-income minorities. According to the U.S. Administration on Aging, which administers the Older Americans Act, the nutrition programs were set up to address the dietary inadequacy and social isolation among older people.

Home-delivered meals and congregate nutrition services are the primary nutrition programs. The congregate meal program allows seniors to gather at a local site, often the local senior citizen center, school or other public building, or a restaurant, for a meal and other activities, such as games and lectures on nutrition and other topics of interest to older people.

The Elderly Nutrition Program

Available since 1972, these programs, funded by the federal, state, and local governments, ensure that senior citizens get at least one nutritious meal five to seven days a week. Under current standards, that meal must comply with the Dietary Guidelines for Americans and provide at least one-third of the Recommended Dietary Allowances for an older person. In practice, the ENP's 3.1 million elderly participants are receiving an estimated 40 to 50 percent of most required nutrients. Often, people receive foods that correspond with their special dietary needs, such as no-added-salt foods for those who need to restrict their sodium intake or ground meat for those who have trouble chewing.

Other nutrition services provided under the Older Americans Act are nutrition education, screening, and counseling. While these nutrition programs target poor people, they are available to other older people regardless of income, according to Jean Lloyd, a registered dietitian and nutrition officer with the Administration on Aging. Although no one is charged for the meals, older people can voluntarily and confidentially donate money, she said. The meals provide not only good nutrition, but they also give older people a chance to socialize—a key factor in preventing the adverse nutritional effects of social isolation.

The services help older participants to learn to shop for, and/or to plan and prepare, meals that are economical and which help to manage or ameliorate specific health problems as well as enhancing their health and well-being. The congregate meal programs also provide older people with positive social contacts with other seniors at the group meal sites.

Volunteers who deliver meals to older persons who are homebound are encouraged to spend some time with the elderly. The volunteers also offer an important opportunity to check on the welfare of the homebound elderly and are encouraged to report any health or other problems that they may note during their visits.

In addition to providing nutrition and nutrition-related services, the ENP provides an important link to other needed supportive in-home and community-based services such as homemaker-home health aide services, transportation, fitness programs, and even home repair and home modification programs.

Program Outcomes

A congressionally-mandated evaluation of the ENP, released in fiscal year (FY) 1996, found that its participants have higher daily intakes of key nutrients than similar nonparticipants and that they have more social contacts as a result of the program.

Among ENP participants, 80 to 90 percent have incomes below 200 percent of the Department of Health and Human Services' poverty level index, which is twice the rate for the overall elderly population.

More than twice as many Title III participants live alone; and two-thirds of participants are either over or under their desired weight, placing them at risk for nutrition and health problems. Title III home-delivered meals participants have twice as many physical impairments compared with the overall elderly population.

In FY 1995, ENP funding neared $470 million and provided 123 million meals to 2.4 million people at congregate meal sites and 119 million home-delivered meals to 989,000 homebound older persons. In FY 1994, 226 American Indian grantees received nearly $17 million, which provided 1.3 million meals to 41,000 congregate meal participants and 1.5 million meals to 47,500 homebound elderly participants.

In FY 1998, total funding for the Title III congregate and home-delivered meal programs was $486.4 million which is 56 percent of the AoA's budget. For every $1 of federal congregate funds, $1.70 additional funding is leveraged; for every $1 of federal home-delivered funds, $3.35 additional funding is leveraged. The leveraged funds come from other sources including state, tribal, local, and other federal moneys and services, as well as through donations from participants. Nationally, total contributions amounted to $170 million.

The average cost of a meal, including the value of donated labor and supplies, was $5.17 for a group meal and $5.31 for a home-delivered meal under Title III. Comparable costs for a meal under Title VI were $6.19 and $7.18, respectively.

Other Assistance

For those who qualify, food stamps are another aid for improving nutrition. Under this program, a one-person household can receive up to $115 a month in food stamps to buy most grocery items.

For the homebound, grocery-shopping assistance is available in many areas. Usually provided by nongovernment organizations, this service shops for and delivers groceries to people at their request. The recipient pays for the groceries and sometimes a service fee. In some communities, private organizations also sell home-delivered meals.

Family members and friends can help ensure that older people take advantage of food programs by putting them in touch with the appropriate agencies or organizations and helping them fill out the necessary forms. Some other steps they can take include:

- looking in occasionally to ensure that the older person is eating adequately

- preparing foods for and making them available to the older person

- joining the older person for meals.

In some cases, they may help see that the older person is moved to an environment, such as their home, an assisted-living facility, or a nursing home, that can help ensure that the older person gets proper nutrition. Whatever an older person's living situation, proper medical and dental treatment is important for treating medical problems, such as gastrointestinal distress and chewing difficulties that interfere with good nutrition. If a medication seems to ruin an older person's taste and appetite, a switch to another drug may help.

A review of basic diet principles may help improve nutrition. Explaining to older people the importance of good nutrition in the later years may motivate them to make a greater effort to select nutritious foods.

Look to the Label

The food label can help older people select a good diet. Revamped in 1992, the label gives the nutritional content of most foods and enables consumers to see how a food fits in with daily dietary recommendations.

Some of the information appears as claims describing the food's nutritional benefits: for example, "low in cholesterol" or "high in vitamin C." Under strict government rules, these claims can be used only if the food meets certain criteria. This means that claims can be trusted. For example, a "low-cholesterol" food can provide no more than 20 milligrams (mg) of cholesterol and no more than 2 grams of saturated fat per serving. A high-potassium food must provide at least 700 mg of potassium per serving.

Less common but also helpful are label claims linking a nutrient or food to the risk of a disease or health-related condition. So far, FDA allows only eight of these claims because they are the only ones supported by scientific evidence. One claim links sodium, a nutrient found in salt and used in many processed foods, to high blood pressure. On the food label, this claim would read something like this:

"Diets low in sodium may reduce the risk of high blood pressure, a disease associated with many factors."

More in-depth information is found on the "Nutrition Facts" panel on the side or back of the food label. This information is required on almost all food packages. Unlike before, this nutrition information is easier to read because it appears in bigger type and is usually on a white or other neutral contrasting background, when practical.

Some nutrition information also may be available for many raw meats, poultry and fish, fresh fruits, and vegetables at the point of purchase. The information may appear in brochures or on posters or placards.

Physical Activity

Besides diet, physical activity is part of a healthy lifestyle at any age. It can help reduce and control weight by burning calories. Moderate exercise that places weight on bones, such as walking, helps maintain and possibly even increases bone strength in older people. A study published in the Dec. 28, 1994, *Journal of the American Medical Association* found that intensive strength training can help preserve bone density and improve muscle mass, strength, and balance in postmenopausal women. In the study, subjects used weight machines for strength training. Also, scientists looking into the benefits of exercise for older people agree that regular exercise can improve the functioning of the heart and lungs, increase strength and flexibility, and contribute to a feeling of well-being.

Any regular physical activity is good, from brisk walking to light gardening. Common sense is the key. But, before a vigorous exercise program is started or started after a long period of rest, a doctor should be consulted.

Taking time out for exercise, using the food label to help pick nutritious foods, taking advantage of the several assistance programs available, and getting needed medical attention can go a long way in helping older people avoid the nutritional pitfalls of aging and more fully enjoy their senior years.

For More Information

To learn more about the food label and nutrition for older people, write for these publications:

Using the New Food Label to Choose Healthier Foods Publication No. (FDA) 94-2276

FDA
5600 Fishers Lane (HFE-88)
Rockville, MD 20857

Healthy Eating for a Healthy Life

AARP (American Association of Retired Persons) Fulfillment
601 E. St., N.W.
Washington, DC 20049
Ask for publication by title and stock number D15565.

To learn about meal programs for senior citizens in your area, call the Administration on Aging's Elder Care Locator, 800-677-1116.

For information about food stamps, contact your county's food stamp office listed in the blue pages of the telephone book.

To find a registered dietitian in your area, call the National Center for Nutrition and Dietetics Consumer Nutrition Hotline, 800-366-1655.

Section 11.2

Medications

"Medications and Older Adults," by Rebecca D. Williams, *FDA Consumer*, September/October 1997, revised January 1999, Publication No. (FDA) 97-3225.

Medications and Older Adults

Mary Parker of Oak Ridge, Tennessee, is quick to joke about her health problems. Her vibrant smile and upbeat attitude belie her 78 years. But last year she had a health problem she didn't find amusing. The medication she took for her swollen sinuses left her so weak and dizzy she couldn't get out of bed. "I felt like I wanted to die," she remembers. "It was awful." She learned an important lesson from the episode.

She thinks twice before taking any medication, questions her doctors and pharmacists, and reviews all her medications regularly with her primary physician. Parker's attitude is a good one for older adults to have, experts say. As people age, they often develop a number of problems taking medications. Being aware that problems may occur is the first way to minimize them.

"You are a partner in your health care," urges Madeline Feinberg, Pharm.D., a pharmacist and director of the Elder Health program of the University of Maryland School of Pharmacy. "This is a partnership between you, your doctor, and your pharmacist. You need to be assertive and knowledgeable about the medications you take."

The Food and Drug Administration is working to make drugs safer for older adults, who consume a large share of the nation's medications. Adults over age 65 buy 30 percent of all prescription drugs and 40 percent of all over-the-counter drugs. "Almost every drug that comes through FDA [for approval] has been examined for effects in the elderly," says Robert Temple, M.D., associate director for medical policy in FDA's Office of Drug Evaluation and Research. "If the manufacturer hasn't done a study in the elderly, we ask for it."

More than 15 years ago, the agency established guidelines for drug manufacturers to include more elderly patients in their studies of new drugs. Upper age limits for drugs were eliminated, and even patients who had other health problems were given the green light to participate if they were able. Also, drugs known to pass primarily through the liver and kidneys must be studied in patients with malfunctions of those organs. This has a direct benefit for older adults, who are more likely to have these conditions.

In several surveys, FDA discovered that drug manufacturers had been using older adults in their drug studies; however, they weren't examining that age group for different reactions to the drugs. Now, they do. Today, new prescription drugs are generally required to have a section in the labeling about their use in the elderly. Says Temple, "The FDA has done quite a bit and worked fully with academia and industry to change drug testing so that it does analyze the data from elderly patients. We're quite serious about wanting these analyses."

When More Isn't Necessarily Better

Of all the problems older adults face in taking medication, drug interactions are probably the most dangerous. When two or more drugs are mixed in the body, they may interact with each other and produce uncomfortable or even dangerous side effects. This is especially a problem for older adults because they are much more likely to take more than one drug. Two-thirds of adults over age 65 use one or more drugs each day, and a quarter of them take three drugs each day.

Not all drug combinations are bad. High blood pressure is often treated with several different drugs in low doses. Unless supervised by a doctor, however, taking a mixture of drugs can be dangerous. For example, a person who takes a blood-thinning medication for high blood pressure should not combine that with aspirin, which will thin the blood even more. And antacids can interfere with certain drugs for Parkinson's disease, high blood pressure, and heart disease. Before prescribing any new drug to an older patient, a doctor should be aware of all the other drugs the patient may be taking. "Too often, older people get more drugs without a reassessment of their previous medications," says Feinberg. "That can be disastrous."

There is also evidence that older adults tend to be more sensitive to drugs than younger adults are, due to their generally slower metabolisms and organ functions. As people age, they lose muscle tissue and gain fat tissue, and their digestive systems, liver, and kidney functions slow down. All this affects how a drug will be absorbed into the bloodstream, react in the organs, and how quickly it will be eliminated. The old adage "start low and go slow" applies especially to the elderly. Older adults who experience dizziness, constipation, upset stomach, sleep changes, diarrhea, incontinence, blurred vision, mood changes, or a rash after taking a drug should call their doctors.

The following suggestions may also help:

- Don't take a drug unless absolutely necessary. Try a change in diet or exercise instead. Ask your doctor if there's anything else you can do besides drug therapy for the condition.

- Tell your doctor about all the drugs you take. If you have several doctors, make sure they all know what the others are prescribing, and ask one doctor (such as an internist or general practitioner) to coordinate your drugs.

- Ask for drugs that treat more than one condition. Blood pressure medicine might also be good for heart disease, for example.

- Keep track of side effects. New symptoms may not be from old age but from the drug you're taking. Try another medication if possible until you find one that works for you.

- Learn about your drugs. Find out as much as you can by asking questions and reading the package inserts. Both your doctor and pharmacist should alert you to possible interactions between drugs, how to take any drug properly, and whether there's a less expensive generic drug available.

- Have your doctor review your drugs. If you take a number of drugs, take them all with you on a doctor's visit.

- Ask the doctor, "When can I stop taking this drug?" and, "How do we know this drug is still working?"

- Watch your diet. Some drugs are better absorbed with certain foods, and some drugs shouldn't be taken with certain foods. Ask a pharmacist what foods to take with each drug.

- Follow directions. Read the label every time you take the medication to prevent mistakes, and be sure you understand the timing and dosage prescribed.

- Don't forget. Use a memory aid to help you—a calendar, pill box, or your own system. Whatever works for you is best.

Medicine and Special Needs

Arthritis, poor eyesight, and memory lapses can make it difficult for some older adults to take their medications correctly. Studies have shown that between 40 and 75 percent of older adults don't take their medications at the right time or in the right amount. About a quarter of all nursing home admissions are due at least in part to the inability to take medication correctly.

A number of strategies can make taking medication easier. Patients with arthritis can ask the pharmacist for an oversized, easy-to-open bottle. For easier reading, ask for large-type labels. If those are not available, use a magnifying glass and read the label under bright light.

Invent a system to remember medication. Even younger adults have trouble remembering several medications two or three times a day, with and without food. Devise a plan that fits your daily schedule. Some people use meals or bedtime as cues for remembering drugs. Others use charts, calendars, and special weekly pillboxes.

Mary Sloane, 78, keeps track of five medications a day by sorting her pills each evening into separate dishes. One is for morning pills, the other for the next evening. Then she turns each medicine bottle upside down after taking the pill so she can tell at a glance if she has taken it that day. "You have to have a system," Sloane says. "Because just as soon as I get started taking my pills, the phone rings, and when I come back to it, I think, 'Now have I taken that?'"

Drug-taking routines should take into account whether the pill works best on an empty or full stomach and whether the doses are spaced properly. To simplify taking medications, always ask for the easiest dosing schedule possible—just once or twice a day, for example. Serious memory impairments require assistance from family members or professionals. Adult daycare, supervised living facilities, and home health nurses can provide assistance with drugs.

Active Lives

Not all older adults are in danger of drug interactions and adverse effects. In fact, as more and more people live active lives well into their 80s or beyond, many take few medications at all. Among healthy older adults, medications may have the same physical effects as they do in younger adults. It is primarily when disease interferes that the problems begin.

To guard against potential problems with drugs, however, older adults must be knowledgeable about what they take and how it makes them feel. And they should not hesitate to talk to their doctors or pharmacists about questions and problems they have with a medication. Says the University of Maryland's Feinberg: "We need to have educated patients to tell us how the drugs are working."

Cutting Costs

The cost of medications is a serious concern for older adults, most of whom must pay for drugs out of pocket. Even those who have insurance to supplement Medicare must often pay a percentage of the cost of their medicines.

For a new prescription, don't buy a whole bottle but ask for just a few pills. You may have side effects to the medication and have to switch. If you buy just a few, you won't be stuck with a costly bottle of medicine you can't take.

For ongoing conditions, medications are often less expensive in quantities of 100. Only buy large quantities of drugs if you know your body tolerates them well. But be sure you can use all of the medication before it passes its expiration date.

Call around for the lowest price. Pharmacy prices can vary greatly. If you find a drug cheaper elsewhere, ask your regular pharmacist if he or she can match the price.

Other ways to make your prescription dollars go further include:

- Ask for a senior citizens discount.

- Ask for a generic equivalent.

- Get drug samples free. Pharmaceutical companies often give samples of drugs to physicians. Tell your doctor you'd be happy to have them. This is especially convenient for trying out a new prescription.

- Buy store-brand or discount brand over-the-counter products. Ask the pharmacist for recommendations.

- Call your local chapter of the American Association for Retired Persons (AARP) and your local disease-related organizations (for diabetes, arthritis, etc.) They may have drugs available at discount prices.

- Try mail order. Mail-order pharmacies can provide bulk medications at discount prices. Use this service only for long-term drug therapy because it takes a few weeks to be delivered. Compare prices before ordering anything.

What to Ask the Doctor

Before you leave your doctor's office with a new prescription, make sure you fully understand how to take the drug correctly. Your pharmacist can also provide valuable information about how to take your medicines and how to cope with side effects. Ask the following questions:

- What is the name of this drug, and what is it designed to do? Is this a generic or a name brand product?

- What is the dosing schedule and how do I take it?

- What should I do if I forget a dose?

- What side effects should I expect?

- How long will I be on this drug?

- How should I store this drug?

- Should I take this on an empty stomach or with food? Is it safe to drink alcohol with this drug?

Section 11.3

Hearing Problems

Reprinted with permission, "Hearing Problems,"
© by Kenneth Hepburn, Ph.D.

Good communication depends a great deal on being able to hear well. Learning if a person has a hearing problem can be hard. Many people may not hear clearly what is being said. Still, they do not ask you to repeat yourself or to make clearer what you mean. Often enough, these people do not themselves know that something is wrong with their hearing. Also, many people, not just those with some hearing loss, "fill in the gaps" of a conversation. They interpret facial expressions and other gestures and read lips.

Poor hearing makes communication harder. It also increases the risk of chance injury (due to not hearing an oncoming car, for instance). Hearing loss combined with the effects of an illness like Alzheimer's disease will make communication even harder. The disease itself isolates the person from you and from the world. Over time, the person has a harder and harder time making sense out of things. Such a situation poses special problems for you, the caregiver.

What if you suspect that the person in your care has a hearing problem? You will need to observe the impaired person carefully. Seek help to get a good evaluation of the person's hearing and to correct problems that might respond to treatment.

Problems may remain which cannot be corrected. As a caregiver, you will have to develop coping techniques that work for you and the person in your care.

Observation and Diagnosis

You may have noticed that the impaired person seems removed from what is going on around him or her. The person may seem distracted or not attentive. Or the person may ask you to repeat what you say.

Keep track of the problems you notice and try to answer the following questions. Discuss this information with the doctor or nurse.

What you observe and recall about the person's hearing can greatly help the doctor in making a diagnosis and in setting up a plan to deal with the problem. The doctor will check to see if the impaired person's hearing is failing. The doctor will try to decide if the problems arise from a source other than hearing loss, such as side effects from drugs or the course of the disease itself.

Questions

- What problems of hearing or attending is the impaired person having?

- When did you first notice the problems?

- Do you see any pattern to the problems? (For instance, does the impaired person seem to have more trouble at certain times and to do better at other times?)

- Has the person ever used a hearing aid? (If so, bring it along with you when you visit the doctor.)

Treatment and Management

You may find that the problem is partly due to a correctable hearing loss. In this case a hearing aid may help. Try to keep in mind, however, that hearing aids do not correct hearing the way glasses correct vision. Hearing aids make all sounds louder. So background noises, like the hum of a refrigerator or the sound of traffic (which people with normal hearing "tune out") are also made louder. These noises can irritate and confuse. People who need and can benefit from hearing aids often object to them at first because background noises become so loud. If this is the case with the person in your care, try using it for just a part of each day at first.

You may learn that a hearing problem exists but that the problem will not respond to treatment. Or you may learn that the impaired person may hear perfectly well and yet still not be able to act appropriately. Communication problems, in this case, result from the disease itself rather than from hearing loss. The disease has made the person's brain unable to understand or recall what the person hears.

In these cases, the problem will have to be managed rather than cured. Your care goals might simply be to keep the person out of harm's way and to help him to act on his own as much as he can. Goals like these promote the person's own sense of well-being and keep your care tasks within reason.

Note: Even if the doctor is unable to find any correctable hearing problem, report any new problems. The doctor or nurse can help you understand what is happening and suggest coping techniques. Also, you want to be sure that any new problem is promptly identified and treated.

Coping Techniques

Here are some tips to help you communicate with a hearing-impaired person. Your doctor or nurse may have specific ideas for coping with the special problems you may be having. Support groups may be a resource to you. Other members may have suggestions, based on their own experiences, for managing the problems you face.

Anticipate problems and be prepared to take extra time. If the impaired person doesn't hear or understand well, you may have trouble even with routine activities. Allow extra time to explain and reassure. Always give yourself extra time when you take the person out of the setting he or she knows well.

Make sure the person can see you well. Approach the person from the front, and face the person directly. Sit close enough for the person to see your face and mouth. Keep your hands away from your mouth while you are speaking. Make sure no bright light is shining in the impaired person's face to distract him or her.

Get and keep the person's attention. Work at getting and keeping the person's attention. Wait to begin what you want to say until the person is focused on you (as much as he or she can). Keep in mind that attention span will be short. Try to get and keep eye contact with the person. Sometimes a gentle touch on the arm or hand, if allowed, will help you make eye contact. Physical contact is a powerful form of communication.

Find out how the person hears best. Perhaps the person has one good ear. If so, you will want to speak on that side. If the person uses a hearing aid, check to be sure it works and is turned on and loud enough.

Be alert to distracting background noises. Turn off the radio or television, for example.

Plan how to express yourself. Think ahead about how to express what you want to say. Short, simple words and sentences will be understood most easily.

Speak slowly, clearly, and distinctly without shouting. A shrill or loud voice will make you sound upset or angry. The person may react by becoming too upset to focus on what you are saying. If your words run together, the person may not be able to keep up with what you are saying. If you speak slowly, it will be easier to pronounce your words more clearly. Lowering the tone of your voice often helps.

Be prepared to repeat yourself. You will no doubt have to repeat yourself many times. Try to keep in mind that the person is not doing this on purpose. On the other hand, don't deny your own feelings. This can be frustrating.

Use gestures to support what you say. If the impaired person can still interpret a nod of the head or shrug of the shoulders, these may be better ways of communicating than words.

Check regularly to see if the impaired person understands. Watch to see what the impaired person does, rather than trusting what he or she says. Impaired people often become very skillful at concealing the fact that they can't understand. If the person doesn't seem to understand, try to find a new, simpler way to say the same thing.

Living with the Problem

If the person in your care has a hearing loss, communication and your caregiving tasks become harder. Managing the day-to-day routine takes more time and effort. You may, as a safety measure, need to keep closer watch over the person's activities.

How well you structure the impaired person's day (and your own) becomes important. A regular routine will be easier for both of you. You especially need to build in time for yourself to take a break. You also need to find helpers who can give you occasional respite from your caregiving duties. Family members and friends can help, or you might want to consider hiring help if you can.

Take care of yourself. Keep in mind that you need to take care of yourself, too. Caregiving can be tiring, frustrating, and irritating. Don't deny your fatigue or your feelings. You may not want to show your feelings of frustration to the impaired person because that might trigger a reaction that could make things worse. Still, you do need to find a way to let feelings like that come out.

Talk with others. Talking with others in similar situations can be extremely helpful. You may want to join a support group. Sharing with others might help you keep in mind that the problems you face do not result from the patient's deliberate refusal to cooperate or from your inadequacy as a caregiver. The problems are part of the disease itself and of the caregiving role.

Section 11.4

Hospitalization Happens

Reprinted with permission, "Planning For Emergencies: What You Need To Do Now," © 1999 North Carolina Division of Aging.

A trip to the hospital with a loved one who has a memory disorder can be stressful for both of you. This information can relieve some of that stress by helping you prepare for both unexpected and planned hospital visits. In it you will find steps you can take now to make hospital visits as easy as possible, tips on making your loved one more comfortable once you arrive at the hospital, and advice on working with hospital staff and doctors.

Share this information with family and friends, copy this section, keep it in a handy spot, and prepare now for the future.

Hospital Emergencies: What You Can Do Now

Planning ahead is the key to making either an unexpected or a planned trip to the hospital easier for you and your loved one. Here is what you should do now:

- Register your relative for a SAFE RETURN bracelet. People who are lost may be taken to an emergency room. The bracelet will speed the process of reconnecting you and your loved one.

- Know who you can count on. You need a family member or trusted friend to stay with your loved one when he or she is admitted to the emergency room or hospital. Have at least two dependable family members, neighbors, or friends you can call on to go with you or meet you at the hospital at a moment's notice so that one of you can take care of the paperwork and the other can stay with your loved one.

Pack an "Emergency Bag" containing the following:

- A sheet of paper listing: the person's name, nickname, address, insurance companies (include policy numbers and pre-authorization phone numbers), Medicare and Medicaid card numbers, doctors (include addresses).

- A list of important phone numbers such as doctors, key family members, minister, and helpful friends.

- A list of all current medicines and dosage instructions. This list should be updated when there is any change.

- A list of medicines taken that have ever caused a bad reaction and a list of any allergies to medicines and foods.

- Copies of important papers such as Durable Power of Attorney, Health Care Power of Attorney, Living Will.

- Extra adult briefs (i.e. Depends) if the person usually wears them. These may not be easy to get in the emergency room if you need them.

- A change of clothes in case the person's clothes become soiled or torn and a plastic bag for the soiled clothing.

- A card that says, "Please Understand—My companion has a memory disorder—Let me help with specific questions." You should avoid talking about your relative's memory changes or behaviors in front of him. This can be upsetting and embarrassing to your relative.

- Moist hand wipes such as Wet Ones.

- A reassuring object, a walkman with a favorite tape, or a portable radio.

- A writing pad and pen so that you can jot down information and directions given to you by hospital staff. You will also want to write down your loved one's symptoms and problems. You might be asked the same questions by many people. Show them what you have written instead of repeating your answers.

- Pain medicine such as Advil, Tylenol, or aspirin. This is for you, the caregiver. A trip to the ER may take longer than you think. Stress can lead to a headache or other symptoms.

- A sealed snack such as a pack of crackers and a bottle of water or juice for you and your loved one. You could wait for quite a while.

- A small amount of cash.

- If you have a cellular phone, put a note on the outside of the "Emergency Bag" to take the phone with you to use outside of the building. Many hospitals ask that cellular phones be switched off before entering the building.

By taking these steps in advance you will greatly reduce the stress and confusion that can often accompany a hospital visit particularly if the visit is an unplanned trip to the emergency room.

At the Emergency Room

A trip to the emergency room may tire or even frighten your loved one. There are some important things to remember:

- Be patient. It could be a long wait if the reason for your visit is not life-threatening.

- Know that results from lab tests take time.

- Offer physical comfort and verbal reassurance to your relative. Stay calm and confident.

- Realize that just because you do not see staff at work, does not mean they are not working.

- Be aware that emergency room staff often has little training in Alzheimer's or dementia disease so help them understand your loved one.

- Do not assume your loved one will be admitted to the hospital.

- Do not leave the ER to go home without a follow-up plan. If you are sent home, make sure you have all instructions for follow-up care.

Before a Hospital Stay

If your loved one is going to the hospital for a planned stay, you have time to prepare and ask your doctor questions. Ask your doctor if the procedure can be done as an outpatient visit. If not, ask if tests can be done before going to the hospital to shorten the hospital stay. Ask if your doctor plans to talk with other doctors. If so, find out if your relative can see these specialists before going into the hospital.

You should also ask questions about anesthesia, catheters, and IVs. General anesthesia can have side effects. Ask if local anesthesia is an option and if you will be allowed in the recovery room.

Before Going to the Hospital

- If your insurance allows, ask for a private room if possible. It is more quiet and calm.

- Let your loved one take part in the planning for the hospital stay as much as possible.

- Don't talk about the hospital stay in front of your relative as if he is not there.

- Plan ahead. Make a schedule with family and friends to take turns sitting with your relative during the entire hospital stay.

- Shortly before going to the hospital, decide the best way to tell your loved one that the two of you are going to spend a short time in the hospital.

- When packing, include a copy of important papers such as a living will and health care power of attorney.

- Pack comfort items. Things to help your loved one feel safe and secure such as favorite clothes or blankets and photos.

During the Hospital Stay

- Have someone with your loved one at all times if possible—even during medical tests. This may be hard to do, but it will help keep your loved one calm and make the hospital stay easier for him.

- Ask doctors to limit their questions to your relative who may not be able to answer. Instead, answer questions from the doctor outside your relative's room.

- Ask the staff to avoid using physical restraints.

- Help your relative fill out menu requests.

- Open food containers and remove trays.

- Talk with your loved one in the way he will best understand.

- Remind your relative to drink fluids. Offer fluids and have him make regular trips to the bathroom.

- Know that a strange place, medicines, tests, and surgery will make a person with Alzheimer's disease more confused. He will need more help with personal care.

- Assume your relative will have problems finding the bathroom and using his call button.

- Sudden confusion can be caused by a medical problem. Ask the doctor if your loved one seems suddenly worse.

Anxiety or Agitation

If anxiety or agitation occurs, try some of the following:

- Remove street clothes from sight.

- Post reminders or cues if this comforts your relative.

- Turn off the television, the telephone ringer, and the intercom.

- Talk in a calm voice and offer reassurance. Repeat answers to questions.

- Give a comforting touch or distract your loved one with offers of snacks.

- Listen to soothing music or try comforting rituals.

- Slow down, try not to rush your loved one.

- Give your loved one something to hold in his hands such as a book, photos, or a favorite item.

Working with Hospital Staff

Remember that not everyone in the hospital knows the same basic facts about memory loss and Alzheimer's disease. You may be their best teacher of what works with your family member.

You can help the staff by giving them a list of your loved one's normal routine; personal habits; likes and dislikes; possible behaviors, what might cause them and how you handle them; and signs of pain or discomfort. You should:

- Make the list easy to read with headings and short, simple statements. Have a copy with the chart and at the nurse's station.

- Decide with the hospital staff who will do what for your loved one. For example, you may want to be the one who helps your family member get a bath, eat, or use the toilet.

- Think about placing a poster above the head of the bed with key information, including names of people important to your loved one and the relationship (spouse, cousin, friend).

- Tell the staff about any unusual behaviors, hearing problems, or communication problems your relative may have and offer ideas for what works best in those instances.

- Make sure your family member is safe, tell the staff about any previous problems with wandering, getting lost, suspiciousness, or falls.

- Do not assume the staff knows your loved one's needs. Tell them in a nice, calm manner.

- Ask questions when you don't understand hospital procedures, tests, or when you have a concern.

- Realize that hospital staff are caring for many people and practice the art of patience.

Chapter 12

Creating a Safe and Workable Environment

An illness like Alzheimer's disease causes steady decline in the patient's abilities. As a caregiver, you will be called on to deal with many problems posed by the impaired person's declining skills. As more and more skills are lost, you will need to take over more and more.

Just what will you need to do? As caregiver, you need to actively manage the person's daily life. At first, you may only have to make daily events simpler. Later, you may need to restrict them. This may well be easier said than done. You also need to look closely at your home setting. Does it make life easier or harder for the person (and for you)?

You have several concerns. You need to see that the impaired person is safe and happy. You need to make sure your caregiving tasks work well for you. You also need some strength and time left for yourself.

This chapter deals with controlling the impaired person's physical surroundings and managing the daily routine. Both are important parts of creating a safe and workable environment for the impaired person, for you, and for everyone else involved. In talking about these

Reprinted with permission "Managing from Day to Day," by Beverly Evans, MPH, OTR and Chief, Occupational Therapy Section of the Department of Veterans Affairs Medical Center, Minneapolis, Minnesota, © Kenneth Hepburn, Ph.D., Geriatric Research, Education and Clinical Center (GRECC) of the Department of Veterans Affairs Medical Center, Minneapolis, Minnesota.

issues, the subject of finding help when you need it comes up too. You can't be alert and on-the-job day and night. You will need to find ways to cope with the increasing need to watch over the impaired person. Family members or social and health agencies might be sources of help.

Assess and Modify Your Home

Conduct a survey of your home to see what you might change or store away while you are caring for this person. Look at your home in great detail to see what might be harmful. Then take steps to prevent harm. The goals of your home survey should be to reduce needless choices, confusion, and danger.

If you ever had to "childproof" your home, the process is somewhat the same. The survey requires you to look at your home and to observe the impaired person in it. Pretend you are a stranger in your home. Put aside your feelings so you can look at your household as a stranger might. Does it make life easier or harder (even dangerous) for the impaired person? Does it help you in your caregiving or not?

Your family and friends, especially members of a support group, can help you with ideas. You can also get outside help from experts in checking the safety and efficiency of the home. Public health nurses (visiting nurses) and occupational therapists are especially good at sizing up a home and suggesting ways to make it work better for an impaired person. Carpenters and handymen may have good, practical tips too. A safety survey should be made in every room of your home. The kitchen and the bathroom are most important. Be sure you check the laundry, workroom, garage, and outdoor areas too. Use these general guidelines:

- **Open up the spaces.** Your work should leave rooms more open. There should be space for wandering and clear pathways from room to room. The fewer things the impaired person runs into, trips over, or feels blocked by, the better. The person shouldn't have to walk around tables or chairs to get from one place to another. Remove items the person could trip over like coffee tables, floor lamps, standing vases, or phone and electrical cords. If you need access to these things, at least move them back out of the impaired person's pathways.

- **Prevent slips and falls.** Do the floors provide good traction for walking? Make sure the floors aren't too slick. If you keep linoleum or vinyl floors polished, use a non-skid wax. Or allow the floor's surface to become dull. (Wash it, but don't wax it, and use a cleaner that doesn't include a waxing agent.) Follow the same routines with wood floors. Are the rugs in your home secure? Do edges stick up so the person could trip? Do you have throw rugs that could slip out from under the person? If so, fasten them down or store them away. Are the surfaces of the bathroom floor and tub or shower slippery? Rough textured strips or decals can be purchased cheaply. They are easy to apply and greatly improve traction. Properly installed grab bars in the right places can make the bathroom safer too.

- **Offer clear contrasts.** Can the impaired person know easily where the floor stops and the wall begins? Where the wall stops and the doorway begins? If you observe the impaired person having problems like walking into walls or being surprised by a doorway, try to make such areas clearer. A number of experts suggest using tape or paint in a contrasting color around borders. Start out with a small experiment to see if the results would be worth the effort and expense to make this change throughout the house. Your neighborhood hardware store can be a resource for you in such projects. Describe what you want to do, and ask for help and suggestions.

- **Remove distractions.** Take away anything you can that seems to upset the impaired person needlessly or to interfere with tasks that must be done. Knicknacks, magazines, mirrors, even certain fabrics or rugs with busy or too bright patterns can be confusing. Some things (like the magazines) are easily removed. Try doing so and see what happens. Other things, like carpeting, drapes, and upholstery, are very expensive. You may not be able to consider changing them. You may suspect that a certain chair or drape pattern is causing problems. Remove the item or use a slipcover for a while to see if you are right. You can then weigh the possible benefit against the expense.

- **Control needless glare off the floors or walls.** Not waxing floors (or using a non-skid wax) and using "flat" rather than "high gloss" or "semi-gloss" paint will reduce glare. As you replace light bulbs, try the "soft light" kind (in the same wattage). Be sure no bare light bulbs are exposed. Draw the drapes if sunlight is too bright. Also, be aware that having the radio or TV on too often or too loud may be stimulating or distracting the impaired person too much.

- **Identify dangerous objects.** Cigarettes, cigars, or pipes may be very unsafe for a forgetful person. In the kitchen, the stove poses the biggest danger. The impaired person could be burned or could start fires. Knives and other pointed utensils such as large meat forks are dangers too. Small appliances like the toaster, toaster/oven, food processor, blender, mixer, can opener, waffle iron, and microwave oven can be very dangerous.

- **Other electrical appliances** (space heaters, electric fans) might pose a threat. Keep in mind that electric appliances must be used with great care around water. There may be a number of items in the bathroom (hairdryer, electric razor, radio, dock, even a telephone) which the impaired person should not use alone. Look carefully at personal grooming items, too. Razors, nail files, clippers, small scissors and such may require more skill to use than the impaired person still has. Are there other sharp or pointed objects lying out in sight like scissors, letter openers, or decorative items? Are there fragile objects like a hand mirror which might be broken, leaving jagged pieces which might injure someone?

- **Look for furniture that can be easily pulled over or toppled** (for instance, a tall, unsecured bookcase). Are there items like stools or stepladders on which the person might climb? Do you have places like stairs where the person might fall? Are there any storm doors or low windows that might be broken? Is the water heater temperature so hot that the water could scald someone? Are there any guns or other weapons in the house?

- **Dispose of dangerous objects.** Throw away old paint thinner or old drugs, for instance. Sell or give away any guns, other weapons, or extra sharp tools. Substitute safe items for dangerous ones whenever possible. Bathroom glasses can be replaced with paper cups or unbreakable plastic glasses. Glass in storm doors or low windows can be replaced with plexiglass or safety glass. Find a safe storage area for dangerous items that you must keep but don't need often. Store such supplies as lawn fertilizer, insect poisons, and gasoline there. If you must keep any guns or other weapons, they should also be locked up (unloaded), and you should have the only key. Be sure to lock up any ammunition too. Your storage area may be a garage or outside shed. You may use a room or area of the house like the attic or basement that you are sure the impaired person can't reach.

Or you may simply use a locked storage closet. You can even try just putting items out of reach (on a top shelf, for instance) if you are sure the impaired person can't climb up to get them.

- **Secure items that might be dangerous.** In each room of the house secure any items that might be dangerous but which you need often. Speak with your local utility company about ways to make the stove safe. For instance, a hidden on-off switch or a cover with a lock may be used. Small appliances which might be misused should be stored in a cupboard or closet with a secure latch on it. Lock up such items as scissors, knives, or pointed kitchen utensils. You can use "childproofing" devices on cabinets and use hooks that are hard to open (or oddly placed) on closet doors. Inexpensive locks can be installed on drawers and cabinets holding especially dangerous items.

- **Store household cleaning supplies safely.** Detergents, polishes, drain and toilet bowl cleaners, shower and tub cleansers are all potential poisons. These should be removed or stored safely. You might want to collect all of the household cleaning materials and store them in one secure place where the impaired person could not get into them. At the very least, make sure you have a secure cabinet in each room where you store such items.

- **Lock up all over-the-counter and prescription drugs.** Off-the-shelf pain relievers like aspirin or Tylenol are quite dangerous in large doses. An overdose of a laxative may not have as serious results as an overdose of Valium, but you don't need either problem. Find a way to lock the medicine cabinet or remove dangerous items to a locked drawer or closet.

- **Consider putting away personal hygiene and grooming supplies.** Mouthwash, toothpaste, cologne, after shave lotions, rubbing alcohol, soaps, and shampoos all look and smell good enough to eat or drink. The impaired person may do just that and become ill. Control access to liquor and even food. A forgetful person may consume more alcohol than is healthful. At times impaired persons may hoard food and become ill from eating an item that has spoiled.

- **Review the laundry room, utility room, and workshop.** You should lower your water heater setting to prevent accidental scalding. Laundry products such as bleach, detergents, and fabric softeners are poisonous if consumed. At the very least, they must be used properly to avoid damaging fabrics or even the washer or dryer. Hide or lock up such products safely. A workshop area may be full of materials that could be very dangerous. Check over the electrical equipment and power tools. Remove what you don't need and make sure that what remains is secure. Remove cutting edges from standing tools such as a band saw, jig saw, or drill press. Paints, paint thinners, and other solvents may be poisonous. Many hand tools can cause injury when used by someone whose coordination or judgment is impaired. Lock up all of these.

- **Check outside as well.** The most dangerous item outdoors is the car. There may also be other things in the garage that could pose a threat (lawn mower, snow blower, chainsaw, axe, charcoal lighter, gasoline, hedge clippers, ladder, etc.). You should carefully control the person's access to all of these. If your home has a swimming pool, you need to be aware that this poses a serious threat. Especially if the person is up and about at night while you sleep, you must be sure he or she can't get out to the pool. Fence off the pool area, and keep the gate locked.

- **Post emergency phone numbers by each phone.** Keep numbers for the doctor, fire department, and police handy. It is a good idea to call the fire station to let them know you have a person at home who might not be able to get out alone in case of a fire. In those areas using the "911" emergency call number, contact the service to inform the staff that an impaired person lives in your home. Then this information will be instantly available in any emergency. Another useful idea is an alert system. An alert system can be used to call certain numbers automatically. As the caregiver, you might carry an electronic paging type of device which will allow you to call for emergency help even if you can't use the telephone. The call may be pre-planned to go to several locations: neighbor, family members, or (in some places) the police or other emergency service. The alarm will continue to repeat its message until such time as someone turns off the system.

Managing the Daily Routine

Managing the daily routine for the impaired person involves three parts. You must simplify, you must structure, and you must supervise.

You want to simplify and structure your care routine as well as the impaired person's activities. To do this you must reduce the number of choices to be made each day by each of you. You must also keep in mind what the impaired person really can do and cannot do. And you must set up priorities for yourself. What really matters? What can you give up? You will need to be ready to compromise your standards in many cases to avoid needless conflict. But you also need to know when to stand firm (about safety issues, for instance).

Simplifying Activities

Reduce the number of choices the impaired person must make. Instead of asking "What do you want for dinner?" you might offer just two choices. If you know there really isn't any choice, don't bring up the subject. You want to allow and encourage the impaired person to make choices, but make sure the choices are within the person's powers. These powers will decline as the disease goes on. If you are aware of changes, you can adapt the choices offered.

Respect the impaired person's likes and dislikes. Be prepared to compromise. This is especially true for the events which must be done each day (eating, dressing, and grooming). If the person becomes attached to a certain plate, cup, glass, placemat, or a certain chair at the table, don't interfere. Even if what the person has chosen is the least attractive old thing you have, this is not a point worth arguing. Compromise will be easier on everyone than needless conflict. Encourage the impaired person to continue self-care as long as possible, but be realistic about the person's ability. This will save you work and help preserve the person's self-esteem. If, for instance, you see that the person has trouble cutting food and using a fork, set the person's place only with a spoon and pre-cut the food. If the person has trouble using a spoon, let the person use his or her fingers. Expect spills and messiness at mealtime. Tie a large napkin around the person's neck, or use a large bib. Use a plastic tablecloth (or a plastic cover) and paper napkins. You may even want to put a large plastic dropcloth under the person's chair. Or think about eating in a room with a vinyl floor rather than one with carpeting.

As long as the person can dress alone, encourage this. As time goes by, the task may take longer and longer. You will then need to help select clothes or remind the person of what to do next. If the person is unsteady, have him or her sit on a chair or use the bed when putting on pants and underclothes. Consider using a tub seat or bench and grab bars to assist the person in moving into the tub or on and off the toilet. Make sure the person's wardrobe suits his or her needs. Scale down the person's wardrobe. This will make choosing something to wear easier. A closet full of clothes on hangers and shelves can be more of a challenge than either of you needs. As the person becomes more and more impaired, a few changes of comfortable and easily laundered clothes are all he or she will need. Ask a friend or a family member to help you choose these, if you like. Don't forget to include the impaired person in making such choices, if possible.

Choose clothes that are practical. Comfort and ease of use are big issues. The clothes you choose should be easy to put on, shouldn't be tight, and should be easy to take off for toileting, bathing, and changing for bed. Two-piece outfits are easy to change, for instance. Consider clothes with elastic waist bands, over-sized pullovers, front closing shirts or blouses, tube socks, reversible shirts, pre-tied, clip-on ties, elastic shoe laces,or velcro fastened shoes. Footwear needs vary with the course of the illness. Running shoes offer good support and traction for the person who does a lot of pacing. If the person is less active, slip-on shoes that fit well will be easier for you when the person is less mobile. If the person prefers bedroom slippers, make sure they have good traction and don't come off easily.

Reduce and simplify grooming tasks. Consider using the shower instead of the tub for bathing. Have the person's hair cut in a way that is easy to wash and comb. If you are caring for a man who cannot shave himself, shave him with an electric razor rather than a safety razor. If you are caring for a woman, consider being less concerned about hair on the legs and underarms. If need be, use an electric razor. Trimmed but unpolished nails are quite adequate. Make-up, if used, can be quite simple. Ask family members or friends to help with some of the special grooming tasks. Have someone come in on a regular basis to give the person a shampoo or to trim the person's nails. If the expense is not too great, a local barber or beauty shop could do a regular shampoo. This combines a pleasure outing with a basic need.

Plan menus for a week or two at a time. Set up a menu pattern that you can follow over the course of a week or two and then repeat. Take into account food likes and dislikes. This may avoid struggles to get the person to eat. Your own tastes also count. Planning meals ahead will make it easier for you to come up with a shopping list. Then, if you need to, you can ask someone else to shop for you. If you are just learning how to plan and prepare meals, the limited menu is doubly helpful. You can ask family members or friends to help you set up the pattern.

Encourage the impaired person to help with household tasks when possible. Simple, repetitive tasks are best. Perhaps the impaired person can still dry dishes even if cooking is too hard. Folding laundry might take the place of doing the wash. Or perhaps raking leaves would be a form of yard work that would still be safe.

Structuring Activities

To structure the day for the impaired person and yourself, you want to come up with a schedule. This, of course, will always depend on the impaired person's abilities. As the disease progresses and these abilities decline, the schedule and what will work may change. At each stage, though, having a repeating pattern of tasks and routines can help both you and the impaired person.

You will need to observe, analyze, and organize the impaired person's activities. This task may require expert help. Consult an occupational therapist or visiting nurse for guidance. Here are some guidelines:

- Observe your days. Start by keeping track for a week or so of what you and the impaired person do on an hour-by-hour basis. Keep track of events and outcomes. What went well and what didn't? When did you feel under strain? When did the impaired person seem upset? When did you feel relaxed? When did the impaired person seem at ease? Are there times of the day when things go well and times when they don't? Are there certain activities that succeed and others that cause a fuss. Are some events such as bathing and getting out of the house happening less often than you wish? Were there any special "high spots?" Were there trouble spots? Were there times when there was little to do, and, if so, how did these times go? Did all the necessary events (eating, dressing, toileting, bathing) take place on time and with as little fuss as possible? How much help did you need to provide so that the person could safely do an activity without becoming confused or upset? For instance, could the person still bathe alone if you drew the bath water? Or could the person put on clothes alone if you selected them?

- Collect your notes and analyze them. Look for patterns. See if you already have a schedule and if it is working for you. Ask for help in examining what you have observed. Your health care team, family members or friends may be more objective. Set up a schedule. The next step is to write out a daily schedule. You must be flexible and keep in mind the impaired person's abilities and interests. The impaired person needs more time than usual to do things. Don't aim for a tight, minute-by-minute plan. Include some "free" time periods too.

- Try to reach a point where you know in advance what will happen each hour of the day. Aim for a regular pattern for each day. Regularity makes things simpler for the person for whom you provide care and for you. The person may not "learn" the pattern of activities, but he or she may be more comfortable and less often surprised in a patterned environment. A patterned day also allows you to spend less time and energy trying to figure out what to do from minute to minute. A patterned day also simplifies the process of using a substitute caregiver once in a while because you can coach that person about what to expect and what to do. Your schedule may, in fact, simply summarize what you are already doing. You might include changes that you have observed. For instance, you may note that the evenings are times when the impaired person is most likely to become upset, while the mornings seem like the calmest times. You may also see that you have often done some activity like bathing in the evening, leading to a lot of fuss. You may decide to switch that activity to the morning, keeping the evenings more calm and pleasant.

- Looking over your notes may also suggest when might be the best time to add a new activity. Try something new during the calm times. Have someone stay with the person while you leave, or try an outing with the impaired person. Try following your schedule for a week. Keep a written record of how it works and what problems arise. Then you can make changes.

- Plan ahead how you will handle those events which occur fairly often but not daily. Think about those events like doctor's visits which occur fairly often but not daily. Plan out how you will handle these too.

- Keep in mind a few "back-up plans" you can use when a planned activity doesn't seem right. You may need alternatives to scheduled activities for those times when the impaired person balks. For instance, if bath time arrives and the person is fussy, try just washing him or her with a washcloth. Offer a milkshake instead of a lunch the person dislikes. If the person won't nap, try a quiet activity instead.

- Finally, keep a written list of simple diversions you can use if you need to distract the impaired person. This is especially important when the person seems to be getting upset. Often you can draw the person out of this mood if you can offer something he or she enjoys doing. For instance, you can offer a cup of tea or coffee or a snack. You might offer to rub the person's neck or back or offer to go with the person on a walk. On your list keep track of activities the person can do (and enjoys doing) alone. This might include such things as playing solitaire, listening to music (especially old favorites), watching TV, knitting, looking through picture magazines or albums, pacing, or even doing a large, simple jigsaw puzzle.

- Add a list of activities you and the impaired person both can enjoy together. Some of these may be at home, and some may be outings. Don't automatically stop going out to public places. Some activities you might use include taking a walk, doing simple chores together, watching TV together, going to a drive-in movie, going to a local coffee shop for a doughnut, or playing simple card games. (Keep in mind that the impaired person may not remember the rules or how to play. You might have to be creative to let the person win from time to time.)

If you find that you can't think of enough things to keep the person occupied and interested, ask for suggestions from a member of your health care team, members of a support group, the director of a senior citizens program, or an activity director or recreational therapist at a nursing home. You could call them, or have someone stay with the impaired person and go visit the nursing home.

Supervising Activities

Even after you have simplified and organized everything you can, you will still need to watch over the impaired person's activities. You may even have to take over or restrict certain activities altogether. Once you have determined that an activity is no longer safe for the impaired person, or poses a threat to others, you have the responsibility and authority to restrict the person's activities, hard though it may be for the person to accept. Here are some suggestions for dealing with typical problems that may arise as the impaired person's powers decline.

- Be prepared to supervise even very personal activities. For instance, bathing alone may become too difficult or dangerous for the impaired person. You will have to take charge more and more. You will want to consider just how often the person needs to bathe. Are there changes in the routine that would help you? You may have to provide help in the form of prompting the person by telling or showing what to do. You may need to help more directly by actually washing the person. As disease progresses, the person's sensitivity to temperature declines. You will have to adjust the water so it will not burn him or her. As coordination and balance decline, you will have to judge whether the person can safely get in and out of the tub or safely stand, unsupported, in a shower. You will need to decide if special equipment like supporting bars or a shower chair might help. At some point you will need to decide if a shower or bath is worth the effort and if it is still safe. Perhaps you will want to switch to sponge baths.

- Be prepared to ban the most dangerous activities. Most experts in the care of dementia patients stress the importance of stopping the patient from driving very early in the disease. Driving is one of the most complex activities most people attempt. Accidents cause an enormous number of deaths and injuries every year. Impaired people should not drive. Other dangerous activities include working with power tools or using firearms. Smoking poses a very real fire hazard. You may want to dispose of all smoking materials. At the very least, the impaired person must be supervised constantly when smoking. Be prepared to have the impaired person resist your efforts. You may find that certain events such as bathing always upset the person. This may be a task that someone else could handle with less stress. At the very least get someone to help you so no one is injured.

- Another problem comes up when the person is still alert enough to get around any measures you may use in trying to prevent a certain activity. For instance, the person may be able to figure out how to start the car by reattaching a wire, but he or she may not have the skills to drive safely. In such a case, you must find some other way to keep the impaired person from the activity. How you do this will vary from person to person and will depend on how much the impaired person is able to understand. You may be able to explain, very simply, that the activity is no longer safe and that the person must not attempt it. You may have to deny access by locking up rooms or equipment and hiding the keys. Or you may have to enlist outside help. Have the doctor, for instance, tell the patient that a certain activity is no longer allowed. The authority of other family members, a health care expert, a police officer, or a clergy member may convince the impaired person he or she is no longer allowed to do something. Sometimes a note from the doctor stating that the person is no longer allowed to do a certain activity may work.

- Be prepared to seek help in supervising the impaired person's activities, around the clock if need be. Family and friends can help you, or you may want to look into the option of hiring help, either in your home or in a care facility. Be sure to seek help early, before you become exhausted or a crisis occurs.

Chapter 13

Older Drivers and Transportation

Older Drivers

Almost any adult with a driver's license can remember that first trip alone in the family car, feeling completely free and independent. Those same emotions complicate the decision faced daily by many older Americans. They must decide whether to keep driving or give up their car.

Maybe driving is not fun any more. Some people may not drive at night because they have trouble seeing. Others might avoid driving on interstate highways. For many older drivers, these are the first signs that driving is becoming a problem.

But, driving is necessary for many. Gone are the days when most could walk a few blocks to the grocery or doctor. Getting around is a problem for the millions of older people who live in the suburbs or rural areas. In cities there are plenty of taxis and public transportation like buses and subways. However, buses and subways may be hard for someone suffering from arthritis or using a cane. Taxis may seem to cost too much.

In 1983 one out of every 15 licensed drivers in America was over the age of 70. By 1995 this had risen to one out of every 11 drivers.

This chapter includes "Older Drivers," National Institute on Aging (NIA), 1999; "Motor Vehicle-Related Deaths Among Older Americans-NCIPC Fact Sheet," National Center for Injury Prevention and Control, 1-15-99; and "Transportation Services: Where to Get Them in Your Community," by Mark Meridy of National Eldercare Institute on Transportation, Administration on Aging (AoA), 2000.

By 2020 one out of every five Americans will be over 65 years of age, and most of them will probably be licensed to drive.

As a group, older drivers are some of the country's safest drivers. Fewer speed or drive after drinking alcohol than at any other age. However, compared to young and middle-age adults, people over 70 are more likely to be involved in a crash while driving and more likely to die in that crash. There are many reasons for this—some can be changed, but others cannot.

How Does Age Affect Driving?

As we grow older, we do not turn into bad drivers. Some of us stay good drivers. Others simply have changes in their ability to handle a car safely. These include:

- Changes in our bodies
- Changes in the way we think
- Health problems
- Medications

Changes in our bodies—As you age, your joints may stiffen, and muscles weaken. Turning your head to look back or steering and braking the car may become hard to do. Movements are slower and may not be as accurate. Your senses of smell, hearing, sight, touch, and taste might grow weaker. Vision, being able to see, is a vital part of driving, but age brings changes in the lens of the eye. Eyes need more light in order to see and are more sensitive to glare. Your ability to see things on the edge of the viewing area, peripheral vision, narrows. Vision problems include cataracts, macular degeneration, and glaucoma. In cataracts the lens of the eye becomes cloudy, causing problems with the ability to see. Macular degeneration is a breakdown of material inside the eye that leads to a loss of vision in the central part of the viewing area. The rise in pressure inside the eye that develops in glaucoma may limit the ability to see things on the edge of the viewing area.

Changes in the way you think—You probably know your body may change with age. You may not be aware of changes in the way your mind works as you age. Some of you find your reflexes are slower. Or, you may have trouble keeping your attention fixed on one situation. You may have a hard time doing two things at once—something you have to do to drive safely. When you drive, you have to take in new information from many sources and then react. Some of you react more slowly when you find yourself in a new situation.

These are all normal changes in how your brain works as you age. There are, however, two forms of mental problems that can also affect your ability to drive. Depression, being "down in the dumps" for a long time, may happen to many older people, but it is not normal. It can, and should, be treated. The attention and sleep problems depressed people of any age sometimes suffer can interfere with safe driving. So can the medicine sometimes used to treat depression. Dementia causes serious memory, personality, and behavioral problems that the person cannot recognize. Someone with dementia may at first remember how to operate an automobile and how to travel to familiar places. However, at some point as the disease progresses, their driving abilities do become impaired. Unfortunately, people with dementia often cannot recognize when they should no longer drive.

Health problems—Other illnesses common among older people can affect your ability to drive safely. For example, having arthritis, Parkinson's disease, or stroke, makes it harder to handle a car safely. Sleep problems or fainting make you less alert at an age when you may already have a hard time focusing your attention. If you have an automatic defibrillator or pacemaker, your doctor might suggest that you stop driving. There is a chance that the device might cause an irregular heartbeat or dizziness while driving. Diabetes may cause nerve damage in your hands, legs, or eyes. The eye damage in diabetes is known as diabetic retinopathy. If you also have trouble controlling your blood sugar level and might be in danger of losing consciousness, you should think about giving up your license.

Medications—Older Americans take more prescription medicines than any other age group. They often have one or more long-term illnesses such as arthritis, diabetes, high blood pressure, and heart disease and may be taking several different drugs. Their bodies may be more sensitive to the effects of medicine on their central nervous systems. The older body may not use up a drug as quickly as a younger body does, so the drug can be active in them for a longer time. Sometimes a combination of medicines increases the effects of each drug on the body.

Several types of medication can make driving harder because they affect the central nervous system. Drugs that might interfere with your driving include sleep aids, medicine to treat depression, antihistamines for allergies and colds, strong painkillers, and diabetes medications.

If you are taking one or more of them, talk to your doctor. Perhaps he or she could change your prescription, or help you decide if the medicine is affecting your driving.

Can I Be a Better Driver?

Perhaps you already know some driving situations that are hard— night, highways, rush hour, and bad weather. You might avoid these types of driving and limit your trips to shopping and visits to the doctor. This lowers your chance of having an accident.

While driving, older drivers are most at risk while yielding right of way, turning, especially left turns, lane changing, passing, and using expressway ramps. Pay extra attention at those times. If there is not a left-turn light, look for alternate routes that do provide such lights.

Most of the advice for older drivers is helpful for all drivers. Plan your trips ahead of time. Stick to streets you know. Don't drive under stress. Keep distractions such as the fan, radio, or talking, to a minimum. Leave a big space between your car and the one in front of you. Don't drive when you are tired.

Think about taking a driving refresher class. Some car insurance companies reduce your payment if you pass such a class. The AARP (American Association of Retired Persons) sponsors "55 ALIVE/Mature Driving." Call 1-888-227-7669 (1-888-AARP NOW) for details about courses in your area. The AAA (American Automobile Association) has a similar class called "Safe Driving for Mature Operators." Contact your local AAA's office for class information. These are 8-hour classroom courses that talk about the aging process and help drivers adjust. You might also check with a local private driving school. Ask if they have an instructor who teaches older drivers. You might want to take such a review every few years.

Certain features on your car can make driving easier. Power steering, power brakes, automatic transmission, and larger mirrors are all helpful. Keeping the headlights on at all times and having a light-colored car helps other drivers see you. Hand controls for the accelerator and brakes might be of use to someone with leg problems. Keep the headlights clean and aligned, and check the windshield wiper blades often. A rear-window defroster is a good way to keep that window clear at all times.

Air bags have saved many lives. Advanced age is not a reason for disconnecting an air bag. However, the National Highway Traffic Safety Administration suggests that air bags may not be as effective in preventing serious injury or death in people over 70 years of age as they are in younger people. Older people are more likely to be injured in a traffic accident. Their bones and blood vessels may be rigid. They might break easily. If the accident is minor, emergency personnel may not realize the possibility of internal bleeding in time. People of any age should push their seats as far back as possible from the air bags in both the steering wheel and the passenger side. Of course, everyone in the car should always wear a seat belt.

Should I Stop Driving?

What if you are doing all you can to be a safe driver and still wonder if you should stop driving. This is a difficult decision. There are questions to ask yourself. Do other drivers often honk at you? Have you had some accidents, even "fender benders?" Are you getting lost, even on well-known roads? Do cars or pedestrians seem to appear out of nowhere? Have family, friends, or your doctor said they were worried about your driving? Do you drive less because you are not as confident about your ability as you once were? If you answered yes to any of these, you probably should think seriously about whether or not you are still a safe driver.

There are books that may help you make this decision. Single copies of the AARP guide, "The Older Driver Skill Assessment and Resource Guide: Creating Mobility Choices," are available free by writing AARP Fulfillment, 601 E Street, NW, Washington, DC 20049, and asking for publication D14957. The AAA Foundation for Traffic Safety has videos and books, including "Drivers 55-Plus: Test Your Own Performance" and "Guide for Families or Friends Concerned About an Older Driver," that may be ordered by calling 1-800-305-SAFE. Some, but not all, are free. See Resources at the end of this chapter for the telephone numbers and addresses.

There are currently no upper age limits for driving. Because people age at different rates, it is not possible to choose one age as the limit. Setting an age limit would leave some drivers on the road too long, while others would be stopped too soon. Heredity, general health, your way of life, and surroundings all influence how you age.

The hard question is whether older drivers should be tested differently and more often. A second question is what would those tests be. The usual road and written tests do not look at the problem areas for older drivers. The useful-field-of-view test is being studied as one possibility. This looks at the amount of viewing area in which someone can absorb information from two different sources and how quickly they respond to it. This area becomes smaller as we age. The smaller the area, the more likely one is to crash. Fortunately, this is a problem that can be improved by training. A doctor who could then certify the driver to the Department of Motor Vehicles would best perform this test.

The Mini Mental Status Exam is also a possible test used to decide if a person is no longer able to drive. This test looks at your ability to perform certain mental tasks. These tasks test those mental skills involved in driving, although they might seem different. You might be asked to copy a particular design or to count backwards from 100 by sevens. Like the useful-field-of-view test, this is not now used for testing drivers.

The aim of these tests is not to get every older driver off the road. Instead, if problem drivers can be identified, some of them could then receive training to improve their driving skills. Unfortunately, others cannot be helped by training and will have to stop driving.

How Will I Get Around?

When planning for retirement, you should think about how you'd get around if you were no longer able to drive. Some communities provide low-cost bus or taxi service for older people. Some offer carpools or transportation on request. Religious groups sometimes have volunteers who take seniors where they need to go.

If such services are not available in your community, taxis may seem too expensive to use often. Remember that you won't have a car to maintain any longer. In fact, the AAA estimates that the cost of owning and running the average car is over $6,500 a year. By giving up your car, you might have as much as $125 a week that could be used for taxis, public transportation, or buying gas for friends and relatives who can drive you places.

Motor Vehicle-Related Deaths among Older Americans

How Large Is the Problem of Motor Vehicle-Related Deaths among Older Americans?

- In 1996, 7,078 people aged 65 years or older died of injuries sustained in motor vehicle crashes.[1] Of those who died, 80% were occupants of motor vehicles and 17% were pedestrians.

- For people 65-84 years old, death rates due to motor vehicle crashes are about 1.7 times higher for men than for women. For those older than 85 years, the rate for men is about three times the rate for women.[2]

- During the past decade, the number of licensed drivers aged 70 years or older has increased by nearly 50%.[3] As the U.S. population ages, that number will continue to increase.

Are Motor Vehicle-Related Death Rates for Older People Higher Than Those for Other Age Groups?

- Motor vehicle-related death rates per 100,000 are higher for people 70 years old or older than for people in any other group except those younger than 25 years.[1]

- Per mile driven, drivers 75 years old or older have higher rates of motor vehicle crashes that result in someone's death than do drivers in all other age groups except teenagers.[1]

What Factors Contribute to Older People's High Rate of Death Due to Motor Vehicle Crashes?

- Age-related declines in sensory (e.g., vision or hearing) and cognitive functions, and physical impairments due to medical conditions may affect some older people's driving ability.[4]

- Older people who are injured in motor vehicle crashes are more likely to die of their injuries than are people in other age groups.[1]

- About half of fatal crashes involving drivers 80 years old or older occur at intersections and involve more than one vehicle.[1]

What Are Older Drivers Doing to Reduce Their Risk of Injury Due to Motor Vehicle Crashes?

- As a group, adults aged 70 years or older wear safety belts more often than does any other age group except infants and preschool children.[5]

- Older drivers tend to drive when conditions are safest.[6] They limit their driving during bad weather and at night, and they drive fewer miles than younger drivers do.

- Older drivers are less likely to drink and drive.[7] In 1996, drivers younger than 70 years old who died in motor vehicle crashes were five times more likely than those 70 years old or older to be intoxicated (blood alcohol concentration of at least 0.10 grams per deciliter).[2]

Do Older Drivers Pose More of a Risk for Injury to Others on the Road Than Younger Drivers Do?

- A study of crashes involving older drivers in Wisconsin found that drivers 65-74 years old did not pose a greater risk of serious injury or death for others than younger drivers did.[8] For drivers aged 75-84, the results were inconclusive.

What Are Our National Objectives with Regard to Older Persons Dying in Motor Vehicle Crashes?

- By year 2000, the Public Health Service aims to reduce motor vehicle-related deaths among people aged 70 years old or older to no more than 20 per 100,000 people.[9] The rate has remained stable at about 23 per 100,000 for more than a decade.[9]

What Measures May Help to Reduce the Rates of Motor Vehicle-Related Deaths for Older People?

Some measures that could benefit older people as well as most other age groups include:

- Improvements in automobile design that simplify driving and increase crash protection. Examples include reduced-glare headlights, improved head restraints, knee bars, and side-interior padding to protect occupants in side-impact crashes.[10]

- Improvements in road design. Examples include wider lanes and shoulders, more one-way roads, better lighting, bigger and brighter signs, and lower speed limits where complex maneuvers are required.[10]

- Increased use of public transportation. This could improve mobility of older people while reducing their necessity to drive.[10]

- Restricted driving privileges when circumstances warrant. For example, some states can restrict driving to a particular time of day, geographic location, or road type.[11] Several states have reduced the length of the license term for older drivers from the usual 4 years to 2 or 3 years.[11]

- Physician reporting. Most states already require that physicians report to the state's licensing agency cases of certain medical conditions that could affect a person's ability to drive.[11]

References

1. Insurance Institute for Highway Safety (IIHS). Facts, 1996 Fatalities: Elderly. Arlington (VA): IIHS; 1997.

2. National Center for Health Statistics. Health, United States, 1996-97. Hyattsville (MD): CDC; 1997. DHHS publication no. (PHS) 97-1232.

3. National Highway Traffic Safety Administration (NHTSA). *Traffic Safety Facts 1996: Older Population*. Washington (DC): NHTSA; 1997.

4. Janke Mk. *Age-Related Disabilities That May Impair Driving and Their Assessment*: Literature Review. Sacramento (CA): California Department of Motor Vehicles; 1994. Report no. RSS-94-156.

5. National Highway Traffic Safety Administration (NHTSA). National Occupant Protection Use Survey 1996. Research Note, Aug 1997. Washington (DC): NHTSA; 1997.

6. Committee for the Study of Improving Mobility and Safety for Older Persons. *Transportation in an Aging Society. Special Report 218, vol 1*. Washington (DC): Transportation Research Board; 1988.

7. Liu S, Siegel PZ, Brewer RD, et al. Prevalence of alcohol-impaired driving. *JAMA* 1997;277:122-5.

8. Dulisse B. Older drivers and risk to other road users. *Accid Anal Prev* 1997;29:573-82.

9. Public Health Service (PHS). Healthy People 2000: Review 1995-96. Washington (DC): PHS, 1996. DHHS publication no. (PHS) 96-1256.

10. Fildes BN, Lee SJ, Kenny D, et al. *Survey of Older Road Users: Behavioral and Travel Issues*. Victoria, Australia: Monash University Accident Research Centre; 1994. Report no. 57.

11. Anapolle J. *Survey of Licensing Procedures for Older, Physically Impaired and / or Mentally Impaired Drivers.* Boston: Registry of Motor Vehicles, Commonwealth of Massachusetts; 1992. Publication No. 17271.

Transportation Services: Where to Get Them in Your Community

Transportation is the critical link that assures access to vital services such as health care and going to the grocery store. The availability of adequate transportation allows older Americans to live independently in their communities and helps prevent isolation and premature institutionalization. For many older people who do not drive an automobile, family and friends provide much of the transportation. However for others, community transportation is the only connection to the outside world.

Where Can I Find Transportation Services in My Community?

The Local Area Agency on Aging or Title VI Program: There are 670 Area Agencies on Aging nationwide. Area Agencies on Aging have an Information and Assistance service providing older persons and their caregivers with specific information about services in the community, including transportation services. These local agencies, monitor and support specialized transportation services for elders in their community. It is also the role of the Area Agencies on Aging to ensure that services are delivered to the older person in need.

There are also 221 programs nationwide that administer Title VI of the Older Americans Act. The Title VI program promotes nutrition and supportive services, such as transportation, to American Indian, Alaskan Natives, and Native Hawaiians. The Title VI Program also has an Information and Assistance service which provides specific information about services in the community.

To contact your local Area Agency on Aging or Title VI Program, refer to the telephone directory in the Blue Pages or government listings and/or in the Yellow Pages under aging, senior citizens, community services, or social services.

If you have difficulty locating your local Area Agency on Aging, call the Eldercare Locator: toll-free at 1-800-677-1116. The Eldercare Locator is a nationwide service to help families and friends find information about community services for older people. The Eldercare

Locator provides access to an extensive network of organizations serving older people at state and local community levels.

The Yellow Pages of the Telephone Book: The Yellow Pages of many telephone books have a special section in the front of the book with the names and addresses of various service organizations. Look under transportation or community services for the names of agencies that provide transportation for special needs.

The National Transit Hotline: The National Transit Hotline can provide the names of local transit providers who receive federal money to provide transportation to the elderly and people with disabilities. Call toll-free 1-800-527-8279.

The State Unit on Aging: The State Unit on Aging is the agency designated by the governor and the state legislature as the focal point for all matters relating to the needs of older persons within the state. The State Unit on Aging is responsible for planning, coordination, funding, and evaluating programs for older persons authorized by both state and federal government. Refer to your state government listings for your state's office on aging or department of human resources.

What Type of Transportation Is Available in My Community?

The type of transportation that is available in your community will vary depending upon where you live. In addition, transportation for the elderly can include door-to-door service, the public bus that travels along a fixed route, or ridesharing in a carpool. The following briefly describes these three general classes of transportation for older Americans.

Door-to-Door/Demand Response: Demand response, also called Dial-a-Ride, refers to a system requiring advance reservations and offering point-to-point or door-to-door transportation from one specific location to another. The door-to-door service provides flexibility, comfort, and potential for adapting to the needs of each rider. Demand response transportation systems usually provide transportation on an advance reservation basis, often requiring payment of fare or donations on a per ride basis.

Fixed Route: Fixed route and scheduled services transport riders along an established route with designated stops where riders can board and be dropped off. Reservations are not required because the vehicles stop at predetermined times and locations. Fixed route services usually require payment of a fare on a per ride basis. Many communities offer discounts to senior citizens.

Ridesharing: Ridesharing programs coordinate people who need rides with volunteer drivers who have space in their automobiles. Typically, this service is scheduled transportation with a specific destination. The destination points can include places of employment, nutrition sites, senior centers, and medical appointments.

Conclusion

A good place to start your search for transportation is your local Area Agency on Aging. Area Agencies on Aging monitor and support specialized transportation services for elders in the community. Although the agency may not provide transportation services directly, its Information and Assistance Service should provide you with information as to where to find transportation.

Resources

American Association of Retired Persons
601 E Street, N.W.
Washington, DC 20049
Toll-Free: 800-424-3410
Tel: 202-434-2277
Website: http://www.aarp.org
E-mail: member@aarp.org

American Automobile Association
1000 AAA Drive
Heathrow, FL 32746-5063
Tel: 407-444-4240
Fax: 407-444-4247
Website: http://www.aaa.com

AAA Foundation for Traffic Safety
1440 New York Avenue, N.W., Suite 201
Washington, DC 20005
Tel: 202-638-5944
Fax: 202-638-5943
Website: http://www.aaafts.org

National Association of Area Agencies on Aging
927 Fifteenth Street, N.W., Sixth Floor
Washington, DC 20005
Tel: 202-296-8130
Fax: 202-296-8134
Website: http://www.n4a.org

National Association of State Units on Aging
1225 I Street, N.W., Suite 725
Washington, DC 20005
Tel: 202-898-2578
Eldercare Locator: 800-677-1116
Fax: 202-898-2583
Website: http://www.nausa.org

The National Institute on Aging (NIA) offers free information on health and aging. For a complete list of publications write or call:

NIA Information Center
P.O. Box 8057
Gaithersburg, MD 20898-8057
Toll-Free: 800-222-2225
TTY: 800-222-4225
Website: http://www.nih.gov/nia/

National Center for Injury Prevention and Control
Division of Unintentional Injury Prevention
Mailstop K59
4770 Buford Highway N.E.
Atlanta, GA 30341-3724
Tel: 770-488-4656
Fax: 770-488-1665
Website: http://www.cdc.gov/ncipc/osp/data.htm

Chapter 14

Evaluating Caregiver Stress

While caregiving can be very satisfying, especially when it is an expression of love and care for someone important to you, it can also be psychologically and physically draining. When demands become overwhelming, your energy, good humor, and coping capacity are taxed.

This can make you feel very stressed out. The stresses you face probably vary from day to day because your caregiving responsibilities shift according to your family member's health and your own energy level.

Maybe you aren't even aware of how much you are doing. To figure out your caregiving tasks, take a minute to complete this list of activities.

Check which of the following kinds of caregiving you currently provide:

__ Household management (cooking, shopping, cleaning, house-keeping)

__ Transportation

__ Personal care (bathing, grooming, toileting)

Reprinted with permission "Why Is Caregiving Often Stressful?" *North Carolina Caregiver's Handbook* pp. 7-12, © North Carolina Department of Health and Human Services, Division of Aging, 1997-1998.

__ Medical care (help with taking medications, applying dressings)

__ Emotional support and companionship

__ Supervision for safety

__ Financial management and decision-making assistance

__ Coordination and management of care provided by others

__ Other (list) _____

Did the number of items you checked surprise you?

Managing stress requires balancing the demands in your life with the resources that can help you cope. Learn to recognize, anticipate and offset the demands and stresses in your life with positive self-esteem, coping skills and adequate social support. This means taking care of yourself as well as spending time and energy with the person(s) for whom you are caring.

Taking care of her father helped Nan Harris learn more about her own strengths and limitations. "From the time I was in grammar school I've taken care of people—my brothers and sisters, nieces and nephews. It's very easy for me to give and give and with Dad I've had to learn to say no," she said. Part of that process happened when she was hospitalized twice for exhaustion last year.

How Am I Doing?

Caring for your older relative or coordinating services for them through community agencies can be overwhelming. Feelings of frustration, depression, anger, or guilt are not uncommon. Many caregivers decide to join a support group to provide emotional comfort. These groups allow people to share feelings and information helping to relieve stress, resentment, and anxiety. Others seek help from their clergy or call their local agency on aging for assistance. Others get their informal support system, such as friends, neighbors and community groups, to work more effectively for them and their older relative.

The questionnaire in Table 14.1 will help you to become more aware of the stresses that you may be under. For each statement, check the column that expresses your situation.

If the response to one or more of these statements is "describes me," it may be time to begin looking for help with caring for your older relative and help in taking care of yourself.

Signs of Too Much Stress

Physical: headache, muscle aches, sleeping and eating problems, getting sick frequently.

Emotional: guilt, anger, loneliness, depression, and anxiety.

Mental: forgetfulness, difficulty making decisions, attention wandering.

Interpersonal: withdrawal, blaming, irritability, impatience, and sensitivity to criticism.

Spiritual: feelings of alienation, loss of hope, purpose, and meaning.

What caregivers need most, say professionals, is a clear sense of their own limits as caregivers.

Table 14.1. Stress Questionnaire

Statement	"Describes me"	"Does not describe me"
I find I can't get enough rest.	_____	_____
I don't have time for myself.	_____	_____
I feel frustrated or angry.	_____	_____
I feel guilty about my situation.	_____	_____
I don't get out much anymore.	_____	_____
I argue with the person I am caring for.	_____	_____
I argue with other family members.	_____	_____
I don't feel I know enough to be an effective caregiver.	_____	_____

You May Want to Try To

- Talk openly with your aging relative and other family members.

- Assess the problems.

- Figure out where to get help.

- Decide how much help you can realistically supply.

Signs of Successful Caregiving

1. Caring for yourself is a priority.

2. Know and respect your limits.

3. Arrange for time for yourself (to be alone).

4. Arrange for time with a spouse, other family, and friends.

5. Give yourself credit for things you do well.

6. Caregiving can be a partnership in which you share responsibilities with others.

All that sounds pretty straightforward, like a good business plan, but it's not always simple.

How to Manage Stress?

Fortunately there are some things that you can do to help manage caregiving stresses.

First Step of Stress Management

Reflect on how you spend your time each day. Imagine a "typical" day. Ask yourself, "How much time do I spend?" (estimate the number or hours each day) [see Table 14.2].

Now that you have sketched out how you spend your time, you can determine how much time you have for yourself and how much time you have with friends or other family members.

Nan Harris felt guilty about asking someone to stay with her father while she did errands but she couldn't find time to go food shopping or keep her own doctors' appointments. Even more troubling, she realized that the only person she was regularly talking to was her sister. Somehow, the challenges of arranging care for dad had taken a priority over keeping up with friends and her own interests.

Second Step of Stress Management

Arrange for a substitute caregiver for short periods of time so that you can get some time away from your caregiving responsibilities.

Nan called her Area Agency on Aging for information about eldercare services in her county. She was fortunate because there was a respite program near her which provides trained volunteers to act as substitute caregivers for short (2-4 hours) periods of time once a week. Nan later related that the "time I spent alone revitalized and recharged me."

Listening to music, reading, taking walks and other forms of exercise, can help you to better handle the stresses you may experience during the day. Taking care of personal business also can help you feel more in control of daily pressures. While most caregivers feel that they can, should, or must provide all the care to their family member, carrying the total burden is not helpful and probably impossible in the long run.

Table 14.2. Typical Daily Activities

Activity	Amount of Time Spent
Eating	_____
Sleeping	_____
Giving care to an older person	_____
Taking part in family activities	_____
Working at my job	_____
Activities with friends & neighbors	_____
Spiritual activities	_____
Being alone	_____
Other	_____
Total Hours	_____

Third Step of Stress Management

Ask for other assistance from family, friends, churches, in-home aide services, and community agencies. Before you dismiss the idea of seeking help consider these three points:

1. Additional help allows you to be a more effective caregiver by giving you time away from the person you are caring for.

2. Your spouse or older relative benefits by seeing and being with someone other than you.

3. Community-based services often allow the older family member to postpone using a nursing home by providing the more difficult and/or skilled care that is needed and can be provided in the home.

Chapter 15

Planning for Long-Term Care

"Long-term care" means helping people of any age with their medical needs or daily activities over a long period of time. Long-term care can be provided at home, in the community, or in various types of facilities. This chapter deals mainly with older people who need long-term care. However, the information also may be useful for younger people with disabilities or illnesses that require long-term care.

When you look for long-term care, it is important to remember that quality varies from one place or caregiver to another. It is also important to think about long-term care before a crisis occurs. Making long-term care decisions can be hard even when planned well in advance.

Quick Check for Quality

Look for long-term care that:

- Has been found by State agencies, accreditors, or others to provide quality care.

- Has the services you need.

- Has staff that meet your needs.

- Meets your budget.

"Choosing Long-Term Care," Agency for Healthcare Research, and Quality, AHRQ Pub. No. 99-0012, December 1998, reviewed July 1999.

Research shows that to make the best choices, you need to think about:

- What your options are.

- Whether they meet your or your family member's needs (physical, medical, emotional, financial, etc.).

- How to find the highest quality care.

Types of Long-Term Care

Research shows that many people do not know about or understand long-term care options. Following are brief descriptions of the major types of long-term care:

Home care can be given in your own home by family members, friends, volunteers, and/or paid professionals. This type of care can range from help with shopping to nursing care. Some short-term, skilled home care (provided by a nurse or therapist) is covered by Medicare and is called "home health care." Another type of care that can be given at home is hospice care for terminally ill people.

Community services are support services that can include adult day care, meal programs, senior centers, transportation, and other services. These can help people who are cared for at home—and their families. For example, adult day care services provide a variety of health, social, and related support services in a protective setting during the day. This can help adults with impairments—such as Alzheimer's disease—continue to live in the community. And it can give family or friend caregivers a needed "break."

Supportive housing programs offer low-cost housing to older people with low to moderate incomes. The Federal Department of Housing and Urban Development (HUD) and State or local governments often develop such housing programs. A number of these facilities offer help with meals and tasks such as housekeeping, shopping, and laundry. Residents generally live in their own apartments.

Assisted living provides 24-hour supervision, assistance, meals, and health care services in a home-like setting. Services include help with eating, bathing, dressing, toileting, taking medicine, transportation, laundry, and housekeeping. Social and recreational activities also are provided.

Continuing care retirement communities (CCRCs) provide a full range of services and care based on what each resident needs over time. Care usually is provided in one of three main stages: independent living, assisted living, and skilled nursing.

Nursing homes offer care to people who cannot be cared for at home or in the community. They provide skilled nursing care, rehabilitation services, meals, activities, help with daily living, and supervision. Many nursing homes also offer temporary or periodic care. This can be instead of hospital care, after hospital care, or to give family or friend caregivers some time off ("respite care").

Another type of long-term care takes place in home-like settings called **Intermediate Care Facilities for the Mentally Retarded.** They provide a wide variety of services to mentally retarded and developmentally disabled people from youth to old age. Services include treatment to help residents become as independent as possible, as well as health care services.

You can learn about long-term care options in your area by contacting:

- The Eldercare Locator (1-800-677-1116, weekdays, 9.00 a.m. to 8.00 p.m., EST). This service can refer you to your Area Agency on Aging.

- Area Agencies on Aging provide information on a wide variety of community-based services. Examples are meals, home care, adult day care, transportation, housing, home repair, and legal services.

- Your State or local Long-Term Care Ombudsman (call the Eldercare Locator for the number). Ombudsmen visit nursing homes and other long-term care facilities to check on and resolve complaints, protect residents' rights, and give emotional support to lonely older people. A call to your area Ombudsman can give you information on: the most recent State survey (inspection) report of the facility; the number of outstanding complaints; the number and nature of complaints lodged in the last year; and the results of recent complaint investigations.

- "Nursing Home Compare" at http://www.medicare.gov/Nursing/ Overview.asp—a Website created by the Health Care Financing Administration, which runs Medicare and Medicaid. This site helps you locate nursing homes in your area. It also has inspection records for nursing homes that receive Medicare or Medicaid funds.

- Hospital discharge planners.

- Social workers (some can be "case managers" or "care managers," who can help you coordinate long-term care services).

- Doctors and other health care professionals.

- Local nursing facilities.

- Volunteer groups that work with older people.

- Clergy or religious groups.

- Family and friends.

There are three important questions to ask yourself when deciding about long-term care for yourself or a loved one:

1. What kind of services do I need?

2. How will I pay for these services?

3. How can I choose the best quality services?

What Kind of Services Do I Need?

Think of long-term care as a menu of services. A person may need only one or a few kinds of services. Or, several kinds may be needed over the course of a person's older years. To help find out what kind of services you or a loved one need, check the items below that apply. Keep in mind that these needs may change over time.

Do you or your loved one need help with daily activities? Health care needs? Both? You can use the following chart to help you identify the type(s) of long-term care that meet your needs. This chart shows which types of long-term care services offer which kinds of help. The "Relative Costs" information shows how costly the settings can be when compared with each other.

Help with Daily Activities

____ Shopping

____ Preparing meals

___ Eating

___ Laundry and other housework

___ Home maintenance

___ Paying bills and other money matters

___ Bathing

___ Dressing

___ Grooming

___ Going to the bathroom

___ Remembering to take medicines

___ Walking

___ Other _____

___ Other _____

*Health Care Needs**

___ Physical therapy

___ Speech therapy

___ Occupational therapy

___ Rehabilitation

___ Medical nutritional therapy

___ Oxygen

___ Care for pressure ulcers or other wounds

___ Alzheimer's disease care

___ Health monitoring (for diabetes, for example)

___ Pain management

___ Nursing care services

___ Other medical services provided by a doctor or other clinician

___ Other _____

*as recommended by a doctor or other health care provider.

How Will I Pay for These Services?

Long-term care can be very expensive. In general, health plans and programs do not routinely cover long-term care at home or in nursing homes. Here is some general information about long-term care coverage:

- **Medicare** is the Federal health insurance program for people age 65 and older and for some disabled younger people. Medicare generally does not pay for long-term help with daily activities. Medicare pays for very limited skilled nursing home care after a hospital stay. If you need skilled care in your home for the treatment of an illness or injury, and you meet certain conditions, Medicare will pay for some of the costs of nursing care, home health aide services, and different types of therapy.

- **Medicaid** is a Federal-State program that pays for health services and long-term care for low-income people of any age. The exact rules for who is covered vary by State. Medicaid covers nursing home care for people who are eligible. In some States, Medicaid also pays for some home and community services.

Table 15.1. Relative Costs Comparison.

	Home Care	Community Services	Supportive Housing Programs	Assisted Living	CCRC*	Nursing Homes
Help with daily activities	X	X	X	X	X	X
Help with health care needs	X				X	X
Relative Costs	Low to High	Low to Medium	Low to Medium	Medium to High	High	High

*Continuing Care Retirement Communities

252

- **Private Insurance**. Medicare beneficiaries may supplement their policy with insurance purchased from private organizations. Most of these policies—often called **Medigap** insurance or by a similar name—will help pay for some skilled care, but only when that care is covered by Medicare. Medigap is not long-term care insurance. Commercial insurers offer private policies called long-term care insurance. These policies may cover services such as care at home, in adult day care, in assisted living facilities, and in nursing homes. But plans vary widely. If you have such a policy, ask your insurer what it covers. If you think you may need long-term care insurance, start shopping while you are relatively young and healthy, and shop carefully.

- **Personal Resources**. You may need to use resources such as savings or life insurance to pay for long-term care. Most people who enter nursing homes begin by paying out of their own pockets. As their personal resources are spent, many people who stay in nursing homes for a long time eventually become eligible for Medicaid.

Your State Health Insurance Program (SHIP) can give you general information about Medicare, Medicaid, managed care plans, and the types of health insurance that can supplement Medicare, including Medigap and long-term care insurance. Counselors also can help you with questions about your medical bills, insurance claims, and related matters. These services are free. To find the phone number of the SHIP office in your State, call the Medicare Hotline at 1-800-638-6833. Or, look at the consumer Website for Medicare services, http://www.medicare.gov.

How Can I Choose the Best Quality Services?

Here are some tips for choosing the kinds of long-term care people most often use: home care (including home health care) and nursing homes.

Home Care

- In many States, home care agencies must be licensed. Check with your State health department to see if your State requires it. If so, be wary if an agency is not licensed.

- Ask if the agency is certified by Medicare. Medicare inspects home health care agencies to assure they meet certain Federal health and safety requirements. Medicare will pay for services only if the agency is Medicare-approved and if the services are covered by Medicare.

- If the home health care agency is certified by Medicare, you can review its survey report. Call the Medicare Hotline at 1-800-638-6833 and ask to be referred to the Home Health Hotline for your State. You can request a copy of the report from that hotline.

- Find out if the agency has been accredited (awarded a "seal of approval") by a group such as the Joint Commission on Accreditation of Healthcare Organizations (630-792-5800); http://www.jcaho.org) or the Community Health Accreditation Program (800-669-1656; http://www.chapinc.org).

- Contact your State or local consumer affairs office to see if any complaints have been filed against a home care agency. Also ask about the outcome of any complaint investigations.

- Whether you work with an agency or hire someone yourself, carefully check the backgrounds of the people who will be coming into your home. Ask for references who have worked with the agency or person. Call them, and ask about their experiences. Would they use the agency or person again?

- Does the home care worker have the necessary skills and training for your needs? Ask to see training certificates. Make sure the worker knows how to safely assist and care for patients.

- Does the agency have supervisors who check on the quality of care its workers provide?

- How does the agency follow up on and resolve complaints?

Nursing Home Care

- All nursing homes that participate in Medicare or Medicaid are visited about once a year by a team of trained inspectors. They check the home and the care provided and prepare a survey report. You have a right to review the report, which must be posted in the nursing home. Speak to the nursing home administrator to learn more about any problems that appear on the report. Ask if the problems have been corrected.

- Call your State or local Long-Term Care Ombudsman. Ombudsmen visit nursing homes on a regular basis and know about each nursing home in their area. You can ask about the latest survey report and about complaints that have been filed. You can also ask what to look for when visiting local nursing homes.

- Compare the inspection records of your top choices by visiting the "Nursing Home Compare" Website: http://www.medicare.gov/nhCompare/home.asp.

- Some nursing homes have been accredited by a national group such as the Joint Commission on Accreditation of Health care Organizations (630-792-5800). It may be helpful to find out if the home participates in this voluntary process and to learn the results.

- Location is very important. Is the nursing home close enough so that family and friends can visit? Close enough for the resident's personal doctor to visit?

- The most important step is to visit—more than once-and look around. Go at different times of the day—for example, first thing in the morning and at mealtimes.

- Do residents seem to enjoy meals? Is there help for those who cannot eat on their own? If possible, eat a meal at the facility.

- Is the home clean and free of odors? Is it pleasant?

- Are residents clean, well groomed, and dressed appropriately for the season and time of day? Are they involved in activities?

- Are staff friendly, helpful, and respectful?

- Talk to staff, residents, and families to find out what they think of the facility.

- Ask to see the area where physical therapy and other rehabilitation services are provided.

- Is the nursing home experienced with special needs—for example, problems with swallowing?

- Who provides the medical care?

- Which hospital(s) does the nursing home use?

Sources of Additional Information

Medicare
Toll-Free: 800-638-6833
Website: http://www.medicare.gov/Publications/Overview.asp

Offers "A Guide to Choosing a Nursing Home," that has sections on gathering information, visiting nursing homes, and residents' rights and quality of life. Includes phone lists for State ombudsmen, State survey agencies, and insurance counseling. 18 pages. Free.

Administration on Aging and National Institute on Aging
Resource Directory for Older People
Website: http://www.aoa.gov/aoa/resource.html

The Administration on Aging and National Institute on Aging offers lists of hundreds of organizations, names, and phone numbers, including State agencies on aging and State long-term care ombudsmen programs. Not available in print.

American Association of Homes and Services for the Aging
Website: http://www.aahsa.org

Offers a series of pamphlets on nursing homes, assisted living, continuing care retirement communities, community services, housing options for older people, and understanding Medicare managed care. Free.

National Association for Home Care
228 Seventh Street, SE
Washington, DC 20003
Tel: 202-547-7424
Fax: 202-547-3540
Website: http://www.nahc.org

Offers "How to Choose a Home Care Provider." Explains who provides what kind of care, the various services offered, who pays for services. Has billing and payment information. Lists patients' rights, accrediting agencies, and State resources and information. Free.

The American Health Care Association
1201 L St., NW
Washington, DC 20005-4014
Tel: 202-842-4444
Website: http://www.ahca.org

Offers for free a series of pamphlets on selecting and paying for long-term care: "Myths and Realities of Living in a Nursing Home," "How to Pay for Nursing Home Care," "What Consumers Need to Know about Private Long-Term Care," and "Circle of Care."

The American Association of Retired Persons
601 E. St., N.W.
Washington, DC 20049
Toll-Free: 800-424-3410
Website: http://www.aarp.org
E-mail: member@aarp.org

"Nursing Home Life: A Guide for Residents and Families," includes first-hand accounts from residents and family members. Topics include adjusting to nursing home life; services and staff; getting what you need; and dealing with poor care. Has useful appendices and resource lists. 44 pages. Free.

Chapter 16

Abuse and Neglect Prevention

What Is Elder Abuse?

There are three basic categories of elder abuse: domestic, institutional, and self-neglect. Domestic elder abuse refers to maltreatment of an older person residing in his/her own home or the home of a caregiver. Institutional abuse refers to the maltreatment of an older person residing in a residential facility for older persons, e.g., a nursing home, board and care home, foster home, or group home. Self-neglect refers to the conduct of an older person living alone which threatens his/her own health or safety.

The four common kinds of elder abuse are:

- **physical abuse**, the infliction of physical pain or injury, e.g., slapping, bruising, sexually molesting, restraining;

- **psychological abuse**, the infliction of mental anguish, e.g., humiliating, intimidating, threatening;

- **financial abuse**, the improper or illegal use of the resources of an older person, without his/her consent, for someone else's benefit; and

---

This chapter contains text from the following Administration on Aging documents: "Elder Abuse Prevention," Fact Sheet; "Conclusions of the National Elder Abuse Incidence Study," 1998; and excerpts from "The National Elder Abuse Incidence Study Final Report," September 1998.

259

- **neglect**, failure to fulfill a caretaking obligation to provide goods or services, e.g., abandonment, denial of food or health-related services.

Service Delivery

State legislatures in all 50 states have passed some form of legislation (e.g., elder abuse, adult protective services, domestic violence laws, mental health commitment laws) that authorizes the state to protect and provide services to vulnerable, incapacitated, or disabled adults.

In more than three-quarters of the states, the services are provided through the state social service department (adult protective services). In the remaining states, the State Units on Aging have the major responsibility. Agencies receive and screen calls for potential seriousness. Some states operate hotlines 24 hours a day, 7 days a week. The agency keeps information received in reports of suspected abuse confidential. If mistreatment is suspected, an investigation is conducted (in cases of an emergency, usually within 24 hours). On the basis of a comprehensive assessment, a care plan is developed which might involve, for example, obtaining a medical assessment of the victim; admitting the victim to the hospital; assisting the victim in obtaining needed food, heat, or medication; arranging for home health care or housekeeping services; calling the police; or referring the case to the prosecuting attorney.

Once the immediate situation has been addressed, the adult protective services agency (APS) continues to monitor the victim's situation and works with other community agencies, serving the elderly, to provide ongoing case management and service delivery. The older person has the right to refuse services offered by APS, unless he or she has been declared incapacitated by the court and a guardian has been appointed.

Where to Go for Help

If, as a concerned citizen or a practicing professional serving the elderly, you suspect that abuse has occurred or is occurring to an older person whom you know, report your suspicions to the local APS agency. In most states, certain professionals are mandated to report abuse. If the suspected incident involves an older person living in an institutional setting, call the office of the local long-term care (LTC) ombudsman.

You can find the telephone number for the APS office by calling directory assistance and requesting the number for the department of social services or aging services. To reach a LTC ombudsman, call the Area Agency on Aging (AAA), which is listed in the government section of your telephone directory, usually under "aging" or "elderly services."

It is essential to call the office with jurisdiction over the geographical area where the elder lives. If you cannot find the number for either of these offices or you are unsure of the office that has jurisdiction over the geographical area in which the older person lives, you can obtain the correct telephone number by calling the Eldercare Locator at 1-800-677-1116, sponsored by the Administration on Aging (AoA). It is helpful to provide the address and zip code number of the older person's residence.

AoA's Involvement in Elder Abuse Prevention

The AoA administers the Older Americans Act (OAA). The AoA's key priority areas are building systems of home and community-based long-term care; promoting consumer empowerment and protection; and serving as a focal point for aging information and education. The OAA supports a nationwide "aging network," consisting of the AoA, including its Regional Offices; the 57 State Units on Aging (SUA's); 655 AAA's; 221 Tribal Organizations, representing over 300 Tribes; and more than 27,000 community service providers.

The OAA provides formula grant funds to SUA's to support state elder abuse prevention activities, authorized by Title VII, Vulnerable Elder Rights Protection Activities. The OAA also funds discretionary project grants, authorized by the Title IV, Training, Research, and Discretionary Projects and Programs.

State Elder Abuse Prevention Activities

The State Elder Abuse Prevention Program, created by the 1987 Amendments to the OAA, was consolidated into the new Vulnerable Elder Rights Protection Activities, Title VII, when the OAA last was reauthorized in 1992. Title VII provides the states discretion in setting priories for spending these moneys. For the most part, states have focused their elder abuse prevention activities in four areas:

- **professional training**, e.g., skill-building workshops for adult protective services personnel; workshops designed to introduce

261

specific professional groups, e.g., law enforcement, to aging and elder abuse issues; statewide conferences open to all service providers with an interest in elder abuse; and development of training manuals, videos, and other materials;

- **coordination among state service systems** and among service providers, e.g., creation of elder abuse hotlines for reporting; formation of statewide coalitions and task forces; and creation of local multidisciplinary teams, coalitions, and task forces;

- **technical assistance**, e.g., development of policy manuals and protocols that outline the proper or preferred procedures; and

- **public education**, e.g., development of elder abuse prevention curriculum for elementary and secondary students; and development and delivery of elder abuse prevention public education campaigns, including radio and television public service announcements, posters, flyers, and videos with training materials suitable for use with community groups.

National Elder Abuse Incidence Study

This final report of the National Elder Abuse Incidence Study (NEAIS) contains estimates of the national incidence of abuse, neglect, and exploitation of older people in domestic settings and information about the characteristics of elder abuse perpetrators and victims, including self-neglecting elders.

Summary of Findings

Victims of Abuse, Neglect, and Self-Neglect

Victims reported to APS resemble the characteristics of victims identified by sentinel agencies, for many categories of abuse and neglect. Women are disproportionately represented as victims, according to reports from both APS and sentinel sources. In APS reports, women represent from 60 percent to 76 percent of those subjected to all forms of abuse and neglect except abandonment, even though, overall, women represent only 58 percent of the elderly population (over 60 years of age). In reports received exclusively from sentinels, from 67 percent to 92 percent of those reported as abused were women, depending on the type of abuse. The greatest disparity between men and women was in reported rates of emotional or psychological abuse, according to APS data. Three-fourths of those subjected to this form of abuse were women rather than men. According to sentinel reports, the greatest disparity between men and women was in the category of financial abuse, in which 92 percent of the victims were women.

A substantial proportion of the victims of neglect was the oldest old (age 80 and over), according to both APS and sentinel reports. APS reports showed that 52 percent of neglect victims were over age 80. Sentinels found 60 percent in this oldest age range. APS reports also suggest that this older category was disproportionately subjected to physical abuse, emotional abuse, and financial exploitation. Overall, our oldest elders are abused and neglected at two to three times their proportion of the elderly population.

Sentinel data show that of those subjected to any form of abuse, fewer than 10 percent were minorities (including Blacks, Hispanics, Asians, Pacific Islanders, and others). On the other hand, higher proportions of victims of most forms of abuse and neglect reported to APS agencies were Black, ranging from 9 percent for physical abuse, the lowest, to 17 percent for neglect. Only small proportions of Hispanics and other minorities are represented in most categories of abuse reported to APS, generally less than 3 percent altogether. These low proportions for these other minorities are supported by the sentinel data. Further research is needed to ascertain whether low rates for Hispanics in particular are due to lower rates of reporting and detection of abuse and neglect, perhaps because of language barriers, or are due to lower rates of actual abuse in these communities.

Elderly self-neglect also is a serious problem, with about 139,000 new unduplicated reports in 1996. (Some of those described as self-neglecting were also subjected to other forms of abuse.) Approximately two-thirds of self-neglecting elders reported to APS were women. In addition, 45 percent of them were over the age of 80. Most victims of self-neglect are unable to care for themselves and/or are confused; many are depressed. This is a difficult and troubling finding, which warrants attention as well as further research.

Perpetrators of Abuse and Neglect

Across all categories of abuse and neglect, the distribution of perpetrators by gender is almost equal, according to reports received by APS. However, this overall equity is due to the preponderance of neglect as a category and the somewhat greater frequency of neglect perpetrated by women (52 percent versus 48 percent by men). For all other categories of abuse reported to APS, men outnumbered women as perpetrators by at least 3 to 2. Among reports by sentinels, which are not broken down by type of abuse because the numbers are too small, male perpetrators outnumbered female perpetrators by 1.8 to 1. This preponderance of abuse by men is significant both in reports obtained from APS and in sentinel data.

According to reports received by APS and data supplied by sentinels, most perpetrators were younger than their victims. According to information supplied by APS, 65 percent of total perpetrators were under age 60; close to the same percentage of perpetrators identified by sentinels were under age 60. Of course, even perpetrators who are older than 60 may still be younger than the persons they abuse. Among reports to APS, the relative "youth" of perpetrators of financial abuse is particularly striking compared to other types of abuse, with 45 percent being 40 or younger and another 40 percent being 41-59 years old.

Table 16.1. Age of Perpetrators of Domestic Elder Abuse for Selected Types of Maltreatment[1]

Age	Neglect	Emotional/ Psycho- logical	Physical Abuse	Financial/ Material	Abandon- ment
40 and under	20.1%	34.3%	20.3%	45.1%	1.4%*
41 to 59	34.2%	42.4%	41.9%	39.5%	67.5%
60 to 69	9.2%*	10.4%*	8.1%*	3.4%*	0.0%*
70 to 79	18.9%*	4.8%*	12.4%*	1.6%*	1.5%*
80 and older	17.7%	8.2%	17.4%*	10.4%*	29.6%*
Total	100%	100%	100%	100%	100%
Percentage of victims experiencing abuse	48.5%	34.8%	26.9%*	30.2%*	4.3%*

[1]Based on an estimated 57,933 substantiated incidents of elder abuse. Some entries have missing values.

*The confidence band for these numbers is wide, relative to the size of the estimate. The true number may be close to zero or much larger than the estimate.

Relatives or spouses of the victims commit most domestic elder abuse according to reports supplied both by APS and sentinels. Approximately 90 percent of alleged abusers, according to both types of sources, were related to victims. APS data suggest that adult children are the largest category of abusers, across all forms of abuse, with proportions ranging from 43 percent for cases of neglect to nearly 80 percent for abandonment, although there were relatively few reported instances of abandonment. Adult children also account for the largest category of alleged abusers in sentinel reports (39 percent). Since family members are frequently the primary caregivers for elderly relatives in domestic settings, this finding that family members are the primary perpetrators of elderly abuse is not surprising.

Table 16.2. Incomes of Elder Abuse Victims for Selected Types of Maltreatment[1]

Income category	Neglect	Emotional/ Psychological	Physical Abuse	Financial/ Material	Abandonment
Less than $5,000	2.4%*	6.2%*	7.6%*	1.9%*	0.0%
$5,000 - $9,999	66.8%	37.8%	49.5%	46.0%	96.1%
$10,000 - $14,999	21.4%	31.0%	18.5%*	29.8%	3.9%*
$15,000 and up	9.5%	25.0%	24.5%*	22.4%	0.0%
Total	100%	100%	100%	100%	100%
Percentage of victims experiencing abuse	51.8%	34.9%	23.9%	30.7%	3.5%*

[1]Based on an estimated 53,667 substantiated incidents of elder abuse. Income was missing for 28.8 percent of reports.

*The confidence band for this number is wide, relative to the size of the estimate. The true number may be close to zero or much larger than the estimate.

Table 16.3. Race/Ethnicity of Perpetrators of Domestic Elder Abuse for Selected Types of Maltreatment[1]

Race/ Ethnicity	Neglect	Emotional/ Psycho- logical	Physical Abuse	Financial/ Material	Abandon- ment
White	76.6%	77.3%	83.0%	77.1%	34.4%*
Black	20.4%	17.8%*	11.3%*	18.7%*	59.0%*
Hispanic	0.8%*	0.8%*	1.4%*	0.8%*	1.4%*
Asian/Pacific Islanders	0.3%*	0.5%*	0.3%*	0.2%*	0.0%*
American Indians/Alaskan Natives	0.1%*	0.0%*	0.1%*	1.5%*	0.0%*
Other/Unknown	1.9%*	3.6%*	3.8%*	1.7%*	5.2%*
Percent of Total Perpetrators	47.5%	35.4%	26.9%	31.0%	4.2%*

[1]Based on an estimated 59,517 substantiated incidents of elder abuse. Some entries have missing values.

*The confidence band for these numbers is wide, relative to the size of the estimate. The true number may be close to zero or much larger than the estimate.

Limitations of NEAIS Research

The NEAIS study design had some limitations that prevented it from making an estimate of all new incidents of elder abuse and neglect in 1996. First, the sentinel approach tends to cause a certain amount of "undercount" in the detection of domestic elder abuse because there are no community institutions in which all elders regularly assemble and from which sentinels can be chosen and elders observed. In the case of child abuse research, on the other hand, schools serve as such a community institution from which primary sentinels are selected. The NEAIS was aware of this inherent limitation in the sentinel research design and tried to ameliorate this challenge by assigning as many sentinels as appropriate from the four large categories of professionals most regularly in contact with elderly people.

A second and related inherent limitation of the sentinel research design is that sentinels cannot observe and report abuse and neglect of elders that are isolated or do not have any (or very limited) contact with any community organizations. The sentinel method is most effective when well-trained sentinel reporters (which NEAIS's were) have opportunities to observe the same elders over a reasonable period of time. If there is minimal contact between the elderly person and sentinels, the opportunities for observing the signs and symptoms of abuse and neglect are lessened.

Finally, limitations in resources available to the NEAIS may have limited the total count of elders and the precision of the results. With more resources, it would have been possible to sample a larger number of study counties and to follow events in each of them for a longer time period. Estimates of child abuse and neglect for the third federally funded incidence study, for example, were obtained in 40 primary sampling units (i.e., counties) using more than 3,000 sentinels over a three-month period, rather than in NEAIS's 20 sampling units, with 1,200 sentinels in two months. One of the effects of the smaller number of counties, sentinels, and months of reporting was the smaller number of total sentinel reports and the resulting relatively large standard errors and wide confidence bands used in calculating the incidence estimates. With smaller standard errors, the NEAIS findings could be more definitive, or precise.

Implications of NEAIS Findings

The findings of the NEAIS raise a number of important issues for policy development, practice, and training in addressing the problems of elder abuse, neglect, and self-neglect. Study findings can provide a basis for designing new and enlightened public policies and practices, which are programmatically responsible, fiscally sound, and compassionate. This report also presents data to support practitioners, caregivers, social researchers, and others in identifying new approaches to reduce and prevent abuse, neglect, exploitation, and self-neglect of the elderly. Because states and localities historically have had responsibility for elder abuse reporting, investigation, intervention, and services, most of the following implications are for state and local governments:

- An important target for policy planners is the abuse and neglect among the oldest elders, which becomes ever more urgent since those aged 85 and over are the most rapidly growing elderly age group.

- Elderly persons who are unable to care for themselves, and/or are mentally confused and depressed are especially vulnerable to abuse and neglect as well as self-neglect. Perhaps our local community organizations and corporations can be mobilized to recognize such potential problems and provide support (e.g., by mobilizing neighborhood programs; by educating and sensitizing employees about elder abuse and neglect).

- Given the large number of incidents of abuse and neglect that are unidentified and unreported, service providers, caregivers, and all citizens who relate to elderly people need to be alerted to the problem of abuse and neglect, taught to recognize it, and encouraged to report suspected abuse.

- Maintain a comprehensive system of services to respond to reports of elder abuse and to provide follow-up services to elder abuse victims.

- Physicians and health care workers may be especially well placed to detect instances of abuse, neglect, and self-neglect given that even the most isolated elderly persons come in contact with the health care system at some point. The education of physicians, nurses, and other health care workers should be focused on how to recognize and report signs and symptoms of elder abuse, neglect, and self-neglect and where to refer victims for other human and support services.

- Increased standardization of state definitions and general reporting procedures for elder abuse and neglect would allow the more meaningful and expedited collection and analysis of data about elder abuse, including monitoring national trends in incidence over time.

- The Western region of the country reported the largest number of reports to APS of any of the regions. With approximately 25 percent of the U.S. population, the Western region was the source of 40 percent of the reports. Additionally, almost 60 percent of the Western region reports were substantiated, in contrast to an overall substantiation rate of 49 percent. More detailed study of these Western states may provide information on promising policies and practices for identifying and reporting abuse that can be replicated elsewhere in the country.

Future Research Questions and Issues for Caregivers and Researchers

The findings of the NEAIS raise a number of questions and issues for researchers and service providers to think about in addressing the problems of elder abuse, neglect, and self-neglect. Clearly some of these complex issues will require additional research:

- The confluence of a high proportion of adult children, spouses, and particularly parents being perpetrators, along with the high proportion of perpetrators being 80 and over, suggests that the following may be important areas for further study:

  - the relationship between abusive family members and caregiving responsibilities;

  - the relationship between abusive spouses and parents and their caregiving responsibilities, particularly for neglect; and

  - the relationship between 80+ year old perpetrators and caregiving responsibilities.

- Are there characteristics of the perpetrators, aged 60 and over, that aging service providers could affect by reaching out and providing services so that abuse committed by perpetrators aged 60+ is reduced?

- Are there characteristics of the caregiving relationships among younger family members who financially exploit their older relatives that could be affected by service interventions for the perpetrators? What are those interventions? Are there services or education for persons aged 60+ that would help them from becoming victims of financial abuse, particularly by younger family members?

- What is the economic condition of victims of abuse and neglect compared with elders overall?

- In-home service providers reported all substantiated sexual abuse cases. Why is this so? What do they know/see that other reporters do not? How can we capitalize on their knowledge?

- Why are black elders more likely to be self-neglecters (18 percent of the substantiated APS reports compared to being 8 percent of the elder population)?

- Why do sentinels recognize abuse among women at a much higher rate than is reflected among APS reports? Do we need to train people better to recognize and detect abuse among men?

- Why do sentinels not see more self-neglect cases than are reported to APS agencies, as sentinels do for abuse and neglect?

- How can employees of banks be educated and encouraged to identify and report incidents of financial exploitation that may come to their attention while serving elderly customers? Although the NEAIS was not very successful in obtaining reports from bank sentinels, banks are in a good position to observe financial abuse and concerted attention should be given to how to better involve them in future research on elder abuse incidence. States and communities with particularly strong bank reporting of financial exploitation (e.g., Massachusetts and San Diego) may provide promising practices for such larger replication.

Conclusion

In conclusion, the NEAIS has documented the existence of a previously unidentified and unreported stratum of elder abuse and neglect, thus confirming and advancing our understanding of the "iceberg" theory of elder abuse. NEAIS estimates that for every abused and neglected elder reported to and substantiated by APS, there are over five additional abused and neglected elders that are not reported. NEAIS also acknowledges that it did not measure all unreported abuse and neglect. Our collective challenge—as policy makers, service providers, advocates, researchers, and society as a whole, is to utilize this information to better the lives of our elder citizens.

Resources

National Center on Elder Abuse
1225 I Street, NW Suite 725
Washington, DC 20005
Tel: 202-898-2586
Website: http://www.nasua.org
E-mail: staff@nasua.org

For information about state elder abuse contacts, call NCEA. The NCEA website also includes a State-By-State Listing of Statewide Toll-Free Telephone Numbers for Reporting/Receiving Domestic and Institutional Elder Abuse The NCEA reports an increase of 150 percent in state-reported elder abuse nationwide over a 10-year period, from 1986 to 1996. However, because abuse and neglect is still largely hidden under the shroud of family and personal secrecy, it is grossly underreported.

Chapter 17

Long-Distance Caregiving

Nearly 7 million Americans provide care or manage care for a relative or friend aged 55 or older who lives at least one hour away, according to a survey cosponsored by The National Council on the Aging (NCOA) and The Pew Charitable Trusts. The survey is the first to focus exclusively on long-distance caregiving.

The caregivers in the survey lived, on average, 304 miles away from the care recipient and spent an average of 4 hours traveling to reach that person. Those respondents who were the primary caregivers for the older person spent an average of 35 hours per month giving care—roughly the equivalent of one week of work each month. One-quarter of all the respondents spent more than 41 hours per month providing care.

Long-distance care is a large and growing concern to baby boomers. The average age of the caregivers interviewed was 46, and nearly half of them were boomers. The survey indicates that approximately 3.3 million boomers are providing long-distance care.

"We expect that the number of long-distance caregivers will more than double over the next 15 years as the baby boomers and their parents age," said James Firman, Ed.D., president and CEO of NCOA. "To deal with this growing phenomenon, employers, consumers, and government will need to foster better ways of helping the caregiver and receiver."

"7 Million Provide Long-Distance Care to Elders, NCOA Study Finds," © 1999 The National Council on the Aging, Inc.

The average care recipient was 78 years old, and 64 percent were women. The care recipient was typically a relative: 53 percent were parents or step-parents of the caregiver; 11 percent were grandparents. "The survey reveals that long-distance caregiving in America is a family affair," said Donna Wagner, Ph.D., vice president for research and development at NCOA. "Most of the caregivers in the study were able to manage their caregiving responsibilities because of the help they received from family and friends. The results demonstrate that policies and programs that help long-distance caregivers also benefit not only care recipients but the entire family unit."

Impact on Workplace: Productivity Losses

As long-distance caregiving grows along with the aging of boomers and their parents, employers in the U.S. may face serious employee leave and productivity issues as a result. More than half of all the respondents said their responsibilities interfere with their professional, social, or family needs. Among the employed respondents, 25 percent said they miss at least one day of work in a typical month because of their caregiving, and 15 percent said they had taken unpaid leave during the past year. NCOA estimates that at least 15 million days of work are missed each year because of long-distance caregiving. Despite the toll that caregiving takes on their personal lives, however, the overwhelming majority of respondents said they plan to continue providing the care indefinitely.

Opportunities for Private Businesses and Voluntary Sector

Given their burdens, long-distance caregivers could benefit from many different forms of assistance. Caregivers report that the greatest unmet needs of the care recipients are for personal care and assistance, companionship, help in coping with an illness, and more family contact. More than 70 percent of the caregivers reported that they would benefit from educational materials about services, and 62 percent said that they would like someone to visit the person and update the caregiver about the recipient's mental and physical health.

"The survey findings confirm a sizeable and growing market for services for elderly people," said Carolyn Asbury, Ph.D., director of the health and human services program at The Pew Charitable Trusts.

"Private businesses and the voluntary sector should begin to look for opportunities to respond to this emerging market." More than half of the survey respondents are already receiving help from formal service providers—often a home health agency or individual.

The survey also suggests that churches and synagogues could be particularly helpful resources for long-distance caregivers. Among care recipients who were affiliated with a faith congregation, 76 percent received some form of help from the congregation. More than 90 percent of the caregivers whose family member or friend had received help from the congregation said they were satisfied or extremely satisfied with this help, and 65 percent of these caregivers said they would like to have or would consider arranging for help from a congregation other than their own or the care recipient's.

In the survey, caregiving was considered "long-distance" if it required travel of at least one hour to reach the care recipient. Caregiving was defined as providing or managing care, services, or financial or legal assistance for a person aged 55 or older. Two hundred respondents were identified as long-distance caregivers and were interviewed in a telephone survey. Respondents were screened from a sample of nearly 1,000 adults representative of the U.S. population.

The National Council on the Aging is a private, nonprofit association of more than 7,500 organizations and professionals in the U.S. who work with an on behalf of older persons.

The Pew Charitable Trusts, a national philanthropy with over $4 billion in assets, support nonprofit activities in the areas of health and human services, culture, education, the environment, public policy, and religion. Through their grant-making in aging, the Trusts seek to promote the ability of elderly people to live independently in their communities.

This information is not intended as a guide to individual health, legal, or financial concerns. It is not intended to replace or substitute for consultation with a qualified health care provider, attorney, certified public accountant, or other professional services provider. No individual should rely on published material for guidance and counsel on specific matters relating to their personal health, legal, or financial concerns. This information is general in nature and at best reflects what are believed to be valid statistical trends which do not necessarily relate directly to any individual's specific situation. No representation is made as to the accuracy or completeness of the information or the analysis thereof. NCOA, its officers, constituent units, and agents assume no responsibility for any damages arising from the use of the information presented.

Chapter 18

Grieving

Overview

Understanding the Problem

- Normal feelings to expect after the death of a loved one

- Each person's reaction to the loss of a loved one is different, and each person must work through grief in his or her own way

- There is no "right" or "wrong" way to feel after someone dies

- Most people who are very upset over someone's death take months to get beyond the most severe emotional stress. Grief beyond a year is common but may require help.

When to Get Help

- Start with your family doctor

- Symptoms indicating the need for professional help

- Information to have ready when you call for help

- What to say when you call

Reprinted with permission, "ACP Home Care Guide for Advanced Cancer–Grieving," © 1997 American College of Physicians.

What You Can Do to Help Yourself

- Allow yourself to experience the pain of grief
- Select a person to share your grief with
- Find what works for you in returning to normal routines
- Read books or poetry on the subject
- Keep a diary or journal
- Encourage others to talk about the deceased
- Talk out loud to the person who has died
- Find out about a bereavement support group

Consider Obstacles

- "People say I should be over this."
- "People give me advice that I don't want to take."
- "Nobody wants to talk about Dad when they're around me."

Carrying Out and Adjusting Your Plan

- Checking on results
- If your plan does not work

Topics with a flag (➤) in front of them are actions you can take or symptoms you can look for.

- The information in this home care plan fits most situations, but yours may be different.
- If a doctor, nurse, or counselor tells you to do something other than what is recommended here, consider all of the information and apply what is meaningful to your own needs.

Understanding the Problem

People who lose a friend or family member to cancer face the same issues as anyone who experiences the death of a loved one, whether by accident or illness. Your feelings and emotions after someone's death can profoundly affect how you relate to others and get through your daily routine. Depending on your personality, you may find it helpful to confide your feelings to another person—sometimes a friend is best, sometimes a family member, and sometimes a professional such as a nurse, a counselor, or a member of the clergy. You may find consolation through sharing or listening at a group—sharing session involving others who have had a recent loss; such groups usually are led by a counseling professional. On the other hand, if you have never been open about your feelings, it is unlikely that you will suddenly change now. Well-meaning people may insist that you must talk it out, but they may not understand you, your past, or your methods of dealing with life's difficult moments.

Each person must work through grief in his or her own way—and it is work (even if not always of the physical kind). Despite the existence of widely published "stages" of grief, each survivor deals with loss as an individual, and the ways in which people handle their loss vary widely. When you are struggling to deal with your own loss, it is useless to worry about whether you are following somebody else's timetable.

The range of reactions to someone else's death is broad. Some people are devastated when it occurs, and others feel very little emotion. Sometimes, people feel their grief only later, and some people never have strong feelings. Different people also may experience different emotions. They may feel guilt, remorse, sadness, or resentment toward others, such as doctors, nurses, hospice workers, or even God. Some people who lose a family member or close friend feel anger and ask questions such as "Why did this happen to him (the one who died)?" and "Why did this happen to me?" Anger also may reach back to events that occurred during diagnosis and care, and you may ask, "Why didn't the doctors find the cancer soon enough?" or, "Why did mother suffer so?"

You may think that you hear the deceased person's voice calling to you, or you may want to have a conversation with that person. You may experience flashbacks, such as remembering the funeral or even the moment of death itself, for no apparent reason. In addition, you may feel as if you are making progress but then suddenly feel worse, and without knowing what triggered it. Although upsetting, these are normal experiences for people who grieve.

Even if the illness was prolonged and you anticipated the death of your loved one, you still may encounter both shock and numbness in the same way as if the death had occurred unexpectedly. During this time, which may last from only a few up to 6 weeks, you may experience a sense of "just going through the motions," as if you were in shock.

When this feeling of numbness and shock begins to subside, you may feel as if you might be overcoming it—thinking "I'm getting back to normal." Just then, however, you unexpectedly may encounter a deeper sense of grief or sadness as reality sets in. When this occurs, you may experience symptoms of grief like those of acute depression—being unable to sleep soundly, losing your appetite, not wanting to get up in the morning, or not wanting to be around other people.

Whatever happens, understand that there is no "right" or "wrong" way to feel after someone's death. Most people's feelings, even if they seem extreme at the time, fall within a range of normal reactions.

Most people who lose someone close to them take months to get over the most severe part of their emotional stress, and for most, it will take at least a year to work through the grieving process. Counselors often consider how a person is doing at the 1-year anniversary of the death as an indicator of how well he or she has adjusted to the loss. Grief that lasts beyond a year is common but may require help.

Remember that life will never again be exactly the way it was before your loved one died. If you are expecting things to "get back to normal" after awhile, you may be disappointed or frustrated to find that the new "normal" is not like the old "normal." Your life will go on, but—precisely because the person was important to you—it will not be the same without him or her.

Your goals

- Know when to get professional help with grief.

- Understand that people handle loss with a wide range of emotions, none of which is "right" or "wrong." Grieve for your loss in your own way rather than feeling that you should be the same as other people you have known or read about.

- Understand that most people who grieve return to their daily routines in 2 to 4 months, but healing often takes a year or longer. Each person's reactions are unique, so be wary of timetables that others may try to force on you.

When to Get Help

The first question you should ask is whether you need help from other people. If you do, an excellent place to start is with your family doctor. He or she may help you directly or aid you in finding the right group session, counselor, or clinic. You should seek help if any of the following is true:

➤ Continued difficulty in sleeping.

If you are losing sleep or feel tired all the time, the first place to go for help is your family doctor. A physician who knows you and your medical history can make an informed decision whether to prescribe medication and, if so, what kind.

➤ Substantial weight gain or loss.

Any substantial change in eating, such as loss of all appetite or a sudden increase in appetite, may be the result of emotional distress. Again, consult your family doctor first, because he or she already knows you and can make an informed judgment about treatment.

➤ Prolonged emotional distress.

If, after 6 months, you do not see a marked improvement of your ability to function in daily life, you should consider seeking help. It is natural to want to withdraw from others after losing a loved one, but if you still cannot enjoy a reasonable quality of life after 6 months, this is a signal that you may need help working through your grief.

➤ If you are overcome by suicidal thoughts.

If suicidal thoughts become central to your thinking and you are encountering them every day, seek help from your family doctor, a counselor, member of the clergy, or a mental health clinic.

Have the answers to the following questions ready when you call your family doctor, counselor, or clinic:

1. How much does grief interfere with my ability to do my job or normal daily activities?

2. Am I having difficulty sleeping?

3. Is my appetite gone, or do I eat significantly more than before the person died?

4. Is suicide an option I would consider?

Here is an example of what someone might say when calling for help:

"I'm David Winters, son of Katherine Winters, who died of cancer 6 months ago. Ever since my mother's death, I've been very upset. I've also been having trouble sleeping through the night since about 2 weeks after she died, and I never had trouble before. I think I may need some help."

What You Can Do to Help Yourself

You can do many things on your own to handle the emotional stress of grief, and you can get help from others as well. You may need one or both forms of help to successfully restore your sense of well-being.

➤ Allow yourself to experience the pain of grief.

What this means is to work through your emotions in the best way you can. If this means crying, screaming, talking to the person who has died, or doing physical activity such as punching a pillow or lifting weights, do that. To heal emotionally, many people need to express their feelings. If you are embarrassed about crying in front of other family members such as your children (whether younger or adult), you may need to tell them: "It may be upsetting to you, but I need to cry and express my feelings. I need to work through this grief."

➤ Select a person to share your grief with.

Find a good listener who has experienced a similar loss, although it probably is best to choose someone who is not grieving over the same person as you are. Someone outside of your immediate family often is a good choice. You want someone who will let you express yourself, not someone who will try to reason you out of your feelings. Candidates might be a member of the clergy or a sympathetic friend or co-worker. Although you may expect family members to be supportive, they most likely are burdened with that very same loss as well. For example, if your spouse dies and you want to share with your adult children, remember that they are grieving the loss of their parent. As a result, they may be unable to give you the compassion you need. In addition, it often is painful for an adult child to see a parent grieving, and they may want you to "get over it" so that their lives can return to some form of "normal."

Be aware that some people, even professionals such as clergy, may not be personally prepared to deal with death—perhaps because of their own grief over someone they have lost or feelings about their own mortality. If you are unable to relate to one person, find another. Many hospice programs offer a one-on-one assignment of a bereavement volunteer to aid families after a death, one of many programs typically extended by hospice to help with grief. Others might include newsletters, a library of books about grieving, or information about bereavement support groups.

➤ Find what works for you in returning to normal routines.

If certain activities such as reading or swimming were relaxing for you before, try to pursue them now. See if that will help you to get back to a normal cycle of living. For some people, losing a loved one is so upsetting that they cannot resume these activities until their grief subsides to some extent.

➤ Read books or poetry on the subject.

Many books, including those with first-person accounts, about working through and overcoming grief are available at your local public library. As with other techniques, however, this will not help everyone. Some people will react by saying, "I have enough to worry about without reading someone else's grief," while others will find direction, a sense of what is normal to experience, and a feeling of connection with others who have had this experience. Similarly, reading poetry, whether alone or aloud in a group, can help by giving artful expression to feelings that often are hard to express or even identify.

➤ Keep a diary or journal.

Some people find it helpful and therapeutic to write their thoughts and feelings in a diary as they proceed through the process of grieving. The British author, critic, and novelist C.S. Lewis (1898-1963), after losing his wife, kept a journal (*A Grief Observed*) of how he was feeling. A private person for whom neither a support group nor reading a book is helpful may find comfort in keeping such a journal. Some people also find it helpful to write their feelings in a letter to the person who has died, which can help to resolve unfinished business or feelings.

283

➤ **Encourage others to talk about the deceased.**

Friends and family frequently avoid discussing the deceased to avoid upsetting the person who is grieving. If you want to talk about the person who has died, you should reassure others that it is okay. All you have to do is say, "I'd like to talk about Dad." Reassure your visitors that while you may cry or become upset, you would rather do that than awkwardly skirt the subject, because he or she was very important to you. Most people can accept your crying or being upset if you are the one who brought up the subject.

➤ **Talk out loud to the person who has died.**

In much the same manner as the letter noted earlier, it is not unreasonable to want to resolve issues with a person who has died by holding a one-sided conversation, aloud, with the deceased. Do this if it makes you feel better.

➤ **Find out about a bereavement support group.**

Bereavement support groups can help to make the process of dealing with loss easier. Signing up for a bereavement support group may be a difficult decision, however, because many people think of their grief as something that is private. You may feel uneasy talking with strangers about your feelings or your loved one. Keep in mind, however, that such groups have helped many people get through their grief and, therefore, may help you.

In a bereavement group, participants learn from each other about normal reactions to grief. Because of their shared experiences, group members often come to care about and to support each other emotionally, and they often share practical ideas for working through their grief as well. In addition, a support group also can help you to get through difficult times like holidays or anniversaries.

Most support groups meet for a limited time, such as six weekly sessions. Others run continuously, and people come in and out as their emotional needs dictate. Most are free; some require a fee. Call a hospice, counseling clinic, member of the clergy, your local Area Agency on Aging, or a hospital to find out about bereavement groups. If that does not work, check your newspaper or the human-services listings of a phone book. It often is good to talk with the leader of a group in advance to learn what is expected and how the group is conducted. Some people attend with a family member or a friend.

If you decide to attend a support group, understand that you may feel worse when you go home after the first session. The reason is that you are dealing with your feelings openly (as well as hearing about everyone else's). In the long run, however, this can be helpful. It also is important to realize that a support group will not restore you to the way you were before the person's death, but it will help you to cope with your new life without the deceased.

Possible Obstacles

Here are some obstacles that other caregivers have faced:

1. "People say I should be over this."

Response: Everyone deals with grief at his or her own pace. You may need to say, "We each go at our own pace. I guess my pace is slower than you expected."

2. "People give me advice that I don't want to take."

Response: Well-meaning advice is not always helpful advice. One example might be if you regularly walked with your deceased spouse and now can no longer bear the thought of walking alone. When people offer advice to take walks, do your best to be gracious and thank them, but then do what you feel is best.

3. "People avoid the subject of Dad when they're around me."

Response: Take charge of the conversation, and reassure them: "I want to talk about Dad, and it makes me feel better to talk about him." Your family and friends may not know that you feel this way, so it is important to tell them.

Think of other obstacles that could interfere with carrying out your plan

What additional roadblocks could get in the way of the recommendations in this plan? For example, will other people help? How will you explain your need for help to other people? Do you have the time and energy to carry out the plan?

You need to develop plans for getting around these roadblocks. The COPE ideas (creativity, optimism, planning, and expert information) are one way of overcoming your obstacles.

285

Carrying Out and Adjusting Your Plan

Carrying out your plan

The process of grieving is unique for each person, so you need to find your own, special way of dealing with it. Experiment, and let your feelings tell you which are helping.

Checking on results

The important thing to remember is that people respond to grief in widely varying ways, and that you will have both ups and downs, good days and bad. Healing takes time. You will know that you are successfully working through grief when your stronger emotions begin to dissipate, such as when you no longer feel anger or deep sadness, and when your interest and involvement in outside activities return to their normal level.

If your plan does not work

Grieving is a difficult but natural process. If you cannot resume some of your normal activities or do not seem to feel better after 6 months, you may want to review "When to Get Help."

Part Three

Caregiving for Specific Conditions and Diseases

Chapter 19

Alzheimer's Disease and Dementia Care

Contents

Section 19.1

Caregiver Role

Reprinted with permission "The Role of the Caregiver," © Kenneth Hepburn, Ph.D., Geriatric Research, Education and Clinical Center (GRECC) of the Department of Veterans Affairs Medical Center, Minneapolis, Minnesota.

A person takes on the role of caregiver to provide for the needs of a close relative or friend during a period of illness or disability. People do not often expect or want to take on this new role. They are seldom well trained for it.

Caregiving can be an occupation with no clear goals. Too often it is an occupation that has no description and no limits. As a caregiver, you will need to think through your goals as frankly as you can and then develop your own "job description" for working toward these goals.

Caring for patients with an illness such as Alzheimer's disease poses special problems. You can only predict parts of what will happen in the course of a dementing illness. There is a steady decline of the patient's abilities to think, remember, and act in appropriate ways. But there is no way to predict what pattern the disease will take, which symptoms will occur, or when these symptoms will occur.

If you are or will be caring for a person with Alzheimer's disease or any other dementing illness, you cannot expect the person to improve. The patient will become less and less able to function. You may be able to learn what ranges of potential care problems exist, but you will not know which ones will arise for you.

You will need to be prepared to adjust your daily routines and your ways of giving care when new symptoms appear. At the same time you will need to avoid thinking about care problems that might be possible but may never occur. The rest of this section discusses what caring for a person with Alzheimer's can mean to you and what skills you will need to develop to cope successfully with your new role. The following ideas will be addressed:

1. Setting goals

2. Changing care needs at each stage of the illness

3. Your tasks as learner/observer/manager

4. Your need for self-care.

Setting Goals

Your most basic care goal throughout the illness will be to ensure, to the extent you can, the patient's physical comfort and safety. You will also want to help the patient preserve a sense of emotional calm and self-esteem.

To do these things, you will have to play many roles. You may have to learn many new skills. You will provide comfort just by being with the person. You will need to watch the person and, perhaps, explain his or her actions to others (for instance, to a friend or doctor). You will have to take control of the places the person goes and the things the person does. You will have to be the person's nurse and his or her advocate. You will decide the person's future—and your own.

Throughout the impaired person's illness, the work of caregiving is largely concerned with watching and problem-solving. To become an accurate observer and effective problem-solver in daily care you will need to learn as much as you can about the disease itself and about the needs, feelings, and reactions of the impaired person. You will also need to learn about yourself. Your own needs, feelings, and reactions to) the impaired person play a big part in how you care for the patient. You're skill at self-care is an important part of ensuring the patient's good care through each stage of the illness.

Care at Different Stages of the Illness

Your basic care goals may not change throughout the patient's illness. Still, your role is a constantly changing one. As each new symptom appears or as an old one fades, the impaired person's needs change. A new set of problems and losses must be taken into account.

Each stage of the illness brings its own special care problems. In the early stages, the patient's main problems might be forgetfulness and impairment of learning ability. Your role might be to help find ways to maintain the person's ability to act on his own, as much as possible. This is the time to put a good health care team in place and to plan for the future. Talk with a lawyer and start a financial plan for yourself and the patient.

Safety is a big concern in the middle stage of the illness. The person's memory is failing and judgment is poor. The person may wander or get into things around the home which pose a danger. You may have to watch very carefully to see that the person doesn't get hurt. During this stage, the job of caregiving may well expand beyond the abilities of any one person. You will need to set up a network of care arrangements to support your efforts.

In the final stages, the patient becomes less and less able to attend to basic activities of daily living, such as bathing and dressing; and more nursing care may be needed. This is the time you will need to consider placing the impaired person in a nursing home. This is a hard choice. Talk about it with people you can trust and who know what you are going through (for instance: family, friends, a social worker, a clergyperson, your doctor). Whether you choose to place the person now or to wait, talking with these people can provide good information and support.

The Caregiver as Learner

You will be better able to cope with the problems Alzheimer's disease causes if you know what an impaired person can and cannot be expected to do. Try to keep in mind that many behaviors of the Alzheimer patient are the result of damage to the brain and are, therefore, beyond the person's direct control.

As a result, the patient may react in ways that seem wrong to you and in ways that trouble you or cause you pain. He may even become so confused by events and be so frustrated by not being able to put things together that he will strike out at you or others (with angry words or actions). You will need to learn how to respond calmly to the person's confusion, how to reassure him, and how to settle his outbursts.

Learning to accept the impaired person's confused actions and respond with kindness may well be easier than learning how to control these actions. A very hard part of this disease is that the impaired person doesn't learn well. You can't teach the person how to act when they are confused or upset.

You will have to learn "tricks of the trade" as you try to find ways to prolong the patient's ability to act on his own. For instance, doing things in a set routine may help the person retain the ability to do them. Praise, rewards, or small treats may also help keep the person in the patterns you want. At different stages of the disease, you may have to do different things. Signs and picture cues may work for some time. Simple spoken commands may also work. Breaking actions into small, step-by-step units may be useful. You may have to help the person start an action.

The Caregiver as Observer

One of the most important things you can do as a caregiver is to observe the impaired person carefully. In effect you become an expert on the person. You become skilled at predicting what the person might do in certain situations, at knowing what will calm the person, catch the person's waning attention, make the person happy, or keep the person busy.

Your observations of the impaired person play a major part in good health care for the patient. Your health care team will rely on you for clear information about the person and his or her state. As observer, you need to be objective, detailed, and nonjudgmental. You are called upon to see and to report promptly any changes in symptoms or actions.

Observing the impaired person can also protect the safety of the patient and of others. You need to watch the impaired person's declining abilities carefully, to remove hazards from the environment and to restrict or supervise activities as needed.

In addition to observing the impaired person, you need to become a good observer of yourself. You need to try to see yourself as the impaired person might see you to be sure your actions don't affect how the impaired person acts. You don't want to trigger troubling or hard-to-handle reactions. This may entail altering or, at least, controlling your natural reactions to the impaired person's actions. You must also watch your reactions to fatigue and to emotional stress so that you can protect your own health and happiness, both for your own sake and for the sake of the person who depends so heavily on you.

The Caregiver as Manager

As the caregiver for a person with Alzheimer's disease or dementia, you become manager of that person. Management skills include relating well, coordinating and supervising the activities of others, delegating tasks when appropriate, and planning for the future. A good manager draws on all of these skills.

A care manager must relate well with the patient and a wide variety of other people, including family, friends, professional advisers, and health care providers. The care manager also needs to work as a team with these others and to coordinate their efforts in providing care and in long-term planning. Finally, the good care manager needs to structure and to supervise the patient's environment and day-to-day activities in a way that meets the changing needs of both patient and caregiver.

The care manager is the major link between the impaired person and family and friends. As such, you will need to let family and friends know what the person's condition is and what help might be needed. As an expert on the impaired person, you may also be able to help the impaired person relate with others, by explaining actions, for example.

The caregiver manages the medical care that the patient receives. As care manager, you find the right help and work with the health care professionals to carry out treatment or care plans.

You may also need to manage legal affairs and finances for the impaired person, with the help of skilled advisers. Current affairs need to be managed, and long-term financial plans must be made to meet the impaired person's future care needs.

The care manager also organizes and directs a network of helpers and an assortment of care arrangements. Perhaps you will simply coordinate family help at first, but later you may need to find and oversee other kinds of help, either at home or in separate care facilities.

Clearly, a good care manager is a very key person in the life of an impaired person. As a care manager, then, you need to pay special attention to your own self-care, too.

The Need for Self-Care

Experts agree that caregiving puts a great strain on body, mind, and spirit. You will need to look after yourself as well as the impaired person.

Physical Health

Caregiving is physically tiring, so you need to pay special attention to your physical well-being. The health care team you consult on the impaired person's behalf should be a resource for you as well. Keep these health care providers informed about how you are, and ask them for suggestions as you need them. Even for people who are not under the strain of caregiving, eating well and getting enough sleep and exercise may be difficult.

As a caregiver, you may well have so many extra demands on your time that you may decide to skimp in these areas. Skimping can take a heavy toll on your ability to function. Try to keep in mind your responsibility to yourself. Your ability to provide care to the person depends on your health. Your ability to pick up the strands of your life when your caregiving tasks are done also depends on your good health.

Emotional Health

Caregiving often brings a large emotional burden. The patient, probably someone close to you, is a victim of an incurable, terminal illness. You may well endure a prolonged period of loss and grief. Other strong feelings may occur: anger, a sense of despair, sorrow, guilt, frustration, a feeling of being alone or overwhelmed. This period can also be a time of considerable anxiety and uncertainty about the future. Many people become very depressed.

One of the harder emotional issues of caregiving is the distance that grows between you and the person in your care. There comes a time when the impaired person is no longer the person you once knew. He or she is no longer reliable and cannot be trusted to remember to do what you ask or to provide you with accurate information. The disease reduces both memory and judgment. Your relationship with the person will surely become different from what it was before the onset of the disease. You will need to give orders and be in charge. You may have to learn how to do things you relied on the person to do. For instance, many men who provide care report they have to learn how to cook or do laundry; many women have to learn how to deal with finances and home repair.

The following ideas may be helpful in caring for your emotional health:

• Don't deny your feelings.

Find ways to let your feelings come out. Don't try to keep them bottled up inside you. People have different ways of expressing their feelings. Some talk with counselors, psychologists, social workers, or members of the clergy. Others are comfortable talking with a doctor or nurse. Still others would prefer to confide in family members and friends. Everyone can benefit from taking time alone to think and sort out feelings.

• Consider joining a support group.

Many caregivers have found emotional support and good suggestions for managing difficult care problems from members of support groups. Such groups bring together people in similar situations, so group members have valuable experience which can be the source of good tips and ideas for you. The group can also offer a safe place to let out your feelings. (Your health care providers or local hospital can refer you to a support group in your area, or you can get information from the Alzheimer's Disease and Related Disorders Association by calling, toll-free, 800-621-0379).

• Make life as easy as possible

During the time you are providing care to the impaired person, you may find many instances which call for compromise. You will need to look closely at standards and values for yourself and for the person in your care. The progress of the disease and the work of caregiving put pressure on these standards. You may find yourself trading off your own ease and comfort against your sense of the way things ought to be. For instance, if you are used to sitting down to dinner in the dining room for a formal meal, there may come a time when the difficulties of doing this offset the pleasure. Serving meals at the kitchen table may well be easier even though less appealing to you personally. There is no easy rule for making these decisions, but, when the time comes, you may find them easier to make than you might have expected.

• Be sure to give yourself credit for the work you are doing.

All the while you care for the impaired person, you are learning and becoming more skilled. You need to see that you have learned new things, have solved problems, and have come up with new ways of managing. While these accomplishments may not prepare you for each new care problem that arises, the knowledge of what you have done so far should give you confidence that you will be able to handle the next problem too.

• Anticipate problems by planning ahead and developing options for alternative care arrangements.

At any point in the illness, you may begin to feel that taking care of the person is too much for you. You will do best for yourself and the impaired person if you have thought through some options for alternative care arrangements. Your health care team can help you get started. Your family and friends can also be a source of help. Community agencies may offer you a wide range of resources and types of help. Nursing homes offer the option of temporary or permanent placement. Explore your options early, and be prepared for your need when it comes.

- Finally, remember that the impaired person doesn't always come first.

Your needs for regular rest, relaxation, and pleasurable activities should be considered important too. An exhausted, depressed caregiver can't provide better care than a person who regularly takes breaks, keeps in touch with friends, and occasionally takes a vacation. Sometimes putting yourself first will actually make you a better caregiver.

Section 19.2

Home Modification Guide

Reprinted with permission, "Alzheimer's-Proofing Your Home," © 1996 Mark Warner A.I.A., and Ellen Warner, M.Ed.. Mark L. Warner, a registered architect and gerontologist, and Ellen Warner, M.Ed., formed Ageless Design, Inc., a consulting firm dedicated to providing information and resources that enable seniors to live longer, safer, and healthier at home.

Caring for a loved one with Alzheimer's Disease may be one of the greatest challenges a family can experience. Until recently, information on how to "Alzheimer's-proof" your home has been difficult to find.

The purpose of this section is to provide information for caregivers and family members of persons with Alzheimer's disease that makes it possible to keep and care for a loved one at home. It is intended to help you create a safer and more sensitive home environment. We will help you discover the steps to take and products that are available to modify your home and tackle the difficulties you may encounter.

Alzheimer's affects the brain and its ability to process information—each case is unique. Logical conclusions should not be expected from a person who is losing their ability to think rationally. There are no rules and every suggestion must be reviewed in terms of your special situation, needs, and abilities of your loved one.

Since each person goes through the stages of Alzheimer's at their own pace, in their own way, what works today may not work tomorrow.

Locks that are effective one day may be figured out the next. Childproof devices are helpful, but remember they were designed for children, not adults. The job of a caregiver is to watch, listen, and constantly adjust to changes.

Adapt the Home for All Family Members

Approach home modifications so that all family members will be safe and comfortable. This includes the person with Alzheimer's, the caregiver(s), the rest of the family, and visitors. We recommend that you divide your home into three areas.

Area One: The Storage Zone

- Two areas of the house are "out of bounds" to the person with Alzheimer's disease. Area One consists of rooms such as the garage, basement, attic, and closets where breakable, dangerous or valuable items are stored. Doors leading to these restricted areas and the outside should be locked, alarmed, or controlled by wander-prevention devices.

Area Two: The Respite Zone

- The second restricted area is dedicated to the caregiver. Anyone caring for someone with Alzheimer's should have a "respite area." "Burn-out" is a big problem for caregivers and there needs to be a place where one can get away, relax and have time alone while someone else provides care.

Area Three: The Safe Zone

- Finally, the remainder of the home is accessible to the person with Alzheimer's. In this area it is okay to roam, rummage, and hide things. "Childproof" plug outlets and remove medicines, dangerous tools, appliances, and chemicals, as well as important documents, bills, and valuable/breakable objects.

Inside the Home

Safe-proofing the home is critical and you will need to examine every situation thoroughly. Remember that eventually people with Alzheimer's lose their ability to think rationally. For example, an electrical plug may appear to be a curious hole to explore or hide something, like a paper clip. Even an aquarium that combines water and electricity creates a potentially deadly situation.

If you live on an upper floor secure the windows and balcony doors. Often the person you are caring for does not realize that they are not on the ground floor—even if it is obvious to you. Easily installed, inexpensive window clamps are available at most hardware stores and will prevent a window or sliding door from opening wide enough to allow a person to walk through.

Remove toxic and seemingly harmless products that, if eaten in excess, could cause illness—like toothpaste or sweeteners. Keep sharp utensils and electrical appliances out of reach. Disconnect the garbage disposal, as it is a popular spot to hide things.

Your entire home should be well lit to help the person with Alzheimer's see where they are going. This is especially important for "dead end" corridors that are often dark and shadowy. An Alzheimer's sufferer may not realize how to turn around and come back.

Lower the thermostat on your hot water heater to its lowest setting or no higher than 120 degrees to prevent accidental burns. You can also install inexpensive anti-scalding devices on the faucets of the sinks, showers, and bathtubs.

Install a seat and a hand-held showerhead in the bath or shower. Showerheads with "on-off" buttons at the hand-held portion offer better control for dealing with those with fears of water or bathing. Grab bars and non-slip bath/shower mats are also advisable.

Remove all electrical appliances from counters and the control knobs from the stove, oven, and inside the refrigerator.

If falling becomes a problem, locate furniture to provide stability when walking across a room. Remove furniture that rolls, moves easily, or cannot support a person's weight. Eliminate throw rugs and low furniture, such as ottomans or magazine racks, that can cause falls or tripping. Remove furniture that is hazardous or difficult to see, such as the ever-popular glass table and glass shelving. Watch out for extension cords and telephone lines that may be tripped over or walked into, pulling an attached lamp or appliance to the floor.

Doors

For doors that lock from the inside, such as the bathroom, either remove the lock or keep an emergency key nearby. For the front door have an extra key well-hidden or give one to a trusted neighbor for emergencies.

Your Backyard

Safe-proof your yard as well. Identify and remove dangerous plants in your yard and home that can be eaten or cause injury. Most yards are landscaped with little or no thought to the toxicity of the plants selected. A simple call or visit to your local poison control center will help you identify the dangerous ones. Move thorned plants that can physically hurt, such as rose bushes or cacti, especially those near wandering paths.

Make sure your yard is enclosed with a fence not easily climbed and locks on the gate. Balconies and porches can be enclosed by installing heavy gauge, impenetrable metal screening that allows a view but not a journey.

Alzheimer's Is a Progressive Disease

Modifications and precautions, appropriate in the earlier stages, may or may not be appropriate for the middle or later stages. For example, mirrors are important to encourage your loved one to continue grooming for as long as possible. However, in later stages many people are confused and agitated by reflections in mirrors—even their own. You will want to remove or cover mirrors if this becomes a problem.

Wandering

Wandering is a serious problem. There are significant differences for dealing with nighttime and daytime wandering.

Night wandering presents unique challenges. While caregivers are asleep it is easier for a person with Alzheimer's to wander off unnoticed. Place a simple door alarm on the knob of the bedroom door. If the knob is turned the alarm will sound alerting the caregiver that someone is on the move. With these alarms in place the caregiver can safely and comfortably get a good night's sleep knowing that movement will not go unnoticed. (Test the alarm to make sure the caregiver can hear it from their bedroom.)

Daytime wandering often involves a continuous "wandering path" that can be a source of stimulating and healthy activity. Look for such opportunities in your home and backyard—often they are created for you. Remember to remove low furniture and anything that your loved one might trip over, bump into, or knock over. Don't overlook higher shelves or wall-mounted fixtures along the way. While the same rules apply to outside paths, it is also a good idea to trim shrubbery and remove any items that prevent a full view of the path.

Patterning

People with Alzheimer's often develop patterns or repeat activities that they find comfortable and enjoyable. By observing their movement around the house you may notice early clues to wandering paths and places where your loved one feels safe. Once these more regularly visited areas become apparent, check them carefully for potential problems. Make sure they are safe, calming, and offer familiar items your loved one will recognize and enjoy.

Simplify Decisions

At the onset of the disease simplify every facet of your loved one's environment. Remove clutter, create predictability, and simplify choices. Instead of six boxes of cereal in the cupboard, have two. Survey your home for any potentially agitating situations. It is important that your home is a calm, safe environment that encourages decisions and tasks that can be completed successfully.

Place large, easy-to-read signs or pictures cut out of magazines on cabinets and drawers to illustrate the contents. Turn this into a family project and make it fun.

Storage for Critical Supplies

As the disease progresses the world shrinks for the Alzheimer's sufferer. More and more time is spent in fewer and fewer rooms. Before this happens, it is important to move supplies and frequently used items to these rooms, close to where they may be needed in times of crisis.

Manufacturers of Helpful Products

Call for a catalogue or local distributor information.

Door Alarms

The Safety Zone
Toll-Free: 800-999-3030

WanderGuard
Toll-Free: 800-235-8085

Secure Care Products
Toll-Free: 800-451-7917
Tel: 603-223-0745

Wander Prevention Systems

WanderGuard
Toll-Free: 800-235-8085

Hand-Held Showerhead with an On-Off or Pause Control

Access with Ease
Toll-Free: 800-531-9479

Alsons
Toll-Free: 800-421-0001

Jaclo
Toll-Free: 800-852-3906
Tel: 908-789-7008

M.O.M.S.
Toll-Free: 800-232-7443

Sears Home Health Care Catalogue
Toll-Free: 800-326-1750

Grab Bars

DSI
Tel: 818-782-6793

Franklin Brass Co.
Toll-Free: 800-829-0089

Häfele
Toll-Free: 800-423-3531

Maxi Aid
Toll-Free: 800-522-6294

Anti-Scalding Devices

Accent on Living
Toll-Free: 800-787-8444

Suggested Reading

The 36-Hour Day, Nancy L. Mace, M.A., Peter V. Rabins, M.D.,
M.P.H., John Hopkins University Press, 2715 North Charles
Street, Baltimore, MD 21218-4319 or call 800-537-5487.

Section 19.3

Communication: Basic Skills and Techniques

Reprinted with permission "Communication: Basic Skills and Techniques," © Kenneth Hepburn, Ph.D., Geriatric Research, Education and Clinical Center (GRECC) of the Department of Veterans Affairs Medical Center, Minneapolis, Minnesota.

Communication means getting across what you really mean and having another person really understand it. This is not always easy under the best circumstances. Communication with a person who has a dementing illness will be even harder. The disease will impair the person's ability to understand words, to find words to use, to put ideas together, and hold them in place.

Loss of the ability to communicate with others may frustrate the patient with Alzheimer's disease. The person may feel cut off from you and others. He or she may feel a loss of control over things. This, in turn, may make the person feel less secure and more anxious or jumpy.

Problems in communication may pose special problems for you, the caregiver. As a caregiver, you are concerned with providing companionship, ensuring the patient's safety, and managing the daily routine. Communicating as well as you can with the impaired person is very important to you in meeting these care goals.

As the caregiver for a person with a dementing illness, you will need to be aware of the person's changing and lessening abilities. You will become an expert in figuring out the impaired person's communications. You will need to judge when the person is or is not fully getting what you and others say. You may well have to set up new ways of communicating with the person.

You will have to be mindful of safety. A person who cannot understand or remember safety warnings runs an increased risk of self-injury and even of injuring others. You must be alert to any problems such as vision or hearing loss which might further impede communication.

Finally, as the person becomes less able to use good judgment, you will need to make all decisions for him or her. The rest of this section offers ideas about where to find help and provides basic guidelines for improving communication.

Improving Communication

Communication means more than talking. Good communication involves three things:

1. active listening
2. the timing and the setting of communication
3. effective self-expression

Active listening: Watching and listening play a big part in good communication. The goal of active listening is to understand not just the words a person says but the meaning the person is trying to get across.

Timing and setting: Some settings make communicating easier, just as certain times seem to be better than others. Be sensitive to potential problems and eliminate distractions.

Effective self-expression: Be sensitive to your own style of communicating. Take note of how you say things. Are you saying what you really mean? Are you saying it clearly and simply? Do you give other messages with your tone of voice, your facial expression, or your body as you talk and listen?

Improving Listening Skills

- **Stop talking.** You can't listen if you are doing all the talking.

- **Be patient.** If a thought is hard or complex, it may take longer for an impaired person to understand or respond. Two or three minutes may be needed before the person can even begin to answer your question. Keep in mind that you can repeat the question or idea after waiting a few minutes for a response.

- **Keep things simple.** Use short sentences and plain words. Avoid complicated questions or directions.

- **Do not interrupt.** The impaired person may need extra time to express what he or she wishes to say. Show interest. Let the person know that you care what he or she is trying to say. Maintain eye contact, and stay near the person.

- **Be gentle and make allowances for poor behavior.** Outbursts are not unusual with this disease, but these are not deliberate. Try to be calm and to use tact, even if the impaired person is loud or abusive. Try to respond to any negative statements with understanding comments until the angry outburst ends. Sometimes the person will say things that hurt you very much, will use language that offends you, or will speak in a way you don't like. At these times, it is important to remember that, while these things do hurt, they are not meant personally.

- **Double-check understanding.** Avoid assuming that the impaired person understands you. The person may even say he or she understands what you have said but still not understand at all. The best way to check understanding is to see what the impaired person does, instead of trusting what he or she says.

Remember: the person will forget. The person will forget things you tell him or her. This can be very frustrating, and there is little that can be done to help it. For your own sake, it is probably best to assume that you will have to repeat many things during the day.

Improving the Setting and Timing

- Make sure the impaired person can see you well. Sit or stand directly in front of the person, and look at him or her when you speak. Avoid glaringly bright or too dark settings.

- Avoid distractions. Communication will be hard, if not impossible, under these circumstances;
  - When the impaired person is involved in some other activity that requires concentration;
  - When the background is noisy (loud street noise, for instance, or the sound of the television or even loud music);
  - When other things or people can attract the impaired person's attention (at shopping centers or restaurants, for example).

- Set aside a quiet place. You may even want to set aside a certain area in your home just for communicating. Try to find a quiet, simple place where you can go when you want to get something across to the impaired person. This could be a separate room or perhaps just a corner.

- Plan ahead, and take extra time. Try to observe the impaired person's daily patterns. Does he or she seem better able to communicate at certain times of day? If so, you can take advantage of good times for important activities and communications. You will also be able to anticipate problems during the bad times, and be prepared to allow extra time for explanations.

Improving Self-Expression

Think ahead about what you will say. Know what information you want to tell or find out, and break this information down into individual parts. You will want to simplify everything as much as possible. For example, give just one direction or piece of information at a time. Ask just one question at a time. Try to think of brief, easy-to-understand words and sentences to explain what you mean, but speak as you would to an adult. Don't talk "baby talk."

Anticipate problems. Be prepared, for example, to repeat yourself many times without losing your temper.

Make eye contact before speaking. Try to sit if the impaired person is sitting or lying down, so you will both be at the same level. Sometimes a gentle touch, if appropriate, can be a way of making sure you have the person's attention before you begin speaking.

Listen to how you sound. Is your voice louder than usual? If so, you may sound angry or upset. Even if the impaired person has a hearing problem, try to speak in a clear, pleasant voice. Speaking slowly and clearly will help. (Once again, though, remember to speak in an adult-to-adult way.)

Watch your "body language." Are you smiling when you speak, or frowning? Are you at ease or tense? If your words and the way you say them do not agree with how you feel and what you really mean, you may very well give a mixed message. Impaired people don't necessarily lose the ability to "read" such non-verbal cues.

306

Living with the Problem

If the person in your care has difficulty communicating, then your role as a caregiver becomes more difficult. You will need to observe closely and adjust to the person's changing abilities. Stay alert to the possible impact on communication of other health, vision, or hearing problems. Managing the day-to-day routine will take more time and effort. Dealing with the person can become frustrating and irritating. If you are upset or angry, the impaired person will almost surely become even more so, making your job even harder. As a result, you will need to develop techniques for coping both with the care problems and with your own feelings.

Retreat from an irritating situation. Try to retreat from an irritating situation for a short break. If that proves impossible, at least promise yourself a reward later for your patience now. It's a good idea to assure the person, over and over, of your love and concern. If you do lose your temper, don't worry needlessly. You may feel sad or guilty about losing your temper in dealing with an impaired person. The impaired person forgets such incidents quickly, and so should you. Just try to make each day go as well as it possibly can for both of you.

Structure the impaired person's day. How well you structure the impaired person's day (and your own) becomes important. A regular routine will be easier for both of you. Be sure to build in time for yourself to take a break. In addition, seek help. Besides working with your health care providers, you will need to create a network of care arrangements to meet both the needs of the impaired person and your own needs. Family members and friends can help, or you might want to consider hiring help occasionally.

Talk with others in similar situations. Finally, remember that talking with others in similar situations can be extremely helpful. Other people may have suggestions, based on your own experiences, for coping with the problems you face. Also, sharing experiences with others should help you keep in mind that such problems do not result from the patients' willful refusal to cooperate. And they don't occur because you are a poor caregiver. The problems are part of the disease itself and of the caregiving role.

You may want to join a support group. The Alzheimer's Disease and Related Disorders Association may be able to help you locate a support group near you. Ask your health care team or a local hospital for a referral. You may not feel at ease in a big group. In this case, you may want to find just one person with whom to talk. This might be someone who is also a caregiver or it might be a professional (like a social worker or a member of the clergy). You might also find smaller groups near you that deal with the problems you are facing.

Section 19.4

Restlessness, Wandering, and Sleep Disturbances

Reprinted with permission "Special Care Problems: Restlessness, Wandering and Sleep Disturbances," © Kenneth Hepburn, Ph.D., Geriatric Research, Education and Clinical Center (GRECC) of the Department of Veterans Affairs Medical Center, Minneapolis, Minnesota.

Many persons with Alzheimer's disease or a related disorder seem to have excess energy. This can show up as restlessness, wandering, and/or disturbed sleep. Each of these can pose special problems for caregivers.

Restlessness and Wandering

Restlessness means fidgeting, not being able to sit still or not being able to stay with one thing for very long. Restlessness is a problem mostly because it may be annoying to others. Wandering, on the other hand, can be a major cause of worry. Wandering poses a real danger. The impaired person might walk out of the house and be hurt or become lost. Restlessness and wandering may have many causes. As the disease progresses, the person's energy level may not decline as fast as his or her abilities do. Restlessness and wandering may result from this excess of energy with nowhere to go. Since the disease damages memory, the person may feel lost and confused most of the time. Wandering and restlessness may be a symptom of the person's anxious search for peace of mind. They may be a sign that the person is frustrated at not being able to express himself or herself. They could also be side effects of drugs the person is taking.

Disturbed Sleep

Most older people no longer need eight hours of sleep each day. Age brings with it a reduced need for sleep. Older persons tend to wake up often and to have lighter sleep. Disturbed sleep may have other direct physical causes. A full bladder, pain, or leg cramps will awaken a person.

When the normal decline in deep sleep mixes with the confusion of dementia, problems may occur. Waking in a dark house, the confused person may wander around and even out of the house. This wandering puts the person at risk of injury. For instance, he or she might fall in the dark. This wandering might also put others in danger. For instance, the person might turn the stove on and then forget to turn it off.

Disturbed sleep has a longer range effect. If an impaired person's sleep is disturbed, the caregiver's sleep is normally disturbed. Both face a serious health threat. Lack of sleep can worsen the symptoms of the illness in the impaired person. It can threaten the caregiver's health and undermine the caregiver's ability to cope and to perform the caregiving tasks.

Some causes of restlessness, wandering, and disturbed sleep will respond to medical treatment. Thus, all problems of this sort should be promptly examined by a doctor. It may be that these behaviors are caused by the progress of the disease and that they will not respond to treatment. Even so, your health care team should have ideas about how to manage and cope with the problem. As a caregiver, you play a key role in helping your health care team look at and solve these problems. You will need to provide detailed reports about the person in your care. You will have to carry out any treatment or care plan and cope with the extra work and worry. You will need to find ways to ensure the impaired person's comfort and safety as well as your own. All these add up to a very hard task. You may need help. Don't be afraid or too shy to ask for it. The rest of this section offers ideas for finding the help you need and for dealing with the problems caused by restlessness, wandering, and disturbed sleep.

Observation and Diagnosis

If the person in your care begins to be restless, wander, or have disturbed sleep, the doctor will want to look at him or her promptly.

This visit will be to make an early diagnosis of the problem. You may then be asked to watch the problem for a while. (Be sure to ask the doctor how you can keep the person safe during this time.) The doctor will tell you what to watch for. You may need to look for signs of a pattern or of a worsening trend. You may be watching for side effects from prescribed drugs. These facts will help the doctor make a final diagnosis. The doctor can then plan the treatment routine with you. As you care for the impaired person, try to observe the patient carefully and answer the following questions. Your doctor may have other questions or comments pertaining to your case.

Questions

- Can you see any pattern in the wandering? (For instance, does the person often go to a certain place or in a certain direction?) Does wandering or restlessness occur at certain times of the day? (Or, does the person normally wake at a certain time of the night?)

- When you first noticed the problem, were there any other changes in the way the person was acting? (For instance, were there changes in mood?)

- Were there any big changes in the home around that time? (Did anyone move in or out? Did anyone in the family die or become ill? Did you acquire new pets or furniture? Were any of the rooms painted?)

- Does anything seem to trigger the restlessness, wandering, or sleep disturbances? (For instance, do they occur when the person needs to go to the bathroom? Do they occur after the person has taken a prescribed drug? What about after having caffeine in drinks like tea, coffee, or cola? Cigarettes or chocolate may also bring on restlessness in some people. Do the problems occur when there are visitors? What about when there is a certain show on TV? Do they seem to have anything to do with the size or timing of meals?)

- Have there been any changes in the kind or amount of food or drink the person consumes? (Keep track of what the person eats and drinks in an average day.)

- Has the person started any new drugs? Has he or she changed the dosage of a drug? Has the person fallen recently?

Note: Be sure your doctor knows all the drugs the person takes, even those bought over-the-counter.

Treatment and Management

Once you have a diagnosis, your doctor can treat any symptoms that can be helped. If a good treatment exists, you may be asked to carry it out at home. Treatment may be simple: cut out all caffeine, for instance. Or you may be asked to give the person drugs and to watch for effects.

The prescribed treatment may not work, or it may solve part of the problem. It may be that there is no real cure for the problem. Times of restlessness or disturbed sleep may just be part of the progressing disease. Still, you and your health care team should work to set up techniques to manage the care problems that remain.

The goal of your caregiving task is to ensure the safety of all and your own peace of mind. A number of techniques which may help you meet this goal are discussed next. These do not involve restraining the impaired person, either with drugs or with physical restraints.

In some cases, your goals may only be achieved by controlling the impaired person's symptoms with the careful use of drugs. Drugs may reduce restlessness or wandering and might help with sleep, but there might be unwanted side effects. Some drugs which slow people down also cause (or worsen) confusion. Discuss this subject with your doctor carefully.

Note: Never give the person over-the-counter medicines or drugs prescribed for you or someone else without talking first with your doctor. The sleeping pill or anti-anxiety pill that works well for you might be all wrong for the impaired person.

Coping Tips

Here are some general ideas for managing problems of restlessness, wandering, and disturbed sleep. Talk these over with your doctor or nurse and make a plan. Then see what works best. If a plan doesn't seem to be working, discuss the problems as well as any new ideas you may want to try. Support group members can also be a valuable source of ideas for managing the problems you are having.

Keep a regular pattern in your life and in the patient's life. Make sure the person gets exercise and eats well. Try to keep the impaired person awake and active during the day. This might help to ensure a

311

restful night. Be sure to include work and recreational activities in the daily routine. For instance, assign sweeping up to the person who is still able to do easy chores around the house. Plan outside events, like taking walks together. Limit the number and length of naps in the daytime. If the person needs rest periods, make them short. In general, try to make the hours before the evening meal the active time and the hours before bedtime the calm time.

Try serving the major meal at midday and avoid large meals at night. Avoid overly fatty or salty foods. To reduce night wakening due to a full bladder, limit the amount the person drinks after dinner. Make sure the person uses the toilet before going to bed. Review the person's problem habits. Use any patterns or cues to predict problems and plan ahead. Do you see any patterns? Does restlessness, for instance, occur at any certain time or in response to any event? Try to cut out any triggering events. Try, also, to figure out ways to distract the person when restlessness or wandering begins.

Set up safeguards in case the person wanders away. Get the person a "medic alert" bracelet. This should include the person's name, address, and phone number. It should also say that the person is "memory impaired."

Let your neighbors and local business owners know that the person may wander. Give them your phone number and ask them to call you if they should see the person out alone. You might want to leave this information (along with a photo of the person) at your local police precinct.

Consider ways to prevent the person from wandering away. There are a number of ways to make it hard to get out of the house or yard. Bells on the doors will let you know when they have been opened. A hard-to-open doorknob (used to childproof doors) may prevent the person from using it. You might want to install on your doors the kind of deadbolt locks that can only be opened with a key. Even an oddly placed latch (up high or down low) may make it hard for the person to use the door. You might put up a sturdy fence around your yard. This would allow the person to wander but keep him or her from wandering off. You might want to try the least costly of these first.

Make sure the person feels safe and at ease. Check the room. Is it too hot or too cold? Is there good light? Is the room calm or noisy? Is too much going on around the person? Think carefully about any changes you make around the house. If the pattern of things changes, the person may become confused and upset.

Seek help. You need to be well and rested. Be sure you take some time away so that you can keep up with your rest. At the very least, take naps when the person in your care naps. Ask friends or family members to take over for you once in a while. Perhaps they can just sit with the person while you sleep. Think about hiring help. Perhaps you can find someone to come into your home, or you might want to arrange for the impaired person to be in a respite care facility for a while.

Living with the Problem

Restlessness, wandering, and disturbed sleep add to your caregiving task. Work with your doctor or nurse to plan coping techniques. If you can, figure out ways to predict and prevent the problem. Also protect your own health and peace of mind. As caregiver, you have a lot on your shoulders. This does not mean you have to do it all yourself. Ask for help.

Don't ignore your own needs and feelings. Dealing with these problems can exhaust you. You may also feel any number of emotions ranging from anger to depression and guilt. Try to keep in mind that these problems are not happening because you are a poor caregiver. These problems are part of the disease itself. Other people have had these problems, so don't feel alone in this. And don't keep these problems and your reactions to yourself. Speak to a friend or family member, a counselor or member of the clergy. Or go to a support group. (The Alzheimer's Disease and Related Disorders Association may be able to help you find a support group near you. Ask your health care team or a local hospital for a referral.) At times like this, sharing what you feel can be very helpful.

Section 19.5

Aggressive and Violent Behavior

Reprinted with permission, "Special Care Problems: Aggressive and Violent Behavior," © Kenneth Hepburn, Ph.D., Geriatric Research, Education and Clinical Center (GRECC) of the Department of Veterans Affairs Medical Center, Minneapolis, Minnesota.

Predicting how an illness like Alzheimer's disease will affect the way a patient behaves is not easy. Some old traits may grow stronger. Others may go away. Sometimes new traits appear. These may be very different from how the person was in the past.

Some of these behaviors or ways of acting may be only odd or annoying. Others may pose very great problems. For instance, sometimes people with dementing illness become hostile and violent. People who have not been violent before may become so for the first time. People who have a history of attacking others may begin to do so even more. Such aggression may take the form of angry shouting or accusing others of wrongdoing. Aggression may also involve physical violence such as breaking household objects or harming others.

Violent behavior is not a frequent symptom of these disorders. It may appear as a phase of the disease and most likely will not go on for the whole course of the disease. Still, phases can last for a long time, sometimes even for years.

Violence seems to be most common in the middle stage of the disease. As the disease progresses, violent outbursts become less frequent. During this middle stage the impaired person is still physically strong, but judgment and memory are failing. The person may be having a hard time doing daily activities, leading to frustration and anger. People with dementing illnesses are easily confused and may be suspicious. They may think that others are trying to do them harm. Other causes of violence include delusions or hallucinations, reactions to drugs, and pain. The person may become violent as a defense against real discomfort (as from being too cold in a bath) or even real abuse (by a substitute caregiver, for instance).

No matter what the cause, outbursts of aggressive or violent behavior are frightening and may be dangerous. They need to be controlled to protect the impaired person and everyone else.

All cases of aggression and violence should be seen promptly by a doctor. Some causes of this behavior may respond to treatment, and the problem may be solved. Even if you learn that the behavior is simply one more part of the disease itself, your health care team may have ideas about how to cope with the problem.

As a caregiver, you play a key role in helping your health care team members learn the nature of this problem and treat or manage it. They rely on your detailed reports about the person in your care. They rely on you to carry out any treatment or care plan.

You are also the one who has to live with the problem. You will have to cope with the extra work, worry, and perhaps embarrassment the problem creates for you. You will need to find ways to ensure the patient's comfort and safety as well as your own. You may even need to restrain him or her.

All these add up to a very hard task. You may need help. Don't be afraid or too shy to ask for it. The rest of this section offers ideas for finding the help you need and for dealing with the problems caused by aggressive or violent behavior.

Observation and Diagnosis

If the person in your care begins to act out of line, the doctor will want to look at him or her promptly. This visit will be to make a tentative diagnosis. Then you may be asked to observe the problem for a period of time. (You should ask the doctor how, during this time, you can ensure your safety and the patient's safety.) The doctor will discuss with you what you should watch for as you observe the patient. You may need to look for signs of a pattern or signs of side effects from prescribed drugs. These facts will help the doctor to make a final diagnosis. The doctor can then plan the treatment routine with you.

As you care for the impaired person, try to observe the patient closely and answer the following questions. Your doctor may have other questions or comments pertaining to your case.

Questions

- Can you see any pattern to the behavior? (For instance, does the behavior occur at any set time of day? Does it occur after the impaired person takes a certain drug? When he or she is hungry? When he or she is frustrated? Or does the behavior seem to come out only with a certain person?).

• When you first noticed the problem, did you notice any other changes in the way the person was acting at that time? (For instance, did the person show a persisting change in mood?).

• Were there any big changes in the home around that time? (Did you move? Did anyone move in or out? Did anyone in the family die or become ill? Did you make any changes in care arrangements?). Has the impaired person started any new drugs or changed drug dosage?

• Has the person suffered a recent injury?

Note: Be sure your doctor knows all the drugs the impaired person takes, even those bought over-the-counter.

Treatment and Management

Once you have a diagnosis, your doctor can treat any symptoms that can be helped. If a good treatment exists, you may be asked to carry it out at home. Treatment may be as simple as setting up rest periods or quiet times or providing small snacks between meals. Or the person may need new drugs to treat a depression which might be causing the combative behavior. You may be asked to watch carefully for the person's responses.

The prescribed treatment may not work, or it may only solve part of the problem. There may be no good treatment for the problem. Outbursts of anger and violence may just be a part of the progressing Alzheimer's disease itself. Even in this case, you and your health care team should work to set up techniques to manage the care problems that remain.

At one level, violent behavior is a care problem like wandering or sleep disturbances. You are faced with a behavior you want to control or change. The behavior is caused by the disease. The person is not acting on purpose or out of spite.

But aggressive or violent behavior may trouble you in ways that other symptoms of the disease don't. In this case, you may find that the person's violent outbursts provoke strong feelings in you. You may feel angry yourself. You may feel guilty, as if you somehow failed or caused the impaired person's reaction. You may be shocked or embarrassed. You may also have to deal with the embarrassment and shock of other people.

Your goal is to ensure the safety—of the impaired person as well as your own safety and peace of mind. A number of techniques are discussed which may help you meet this goal. These do not involve restraining the impaired person, either with drugs or with physical restraints.

In some cases, these goals may only be achieved by resorting to careful use of drugs. Drugs may reduce aggression and violence, but there might be unwanted side effects from some of them. Drugs which calm the patient may also produce sleepiness or increase confusion. Some have more physical side effects, like constipation or dizziness. Usually, doctors prescribe the lowest useful dose of appropriate drugs and attempt to minimize side effects. Discuss this subject with your doctor carefully.

Coping with the Problem

Here are some general ideas for managing problems of aggression and violence without using drugs. Discuss these ideas with your doctor or nurse, and make a plan. Then see what works best. If a plan doesn't seem to be working, call the doctor or nurse back right away to discuss the problems you are having. You should also discuss any new ideas you may want to try. Support groups offer another valuable resource to you. Other members may have good ideas, based on their own experiences, for managing the problems you are facing.

Check the Entire House

Remove from reach any object the person might use as a weapon.

Review the Person's Daily Habits

Take advantage of any patterns or cues to prevent the problem from happening. Some outbursts may just happen, with no pattern or warning. Others may be the endpoint of a slow build-up of tension. Do you see a pattern? Do such behaviors occur at certain times or in reaction to certain events? You may feel more in control if you can predict when problems may occur and avoid things that might trigger the behavior.

Distraction

Set up ways to distract the person when you see a violent outburst coming. Keep a written list of things the person likes (such as going for a walk, listening to music, having a snack) and offer these as diversions.

Seek Help

If you see that these behaviors come on during certain activities (like bathing or dressing), try to get others to help you at these times. Keep handy the phone numbers of neighbors or family members who can help you on short notice. Keeping a list of other emergency phone numbers (police, fire department, doctor, ambulance) by the phone is also a good idea. You may want to look into hiring help, either in-home help or a respite care facility.

Self Protection

If all else fails, protect yourself. Stand out of range and, if you feel that the person may injure you, leave the room.

Physical Restraints

Experts do not agree about physically restraining an impaired person during a violent outburst. If you are strong enough to hold the person and restrain the violent outburst, you might try doing so. The danger is that you might frighten or further anger the person. This could make the situation worse. If the person struggles, there is the chance that one or both of you could be hurt. This matter is best treated case by case. Discuss the matter with your health care team.

Living with the Problem

If the person in your care becomes aggressive or violent, your caregiving role has been enlarged. This is even more the case if the problem cannot be helped by treatment. You need to observe the patterns of the problem and to work with your doctor or nurse to plan techniques for coping. You need to figure out ways to predict and prevent the problem, if you can. Also, you need to protect your own safety and peace of mind and that of others.

Your role of caregiver does not include allowing yourself to be hurt by an impaired person who has become violent. You must be the one who plans, manages, and oversees all care arrangements. Still, your role does not require that you do all of the caregiving. As with other parts of your caregiving task, seek help.

Don't Ignore Your Own Needs

As in all aspects of caregiving, don't ignore your own needs and feelings. Dealing with aggression or violence can frighten and exhaust you. You may feel any number of emotions ranging from anger to depression and guilt. Try to keep in mind that these problems are not happening because you are a poor caregiver. The problems are part of the disease itself. Other people have had these problems, so don't feel alone in this. And don't keep these problems and your reactions to yourself. Speak to a friend or family member, a counselor or member of the clergy. Or go to a support group. (The Alzheimer's Disease and Related Disorders Association) may be able to help you find a support group near you. Ask your health care team or a local hospital for a referral.) At times like this, sharing what you feel can be very helpful.

Chapter 20

Brain Injury

Susan's Story

Susan was 7 years old when she was hit by a car while riding her bike. She broke her arm and leg. She also hit her head very hard. The doctors say she sustained a traumatic brain injury. When she came home from the hospital, she needed lots of help, but now she looks fine.

In fact, that's part of the problem, especially at school. Her friends and teachers think her brain has healed because her broken bones have. But there are changes in Susan that are hard to understand. It takes Susan longer to do things. She has trouble remembering things. She can't always find the words she wants to use. Reading is hard for her now. It's going to take time before people really understand the changes they see in her.

What Is Traumatic Brain Injury (TBI)?

A traumatic brain injury (TBI) is an injury to the brain caused by the head being hit by something or shaken violently. This injury can change how the person acts, moves, and thinks. A traumatic brain

"Traumatic Brain Injury Fact Sheet," Fact Sheet Number 18, National Information Center for Children and Youth with Disabilities (NICHCY), March 2000; and reprinted with permission "The Positive Approach to Coping with Life after Brain Injury," by Carolyn Rocchio, © *Family News & Views*, Vol. 4, No. 6, June 1997.

injury can also change how a student learns and acts in school. The term TBI is used for head injuries that can cause changes in one or more areas, such as:

- thinking and reasoning,
- understanding words,
- remembering things,
- paying attention,
- solving problems,
- thinking abstractly,
- talking,
- behaving,
- walking and other physical activities,
- seeing and/or hearing, and
- learning.

The term TBI is not used for a person who is born with a brain injury. It also is not used for brain injuries that happen during birth.

The following definition of TBI comes from the Individuals with Disabilities Education Act (IDEA). The IDEA is the federal law that guides how schools provide special education and related services to children and youth with disabilities.

IDEA's Definition of TBI

Our nation's special education law, the Individuals with Disabilities Education Act (IDEA) defines traumatic brain injury as

"...an acquired injury to the brain caused by an external physical force, resulting in total or partial functional disability or psychosocial impairment, or both, that adversely affects a child's educational performance. The term applies to open or closed head injuries resulting in impairments in one or more areas, such as cognition; language; memory; attention; reasoning; abstract thinking; judgment; problem-solving; sensory, perceptual, and motor abilities; psycho-social behavior; physical functions; information processing; and speech. The term does not apply to brain injuries that are congenital or degenerative, or to brain injuries induced by birth trauma." 34 Code of Federal Regulations §300.7(12).

How Common Is TBI?

More than one million children receive brain injuries each year. More than 30,000 of these children have lifelong disabilities as a result of the brain injury.

What Are the Signs of TBI?

The signs of brain injury can be very different depending on where the brain is injured and how severely. Children with TBI may have one or more difficulties, including:

- **Physical disabilities:** Individuals with TBI may have problems speaking, seeing, hearing, and using their other senses. They may have headaches and feel tired a lot. They may also have trouble with skills such as writing or drawing. Their muscles may suddenly contract or tighten (this is called spasticity). They may also have seizures. Their balance and walking may also be affected. They may be partly or completely paralyzed on one side of the body, or both sides.

- **Difficulties with thinking:** Because the brain has been injured, it is common that the person's ability to use the brain changes. For example, children with TBI may have trouble with short-term memory (being able to remember something from one minute to the next, like what the teacher just said). They may also have trouble with their long-term memory (being able to remember information from a while ago, like facts learned last month). People with TBI may have trouble concentrating and only be able to focus their attention for a short time. They may think slowly. They may have trouble talking and listening to others. They may also have difficulty with reading and writing, planning, understanding the order in which events happen (called sequencing), and judgment.

- **Social, behavioral, or emotional problems:** These difficulties may include sudden changes in mood, anxiety, and depression. Children with TBI may have trouble relating to others. They may be restless and may laugh or cry a lot. They may not have much motivation or much control over their emotions.

A child with TBI may not have all of the above difficulties. Brain injuries can range from mild to severe, and so can the changes that result from the injury. This means that it's hard to predict how an individual will recover from the injury. Early and ongoing help can make a big difference in how the child recovers. This help can include physical or occupational therapy, counseling, and special education.

It's also important to know that, as the child grows and develops, parents and teachers may notice new problems. This is because, as students grow, they are expected to use their brain in new and different ways. The damage to the brain from the earlier injury can make it hard for the student to learn new skills that come with getting older. Sometimes parents and educators may not even realize that the student's difficulty comes from the earlier injury.

What about School?

Although TBI is very common, many medical and education professionals may not realize that some difficulties can be caused by a childhood brain injury. Often, students with TBI are thought to have a learning disability, emotional disturbance, or mental retardation. As a result, they don't receive the type of educational help and support they really need.

When children with TBI return to school, their educational and emotional needs are often very different than before the injury. Their disability has happened suddenly and traumatically. They can often remember how they were before the brain injury. This can bring on many emotional and social changes. The child's family, friends, and teachers also recall what the child was like before the injury. These other people in the child's life may have trouble changing or adjusting their expectations of the child.

Therefore, it is extremely important to plan carefully for the child's return to school. Parents will want to find out ahead of time about special education services at the school. This information is usually available from the school's principal or special education teacher. The school will need to evaluate the child thoroughly. This evaluation will let the school and parents know what the student's educational needs are. The school and parents will then develop an Individualized Education Program (IEP) that addresses those educational needs.

It's important to remember that the IEP is a flexible plan. It can be changed as the parents, the school, and the student learn more about what the student needs at school.

Tips for Parents

- Learn about TBI. The more you know, the more you can help yourself and your child. See the list of resources and organizations at the end of this chapter.

- Work with the medical team to understand your child's injury and treatment plan. Don't be shy about asking questions. Tell them what you know or think. Make suggestions.

- Keep track of your child's treatment. A 3-ring binder or a box can help you store this history. As your child recovers, you may meet with many doctors, nurses, and others. Write down what they say. Put any paperwork they give you in the notebook or throw it in the box. You can't remember all this! Also, if you need to share any of this paperwork with someone else, make a copy. Don't give away your original!

- Talk to other parents whose children have TBI. There are parent groups all over the U.S. Parents can share practical advice and emotional support. Call NICHCY (1-800-695-0285) to find out how to find parent groups near you.

- If your child was in school before the injury, plan for his or her return to school. Get in touch with the school. Ask the principal about special education services. Have the medical team share information with the school.

- When your child returns to school, ask the school to test your child as soon as possible to identify his or her special education needs. Meet with the school and help develop a plan for your child called an Individualized Education Program (IEP).

- Keep in touch with your child's teacher. Tell the teacher about how your child is doing at home. Ask how your child is doing in school.

Tips for Teachers

- Find out as much as you can about the child's injury and his or her present needs. Find out more about TBI. See the list of resources and organizations at the end of this chapter.

- Give the student more time to finish schoolwork and tests.

- Give directions one step at a time. For tasks with many steps, it helps to give the student written directions.

- Show the student how to perform new tasks. Give examples to go with new ideas and concepts.

- Have consistent routines. This helps the student know what to expect. If the routine is going to change, let the student know ahead of time.

- Check to make sure that the student has actually learned the new skill. Give the student lots of opportunities to practice the new skill.

- Show the student how to use an assignment book and a daily schedule. This helps the student get organized.

- Realize that the student may get tired quickly. Let the student rest as needed.

- Reduce distractions.

- Keep in touch with the student's parents. Share information about how the student is doing at home and at school.

- Be flexible about expectations. Be patient. Maximize the student's chances for success.

Resources

DeBoskey, D.S. (Ed.). (1996). *Coming home: A discharge manual for families of persons with a brain injury.* Houston, TX: HDI. (Telephone: 800-321-7037; 713-526-6900.)

DePompei, R., Blosser, J., Savage, R., & Lash, M. (1998). *Special education: IEP checklist for a student with a brain injury.* Wolfeboro, NH: L&A Publishing/Training.

DePompei, R., & Cluett, B. (1998). *All about me!* Wolfeboro, NH: L&A Publishing/Training. (For use by elementary school children with TBI.)

Glang, A., Singer, G.H.S., & Todis, B. (1997). *Students with acquired brain injury: The school's response.* Baltimore, MD: Paul H. Brookes. (Telephone: 800-638-3775.)

Lash, M. (1998). *Resource guide: Children and adolescents with brain injuries.* Wolfeboro, NH: L&A Publishing/Training.

Lash, M., Wolcott, G., & Pearson, S. (1995). *Signs and strategies for educating students with brain injuries: A practical guide for teachers and schools.* Houston, TX: HDI. (Telephone: 800-321-7037; 713-526-6900.)

Savage, R. (1995). *An educator's manual: What educators need to know about students with TBI (3rd ed.).* Houston, TX: HDI. (See phone number above.)

Snyder, H. (1998). *Elvin the elephant who forgets.* Wolfeboro, NH: L&A Publishing/Training. (A 16-page picture book for children.)

Ylvisaker, M. (1998). *Collaborative brain injury intervention: Positive everyday routines.* San Diego, CA: Singular Publishers. (Telephone: 800-521-8545.)

The Positive Approach to Coping with Life after Brain Injury

Brain injury is a major public health problem worldwide, and when it occurs, it intrudes upon the lives of every member of an extended family. Just as the person who is injured is changed, all others who care about that individual are affected in a variety of ways, some positively, while others negatively. What are some of the forces at work that help people cope with these inevitable changes? When speaking with survivors of brain injury and their families, I found that there are many commonly shared ideas about getting through catastrophic situations in an emotionally and physically healthy manner. Some recommendations worth considering follow.

Many families immediately respond that faith helped them through the recovery of a loved one. Some families with no religious affiliation and little or no experience with prayer found that when faced with tragedy involving a family member or dear friend, they found themselves praying, possibly for the first time.

The healing power of prayer is universally accepted as the first line of defense for "believers," and recent studies support the theory that faith influences the body. "The mind and body used to be considered separate realms," says S. Bryant Kendrick, associate professor of internal medicine at Bowman Gray School of Medicine, Wake Forest University in Winston-Salem, N.C. (Goodwin p. 83). Just as stress increases the production of hormones that affect the immune system, so also does the mind over body theory hold true when dealing with other life events.

327

The federal government has funded 43 medical studies on spirituality and religion as therapy, and even the prestigious *Journal of the American Medical Association* has shown interest in the subject by asking its readers if prayer or participation in religious observances should be recommended when prescribing for patients. The National Institute of Health care Research (NIHR), a think tank, has initiated a project called "Faith and Medicine" to educate medical students in the value of spirituality in patient care and promote additional research in this area. Thirty of our 126 medical schools now offer courses in faith and medicine. We are coming closer to a time when the two previously diverse subjects are becoming recognized as equal components for improving health and well-being.

A San Francisco cardiologist conducted a study in 1988 of patients admitted to his cardiac care unit. In a double-blind study, half of the patients were randomly selected to be prayed for by persons they had never met. All patients were receiving standard cardiac care, but the other half were not prayed for by large numbers of persons other than their families. The recovery was astounding in the group receiving prayers—they experienced fewer complications, fewer cardiopulmonary arrests, and less pneumonia.

An interesting statistic compiled by the Gallup Poll in 1994 indicates that 96 percent of Americans believe in God; however, the American Psychiatric Association published a report in 1989 indicating that only 43 percent of therapists believe in God. And the *Journal of Family Medicine* reported in 1990 that 50 percent of individuals polled wanted their doctors to pray with them.

In addition to faith as a major component promoting healing, many families talked about humor and a positive attitude as a force that sustained them through difficult times. There is certainly nothing funny about brain injury, but finding reasons to smile each day is a factor in health and raises the level of optimism. Experts in child behavior agree that laughing and having fun with your kids increases their self-esteem, teaches them social skills, and helps them establish positive peer relationships. (Ford) If in fact that statement is true, then it stands to reason that finding ways to approach our problems with humor and greater optimism should reduce the negative impact and allow us to deal more effectively with them. I know that humor is a significant factor in my son's ability to cope with his life changes after brain injury. Always a laid-back casual guy, he found many opportunities to laugh at himself during his recovery and throughout the last 15 years of living with brain injury.

He was the family comedian with a knack for the ridiculous; he was an uninhibited show-off, but also very manipulative. For example, in the midst of having the riot act read to him for some indiscretion, he would envelope me in a bear hug and plant a sloppy kiss on my forehead. It was hard to stay mad at him for any length of time, even while being manipulated.

As he lay in a coma after his brain injury, I tried to find ways to stimulate him, to coax him into consciousness, but most of all maintain my own sanity by feeling I was fulfilling an important mission at his bedside. I told him jokes, read MAD magazine, and told him about the latest skit from Saturday Night Live, a show he faithfully watched with his sisters. Once he moved out of the ICU and could have visitors, I made sure his friends were prepared for his appearance (trach, G-tube, and a variety of other unfamiliar medical trappings), and that they came often and always with an upbeat attitude. Whether or not the atmosphere we created changed the course of Tim's recovery remains to be seen, because there is little evidence that persons can be awakened from coma by external means. However, we were rewarded when he smiled for the first time on the 71st day post-injury. The smile gradually took shape as he thumb-wrestled with a visiting friend. We played finger games frequently to keep his hands and fingers from contracting. I recorded this event in my daily journal as a red letter day. Although no sound accompanied the smile, it encouraged us immensely. We hoped it was the beginning of the return of the Tim we knew best—always smiling.

One of the most talked about examples of the healing quality of humor is the story of Fulton Oursler, a former editor of *Reader's Digest*, who when diagnosed with an incurable illness simply decided that he wasn't ready to die. He rented a suite at a hotel, assembled all of the films of the Marx Brothers, Abbott and Costello, Ritz Brothers, Charlie Chaplin, and all other comedians, shut himself off from the rest of the world, laughed and put all cares of the world aside. His health gradually improved.

Over the years, I have been amazed about ways families manage catastrophic events. Those whose energies are spent in more positive and upbeat ways, such as praying for survival and hopeful outcomes, viewing life from the perspective of the half-full versus half-empty glass, seem to survive with less emotional scars than others whose negativity seems to sabotage efforts to improve outcome. In the 15 years I have dealt with my son's injury, and my 14-year involvement with the Brain Injury Association, I have been privileged to meet and form friendships with some of the most optimistic and fulfilled people

I know. They are the movers and shakers of the brain injury movement, and they are the backbone of support group development and advocacy. You won't find sad faces at a brain injury conference. You'll find people from all walks of life pursuing their goals in a positive and forward-thinking mode.

It's not to say that all prayers are answered, or that feeling the need to act happy when you're not will result in the good life. However, the "whatever works for you" strategy does make one an active participant in the outcome. Problems will accompany us wherever we go, but it's a less-rocky road if we trod it with faith and find ways to laugh off the heartaches we experience.

References

1. Ford J: The family that laughs together. *Family Circle*. 2/18/97:86.

2. Goodwin J.: The healing power of prayer. *Family Circle*. 1/9/96:82-85.

Organizations

Brain Injury Association
(formerly the National Head Injury Foundation)
105 North Alfred Street
Alexandria, VA 22314
Toll-Free: 800-444-6443; Tel: 703-236-6000
Website: http://www.biausa.org
E-mail: FamilyHelpline@biausa.org

Emergency Medical Services for Children–
National Resource Center
111 Michigan Avenue N.W.
Washington, DC 20010-2970
Tel: 202-884-4927

Epilepsy Foundation–National Office
4351 Garden City Drive, Suite 500
Landover, MD 20785
Toll-Free: 800-332-1000; Tel: 301-459-3700
TTY: 800-332-2070
Website: http://www.efa.org
E-Mail: postmaster@efa.org

Family Caregiver Alliance
690 Market Street, Suite 600
San Francisco, CA 94104
Tel: 415-434-3388
Website: http://www.caregiver.org

Family Voices
P.O. Box 769
Algodones, NM 87001
Tel: 505-867-2368
Website: http://www.familyvoices.org
E-mail: kidshealth@familyvoices.org

Head Injury Hotline
212 Pioneer Building
Seattle, WA 98104-2221
Tel: 206-621-8558
Website: http://www.headinjury.com
E-mail: brain@headinjury.com

National Information Center for Children and Youth with Disabilities
P.O. Box 1492
Washington, DC 20013
Toll-Free (Voice/TTY): 800-695-0285
Fax: 202-884-8441
Website: http://www.nichcy.org
E-mail: nichcy@aed.org

Chapter 21

Cancer

Overview

Understanding the Problem

- Caregivers are problem-solvers
- Caregivers work as team members
- Caregivers work to have a positive attitude
- Caregivers take care of themselves

When to Get Professional Help for Yourself

- If you are experiencing severe anxiety or depression, feeling overwhelmed, or don't know who to call for help
- If communication between you and the patient with advanced cancer has broken down
- If your relationship with the patient has a history of abuse, addiction, or conflict

What You Can Do to Be a Supportive Caregiver

- Work and communicate effectively with the patient

Reprinted with permission, "ACP Home Care Guide for Advanced Cancer–Caregiving," © 1997 The American College of Physicians; and excerpts from "Advanced Cancer," National Cancer Institute, NIH Publication #98-856, revised September 1998.

- Support the patient's spiritual concerns
- Help to resolve the patient's unfinished business
- Work with health professionals
- Work with family and friends
- Take care of your own needs and feelings

Possible Obstacles

- "He doesn't want to talk about feelings."
- "What if she talks about things that I don't want to hear?"
- "She won't follow my advice."
- "I don't have time to take care of my own needs."
- "If I don't do it, it won't get done."
- "I hate asking other people to help me."
- "The person I'm helping doesn't want anyone else to help."

Carrying Out and Adjusting Your Plan

- Use the strategies in this guide
- Be realistic in your expectations for sharing feelings
- Be realistic in your expectations about yourself
- Ask for help before you feel overwhelmed

Topics with a flag (➤) in front of them are actions you can take or symptoms you can look for.

Understanding the Problem

- The information in this chapter fits most situations, but yours may be different.
- If the doctor or nurse tells you to do something other than what is recommended here, follow what they say.
- If you think that there may be a medical emergency, see "When to Get Professional Help for Yourself."

Caregivers Are Problem-Solvers

Caregiving involves solving problems. You have been solving problems throughout your entire life, but many of the problems that come with advanced cancer are new to you and the person you are helping. This chapter will help both of you to solve these new problems, giving information and guidance that are organized into specific steps for you to take.

The individual plans in this chapter are designed to help you solve problems, but you, the patient, and his or her family and friends will actually solve the problems yourselves. You decide what actions to take. You adjust the plans to meet your special situation. You carry out the plans, and you monitor how well they are working and make changes as they are needed. You also must develop new plans on your own to deal with any problems not mentioned here.

You and the person you are helping are in charge of dealing with your problems. You are not people simply following instructions; you are people making decisions and taking actions.

You Are a Member of a Team

Good palliative care requires a team of people with different skills and perspectives. Nurses, physicians, social workers, and clergy make important and unique contributions to palliative care, but family members, friends, and hospice volunteers also are important contributors. You already have (or will develop) a close, personal relationship with the person who is ill—so you will play a key role when involving this person in his or her own care. Your relationship will help you to understand and interpret the feelings, desires, and needs of the person who is ill. You will be the first to become aware of many physical and emotional problems, the first to deal with those problems, and often the person who will carry out the plans that you and other team members develop.

As a team member, your job is to work cooperatively with other members to solve caregiving problems. To do this, you need to use the COPE problem-solving method. You need to collect facts, get expert information and guidance about what to do, develop a plan for dealing with the problem, and then carry out that plan while keeping the other team members informed. You need to have an optimistic and a realistic attitude, and as much as possible, you need to keep the patient both informed and involved in what is done.

Work to Have a Positive Attitude

Emphasize the positive parts of caregiving. For example, some successful caregivers see their work as helping someone they love and care for deeply. Others see caregiving in a spiritual way—"I think this is part of God's plan for me." Still others feel that caregiving has enriched their lives, and some see it as a challenge and want to do the best job they can. In addition, some people view caregiving as a way of showing appreciation for the love and care they have received from those who now need their help. Caregiving can have important benefits. It can give you a sense of satisfaction and confidence, and families who perform caregiving often feel closer to each other and to the person who is ill. You also may discover inner strengths you never realized you had.

You can use the illness to open doors to new friends and relationships as well. This can happen through talking with other people who have faced the same problems, meeting people at a support group, meeting people who have volunteered to help with caregiving, and from family members and old friends who have grown distant but are drawn together again because of the illness.

Take Care of Yourself

Helping someone with advanced cancer can be difficult and stressful, but the more you take care of your own needs for rest, food, enjoyment, and relaxation, the better you will be able to help.

Your goals

- To be an effective team player working not only with the patient but with health professionals, family members, and friends in solving home care problems.

- To care for your own needs during the illness so that you will have the emotional strength to be an effective caregiver.

When to Get Professional Help for Yourself

Many people need help with caregiving. Some prefer family and friends for this, but others want hired help from local agencies or private duty services. Even with additional helpers, however, you may find that keeping someone with advanced cancer at home is not the best idea. Ask health professionals, clergy, or other professionals for help if any of the following conditions exist:

➤ **You are experiencing severe anxiety or depression.**

➤ **Communication between you and the patient has broken down or become painful and difficult.**

The stresses that come with advanced cancer—physical, psychological, financial, and emotional—can hamper your ability to communicate with the person you are caring for. If the levels of anxiety and stress have risen to the point where you cannot talk openly about important issues, get professional help from a member of the clergy, a hospice staff member, home health staff member, counselor, or social worker.

➤ **Your relationship with the patient is affected by a history of abuse, addiction, or conflict.**

Caregivers who have suffered through verbal, mental, physical, or sexual abuse from the person they are caring for, or for whom alcohol or drug addiction has affected their relationship, are likely to have serious problems in caregiving. They already have strong and deep-seated negative feelings, usually built up over many years, and this situation calls for professional help from the start.

➤ **You feel overwhelmed and unsure if you can manage at home.**

This is a common concern. Ask for help from nurses or social workers at the hospice, clinic, or doctor's office you have visited. They can assist you in getting the help that you need.

➤ **You don't know who to call for extra help at home.**

Call the hospice, home health agency, or department of social work at the hospital you use, and explain your concerns. They may refer you to a local agency or have a visiting nurse or social worker come out and speak with you.

➤ **You want to know the pros and cons of moving someone to a nursing home or other setting.**

➤ **You feel badly yourself, or very "down" and alone.**

What You Can Do to Be a Supportive Caregiver

Work and Communicate Effectively with the Patient

This is your most important and challenging job. The person you are caring for must deal with the physical effects of the disease and medicine as well as the psychological and social challenges of living with advanced cancer. This may make it difficult for the patient to participate in the home care plan. Nonetheless, your job is to involve as much as possible the person you are caring for in making decisions and carrying out the plan. You should support the person's efforts to deal with the reality of the prognosis emotionally, and this includes efforts to:

➤ Help the person to accept that he or she has advanced cancer.

Some people with advanced cancer deal with upsetting news by pretending that it simply did not happen. This can be healthy when it helps them to live as normal a life as possible. It can be harmful, however, if they do things that make the illness worse, such as avoiding medicine or engaging in activities that are physically harmful.

Sometimes, what looks like "denial" is the patient's attempt to protect loved ones from what is really happening. If this is the case, reassure the person that you are willing to listen and talk about all aspects of the illness—even though it may be hard for both of you.

Support the patient's efforts to live as normal a life as possible, but if he or she is pretending that nothing is wrong, you need to be clear in your own mind about what is really happening. This is when your own objectivity is important in making sure that the patient is benefiting from his or her pretending and not doing things that could be harmful.

➤ Create a climate that encourages and supports sharing feelings.

Talk about important or sensitive topics in a time and place that is calm and conducive to open communication—not in the midst of a crisis or family argument. If your family usually talks around the dinner table, that is the proper time. Think about when you have had important talks in the past, and try to recreate that setting.

Communicate your availability. One of the most important messages you can give to the person you are caring is this: "If you want to discuss this uncomfortable issue, I'm willing to do it." Leave the timing up to the patient, however. To the greatest extent possible, leave decisions on what feelings to share as well as when, how, and with whom to share them up to the patient. By not pressing the issue, you allow the person with advanced cancer to retain control over part of his or her life at a time when many issues and decisions no longer are.

➤ Understand that men and women often communicate in different ways, and make allowance for those differences.

Although there are many exceptions, women often express their feelings more openly than men in our society. If you are a male caregiver and the person you are caring for is a woman, be aware that when she shares her feelings, you may find yourself giving advice when she wants support and understanding instead. If you are a female caregiver and the person you are caring for is male, be aware that he may express his feelings differently than you would, and pay special attention when he talks about things that are important to him.

➤ Be realistic and flexible about what you hope to agree on or communicate.

People with advanced cancer want to share many things, but they may not share them all with just one person. Let the patient talk about whatever he or she wants with whomever he or she wants. If the patient isn't telling you everything, this is fine as long as he or she is telling somebody the rest. Also, remember that a person may have spent a lifetime developing a particular style of communication, and this will not change overnight. Some people, both men and women, have never talked about their feelings. Try to accept that this pattern most likely will not change even now.

Sharing does not always mean talking, either. The person with advanced cancer may feel more comfortable writing about feelings or expressing them through an activity. He or she may express feelings in other nonverbal ways as well, such as through gestures or expressions, touching, or just asking that you be present.

➤ Help the patient to deal with anxiety and depression.

People with advanced cancer may become anxious because of worries about medical procedures, their cancer, or the future. Their anxiety also may be a side effect of medicine they are taking or even of the cancer itself.

Many people feel depressed at some time during their illness. Seek advice on how to control depressing thoughts and feelings, especially when they are just beginning.

When You and the Patient Disagree on Important Issues

Remember that you and the person you are caring for do not always have to agree. You may disagree on issues such as when, how, and what to share, but remember that this is one of the patterns of life and cannot always be resolved. Then this is the case, the following suggestions may prove useful:

➤ Explain your needs openly.

Sometimes, you may need to ask the patient to do something that will make your own life easier or your caregiving responsibilities more manageable; for example, you will want to know when any pain begins rather than when it becomes very severe. These situations can create conflict, and you should understand that conflict resolution does not always mean that everybody is happy. On some issues, you will have to give in. On others, you will have to ask the person you are caring for to give.

➤ Suggest a trial run or time limit.

If you want the person you are caring for to try something, such as a new bed or a certain medication schedule, and he or she is resisting, ask the person to try it for a limited time, such as a week, and then evaluate the situation. This avoids making the patient feel locked into a decision. If the person resists writing a will or power of attorney, ask if he or she will at least read one over and discuss it.

➤ Choose your battles carefully.

Ask yourself what is really important. Are you being stubborn on an issue because you need to win an argument or be in control? You can save both time and energy by skipping the minor conflicts and using your influence on issues that really count.

➤ Let the patient make as many of his or her decisions as possible.

A good example of letting a patient make his or her own decisions is when adult children living some distance away from the person with cancer want to move him or her into a nursing home. Although moving to a nursing home may make the adult children feel better, it may not be what the person with cancer wants. If the patient understands the consequences, such as that no one may be around to help if he or she falls, then the caregiver should accept the patient's right to make that decision. Taking away someone's ability to make decisions can undermine his or her feelings of control, which in turn interferes with the person's ability to deal with other aspects of this stressful illness.

Support the Patient's Spiritual Concerns

Spiritual concerns raise fundamental questions about life. Why are we here? What is a good life? What happens after death? These profound questions become especially important as life nears its end. As a caregiver, you can support the patient in thinking about his or her own answers to these questions.

Spiritual questions are not answered easily, of course. For those people whose faith gives answers and comfort, your support of that faith will be both helpful and appreciated. For those who are troubled by uncertainty, you can help by sharing your own questions and uncertainties—showing that their concerns are normal and reasonable. If you can admit to the possibility, it may be helpful to say that not all spiritual questions can be answered. It also may useful to ask about beliefs that were helpful to the patient before this illness and if they can be helpful again now.

Professionals such as clergy or counselors who have experience helping people with spiritual problems near the end of life can be very comforting to the person you are caring for—provided that he or she wants their help. Spiritual questions are very personal; therefore, the person with these concerns is the one who knows best who can help. Bringing in someone who is not wanted can backfire and cause rather than resolve problems. Let the person you are caring for know that you will be happy to arrange visits by clergy or others who could help—but that this decision is entirely up to him or her. Do not expect all clergy to be equally skilled in working with people during the last stage of life, however. If one is not helpful, keep looking until you find one who is. Hospice or palliative care staff can help you locate someone with the necessary skills, and hospital chaplains usually are experienced in working with people near the end of their lives and may be able to help.

If the patient is seriously depressed because of spiritual concerns, seek help from a mental health professional or clergy with training in mental health care. Also, be available to listen. Speaking with another person who is understanding helps to put one's thoughts in perspective and also to see that others appreciate and understand them. The person with advanced cancer may want to make sense of life his or her experiences—to reminisce, talk about the past, and look for meaning in what has happened. As a caregiver, listening is the most important thing you can do to help. Let the person you are caring for know about your willingness and availability for these discussions when and if he or she wants them. If you find it very difficult to listen to the patient's concerns, then find someone, such as a member of the clergy, family member, or friend, who can.

For people whose religion is very important and gives meaning to both their lives and their dying, you can help by asking questions that allow them to tell you, if they wish, what about their faith has helped them through life and is helping them now. You must be careful to accept and respect views that are different from your own, however. Let them tell you if there are ways you can encourage and support them in their faith. Would they like to listen to a tape of hymns or other religious music? Is there a religious symbol that would bring them comfort? Would they like to share with clergy from their faith one of their traditions, such as a bedside prayer service?

Share your views and feelings when you are asked or think that he or she would like to ask. Hearing another person's thoughts and feelings can be helpful to someone who is troubled by spiritual problems, but always let the person you are caring for be your guide— never impose. Sometimes, reading together from spiritual writings can be comforting and may help to resolve unanswered or unresolved questions. These readings also can provide an opportunity to share how you feel about these issues as well.

You may be worried yourself about spiritual questions. Watching and helping someone who is dying sometimes can bring up very difficult issues. These may be about the unfairness of the situation, fear about what will happen to the person you are caring for after his or her death, fears about your own death, and general confusion and anxiety about what life is about. Talking with clergy, counselors, hospice staff, or health professionals who work with the family and friends of dying people can be very helpful. They have experience helping those like yourself. They will listen and help you to think through these issues. You may find it easier to talk to some people more than others, and you also may find that some are more helpful than others. If the first people you talk to cannot help you, keep looking until you find the person who can.

Help to Resolve the Patient's Unfinished Business

People near the end of their life commonly want to take certain actions or have certain experiences before they die. Sometimes, it is to do or see something important or pleasant again, such as being with friends or visiting an especially meaningful place. Sometimes, it is to say things to someone that have been unsaid in the past or to resolve some old misunderstanding or conflict. Arranging for these experiences can be substantial undertakings, involving contacting other people and organizing long-distance travel.

Do not expect that the experiences you arrange will always be successful. Even with the best of intentions, things may not happen as you or the person you are caring for would like. The weather may be less than ideal for the trip. The people you work hard to bring together may not say helpful things once they arrive. When it is over, both of you may be disappointed. The fact that you tried, however, can be very important—and this may make all of the effort worthwhile. Before committing to such a major undertaking, ask yourself how you and the person being cared for would feel if the experience is less than you hope. Would it still be worth the time and resources? If your answer is no, ask what you could do that would be less costly or stressful. If your answer is yes, then move ahead (with realistic expectations).

Working with Health Professionals

Here are some practical suggestions to keep in mind when you need information and help from health professionals:

➤ **Be clear about what you want, and get to the point as soon as possible.**

Make lists of questions and concerns, and have them in front of you when you talk with health professionals.

➤ **Have all the information that health professionals may need ready when you call.**

Try to think ahead about what information medical staff may need, and try to have it ready when you call.

➤ **Write down the answers.**

This will ensure that you have the information correct and do not forget it. Have paper and a pencil ready when you call. It is good to keep your questions and answers together in a file or drawer where you can easily find and review them.

▶ **Be firm and straightforward about getting the information and the help that you need.**

Health professionals are there to help you be a good caregiver, so make your requests with confidence that you will get the help you need. Feel free to tell them when you do not understand. Remain calm, and speak in a pleasant, polite voice. Being angry usually is not helpful. Being pleasant, firm, persistent, and showing your appreciation usually are the best strategies.

Working with Family and Friends

▶ **Do not try to do everything yourself. Ask for help.**

Family members, friends, clergy, and people who belong to community organizations all can help you. Some can help with planning, and others can help with carrying out those plans and giving support.

People who live in the same household or are going to be very involved in carrying out a plan should help in developing it, and they should read and understand this guide. Then, they will be able to work with you and the patient as a team. If they have had a hand in its development, they will be more committed to carrying out the plan.

Others may want to help but need to be told how. It is important to be clear with these people about what you would like them to do as well as the limits of what is expected of them.

Taking Care of Your Own Needs and Feelings

You need to be at your best if you are to provide the best care. Therefore, pay attention to your own needs as well as those of the person you are helping. Set limits on what you can reasonably expect yourself to do. Take time off to care for yourself, and ask for help before stress builds.

It is natural to have strong feelings when you are helping someone with a serious illness. Some common feelings that caregivers have as well as strategies for dealing with them if they become severe are:

Feeling Overwhelmed

Caregivers as well as the person being cared for can feel overwhelmed and confused when they learn that the disease is not responding to treatment or is progressing. Here are some ways to deal with feeling overwhelmed:

➤ Try not to make important decisions while you are upset.

Sometimes, you must make decisions immediately, but you often do not have to. Ask the doctor, nurse, or social worker how long before a decision needs to be made.

➤ Take time to sort things out.

➤ Talk over important problems with others who are feeling more level-headed and rational.

If you are feeling very upset or discouraged, ask a friend, neighbor, or family member to help. They can bring a calmer perspective to the situation as well as new ideas, and they can help you in dealing with the problems that you face.

Anger

There are plenty of reasons for you to become angry while caring for a person with advanced cancer. For example, the person you are caring for may be demanding or irritating at times. Friends, family members, or professionals may not be as helpful or understanding as you would like. Some people grow angry because they feel their religion has let them down. It is natural to be angry when your life has been turned inside out, which often happens with a serious illness like cancer.

These feelings are normal. What is important is what you do with them, not that you feel them in the first place. The best way to deal with angry feelings is to recognize them, accept them, and find some way to express them appropriately. If you do not deal with your anger, it can get in the way of almost everything you do.

Here are some ways to deal with your anger:

➤ Try to see the situation from the other person's point of view, and understand why he or she acted that way.

Recognize that other people are under stress as well, and that some people deal with stressful situations better than others.

➤ Express your anger in an appropriate way before it becomes too severe.

If you wait until your anger is severe, it will impair your judgment, and you are likely to make other people angry in return.

➤ Get away from the situation for awhile.

Try to cool off before you go back and deal with what made you angry.

➤ Find safe ways to express your anger.

This can include beating on a pillow, yelling out loud in a car or closed room, or doing some hard and vigorous exercise. Sometimes, it helps to vent anger with someone who is "safe"—someone who will not be offended or strike back, like a friend or member of the clergy.

➤ Talk to someone about why you feel angry.

Explaining to another person why you feel angry often helps you to understand why you reacted as you did, allowing you to see your reactions in perspective.

Fear

You may become afraid when someone you care for deeply has a serious illness. You do not know what is in store for this person or for yourself, and you may fear that you will not be able to handle what happens. Here are some ways to deal with your fears:

➤ Learn as much as possible about what is happening and what may happen in the future.

Knowledge can help to reduce fear of the unknown, and it can help you to be realistic so that you can prepare for the future. Talk with health professionals and other people who have cared for someone with cancer to see if you are exaggerating the risks.

➤ Talk with someone about your fears.

It often helps to explain to an understanding person why you feel afraid. This allows you to think through the reasons for your feelings. Also, talking with an understanding person will show you that other people realize and appreciate how you feel.

Loss and Sorrow

A serious, life-threatening illness can bring on a great sense of loss and sorrow. You may feel sad that plans you had for the future might not be fulfilled. You may feel the loss of the "normal" person and the "normal" things you did together before the illness. Memories of how he or she used to be may make you sad, and you may feel burdened by more responsibilities that you must handle alone. Here is a way to deal with feelings of loss and sorrow:

➤ **Talk about your feelings of loss with other people who have had similar experiences.**

People who have been caregivers for persons with a serious illness usually will understand how you feel. Support groups are one way to find people with similar experiences.

Guilt

Many people who care for someone with advanced cancer feel guilt at some time during the illness. They may believe they did something to cause the cancer or that they should have recognized the disease sooner. They may feel guilt about not doing a better job of caring for the person with cancer or because they are angry or upset with him or her. They also may feel guilt because they are well and a person they care for deeply is sick. Some people even feel guilt almost out of habit, having learned from childhood to feel that way whenever something goes wrong.

Although feelings of guilt are understandable, they can interfere with doing the best possible job of caregiving. Guilt makes you think only about what you did wrong. Most problems have many causes, and what you did most likely is only part of the reason (assuming it even has anything to do with the problem at all). To solve a problem, you must look objectively at all of the causes and then develop a plan to deal with the entire situation. For example, if you feel anger toward the person you are caring for, this is partly because of what he or she did as well as what you did. To deal with the cause of that anger, you need to talk openly with the person you are caring for about what both of you did—not just feel guilt about what you did or feeling angry.

Your goal here is to work toward forgiveness, both for yourself and for the other person. Dwelling on feelings of guilt about the past will rob you of the precious energy you need to cope with the present.

Here are some ways to deal with feelings of guilt:

➤ **Do not expect yourself to be perfect.**

Remember that you are human and will make mistakes from time to time.

347

➤ **Do not dwell on mistakes.**

Accept your mistakes, and get beyond them as best you can. Repetitive, negative thoughts such as guilt can be controlled by pushing them aside with positive, constructive thoughts.

Possible Obstacles

Think about what could prevent you from carrying out your plan for being an effective caregiver. Here are some obstacles that other caregivers have faced:

1. "He doesn't want to talk about feelings."

Response: He is the best judge of that. Your job is to make sure that opportunities to listen are there when and if he decides to talk about his feelings.

2. "What if she talks about things that I don't want to hear?"

Response: Even if what are hearing hurts you, consider it in the larger picture of what it means for the patient to be able to express it. Remember that you do not have to resolve everything. You are helping even if you only listen.

3. "She won't follow my advice."

Response: If you are feel frustrated because the person you are caring for will not follow your advice, try to understand how important it is for the patient to retain some control over her life. You may know what is best for her, but realize that your job is to support, not to make decisions for her. If you have a dominant personality or usually have been the one to make decisions in your family, be prepared to practice letting go.

4. "I don't have time to take care of my own needs."

Response: This is the most common reason that caregivers become exhausted. They become preoccupied with problems and do not pay attention to themselves. You will be a better caregiver in the long run if you take the time (especially when stress is high) to get help so that you can do things that you enjoy and relax you.

5. "If I don't do it, it won't get done."

Response: Yes, it will. No one is indispensable. You also should sort out things that really need to be done versus those you would like to see done. It is perfectly acceptable to let some things, such as housework, slide a bit when you take on new responsibilities.

6. "I hate asking other people to help me."

Response: There are two ways around this problem. First, you can get together socially with people who could help and let them volunteer. Second, you could have someone else ask for help for you. Try to make the times when others visit both pleasant and rewarding, then they will want to visit and help.

7. "The person I'm helping doesn't want anyone else to help."

Response: Suggest trying to get help for just a short time, after which you can talk over how it worked. Also, explain to the person you are caring for that you need the help, not him or her.

Think of other obstacles that could interfere with carrying out your plan.

What additional roadblocks could get in the way of your being a successful caregiver? For example, will the person with advanced cancer cooperate? Will other people help? How will you explain your needs to other people? Do you have the time and energy to carry out these responsibilities?

You need to develop plans for getting around these road blocks. The four COPE ideas (creativity, optimism, planning, and expert information) can help.

Carrying Out and Adjusting Your Plan

Carrying Out Your Plan

Start using the ideas in this guide immediately. Do not wait until you feel overwhelmed. It is easier to develop good caregiving habits and attitudes early, before problems get out of hand.

Checking on Results

Every week or so, take the time to think about how you are doing as a caregiver. Look through this plan, and ask yourself how closely you are matching the "successful caregiver" that is described.

If Your Plan Does Not Work

Be realistic about what you expect from yourself. Do not expect to be perfect. Everyone makes mistakes, and learning to be a caregiver for someone with cancer takes time. If there are some parts of caregiving that are especially difficult for you, ask others for help.

Be realistic in your expectations about feelings being shared. Most people do not change their styles of communicating quickly. If you cannot do the things that are essential for the person you are helping, talk with the doctor, nurse, or social worker about getting the help that you need. If you become so upset that it interferes with your ability to do what needs to be done, or you are experiencing severe depression or anxiety, talk with the doctor, nurse, or social worker about getting help.

What the Cancer Patient Can Do for Themselves

Feelings of Isolation

Living with a serious illness can be discouraging. You will have good days and bad days, just as you did before, and your ability to deal with these changes may vary. In the morning you may feel down, but by afternoon your outlook may improve. On one day, you may have little energy, but on another, your mood and spirit may rebound. During the bad times, try to remember the good moments and remind yourself there can be more good times ahead.

Taking charge of your life is one way to help yourself. Take an active role in the kind of care you receive. Participate in daily activities with your family and friends.

Do things for yourself that make you feel good, such as attending religious services or encouraging visits from friends. Let others help you. Let them know what they can do for you and what you can do for yourself. They will be grateful for specific suggestions. Your caregivers may recommend things that don't seem as important to you now, such as exercise, medications, and food. But these measures will help you keep your strength and independence for as long as possible. Working with your caregivers and family helps you maintain a sense of control, purpose, and hope.

Set the tone for those around you. Making those around you feel comfortable now will help them to be comfortable around you throughout your illness. As one patient said: "You have to do this because no one knows how you want to be treated, and they may be waiting for a cue. No one else will talk about it unless you do."

At the same time, remember that you don't have to be noble and heroic if you don't feel that way. Sometimes loved ones may want you to try to keep your feelings of sadness or anger inside because they can't face their own painful emotions; however, your feelings are important and need to be shared.

Facing the Challenge

It may be very hard to accept that your body is no longer as strong and reliable as it once was. As cancer progresses, you will not be as independent as you once were. This new dependence on others may affect your self-respect. Your role in the family and at work will change as well. When this happens, remember that the qualities that made you a good friend, loving parent, caring mate, or responsible worker haven't changed.

You may be able to continue many of your regular activities, such as playing sports, doing volunteer work, or traveling. Advances in the ability to control pain and to administer needed medications and treatments outside the hospital can give those in the later stages of cancer more independence while receiving medical care.

Arranging family albums, scrapbooks, or hobby collections; working on a computer; or keeping a daily journal of your feelings and experiences are activities you can do if you are less active. Just remember to conserve your strength for the activities you really want to pursue.

Keep in mind that you can have control over many aspects of your life whether you are bedridden or not. You can make decisions about your care, your activities, food preferences, and what you need to make yourself comfortable. In the hospital, for example, you can wear your own clothes or use your own blanket and pillow. In some cases, you also may be able to participate in decisions about your schedule for resting, bathing, and so on.

Maintaining independence makes many patients feel better about themselves. However, well-meaning family and friends may try to make decisions for you, and sometimes you must rely on others for your care. When you face situations such as these, just remember: You know better than anyone what you need to make the most of each day.

Handling Emotions

People who are dying from cancer may be sad, depressed, angry, scared, or all of these. These feelings are very human and natural. You already may be grieving for the loss of the person you were before

351

you had cancer. As your friends will grieve for you, you now may be grieving for your loss of them.

You may be wondering what experiences you will miss in life, what the moment of death will be like, and whether you will continue to "be" after death. You may think about what will become of your family and friends and how these people will react to your death.

Don't bottle up your emotions. Letting feelings out will help relatives, friends, and caregivers understand your needs; may relieve some of your sadness, depression, or anger; and even may reduce physical discomfort. For some people, writing about emotions can help, and occasionally you may want to punch a pillow, scream, or have a good, long cry. Go ahead and express your feelings.

If you are feeling angry, it will help both you and others to understand that your anger may not be meant for them. You might even think of ways to make your anger work for you. For example, perhaps you can focus your energy on changing some aspect of your care that displeases you.

Many people with a terminal illness develop an interest in expressing or trying to resolve spiritual or religious issues. Even if you don't consider yourself a "religious person" or haven't taken part in religious services, you may find comfort in exploring spiritual matters with a friend, family member, or member of the clergy. For some, prayer and/or meditation can be a positive spiritual boost.

Talking It Over

Honest and open communication about your illness can help you in several ways. It can help those close to you understand how you want to be treated, and the weight of your problems may be lightened just by talking them over with a family member, a friend, or other cancer patients who may think of ideas to help comfort you. Sharing your feelings also may reduce stress.

You may find this kind of communication difficult, and it may be hard for others. Still, talking over your worries and concerns and knowing how your loved ones feel can give you strength and reassurance. To discuss these issues, try to choose people who are comfortable with your illness.

Keep in mind, not everyone can handle your suffering and loss. Friendships and family relationships may change—not because of you but because others may not be able to cope with their own emotional pain about your illness. If this is the case, you might want to talk to a member of your medical team or to someone trained in counseling, such as a nurse, social worker, psychologist, member of the clergy, or, if you are receiving care at home, a professional home health care worker. Also, you may find support by attending self-help groups where people meet to share common concerns. Your caregivers, hospital, or a hospice can help find the right person or group for you.

Making the Unknown Known

Some say it is not death people fear but the days, weeks, or months that precede it. Many are afraid that there will be pain during this time and wonder if they will become a burden. Patients with a serious illness fear the unknown, isolation, abandonment, and loss of physical and emotional control. They worry about the future of those who will outlive them.

Understanding your condition can help you and your family resolve these fears. The more you learn about your condition and treatment, the more your fears of the unknown are reduced. Don't hesitate to ask your doctors, nurses, and other caregivers if there is something you want to know. Remember: It is your right to receive answers, even to the most direct questions about your future.

Sometimes your health care providers will seem hesitant to offer information. They may not be able to explain exactly what to expect. Or they may wait until you seem ready for the information. You can signal your readiness by asking specific questions—about your life, your illness, and about dying.

Try to include one or more relatives, friends, or others who are supportive in talks with your health care providers. If the health providers explain matters directly to your caregivers, your caregivers gain a clearer understanding of how they can help you, and their concerns can be eased.

Relieving Pain and Discomfort

Many people with cancer fear physical pain. However, not everyone with cancer has pain. And those who do have pain are not in pain all the time. If you have pain, it can be treated. Talk to your doctor or nurse about pain control. Don't wait until your pain is severe. Pain almost always can be lessened.

Cancer patients may have pain for a variety of reasons. Pain may be due to the cancer itself, or it could result from treatment methods. For example, after surgery, a person feels pain as a result of the operation itself. Sometimes, the pain is unrelated to the cancer, such as a muscle sprain, a toothache, or a headache. Whatever the cause, pain can be relieved. The best way to manage pain is to treat its cause. Whenever possible, the cause of the pain is treated by removing the tumor or decreasing its size. To do this, your doctor may suggest surgery, radiation therapy, or chemotherapy. However, your doctor may be more likely to recommend pain relief methods to control your pain. These methods include pain medicines, operations on nerves, nerve blocks, physical therapy, and techniques such as relaxation, distraction, and imagery.

Many people are reluctant to use pain medications for fear of becoming addicted. But taking medication to relieve pain will not make you an "addict." In fact, studies show that medically supervised use of narcotics (also known as analgesics) to control cancer pain does not cause addiction. Also, research shows that patients who take medication to prevent rather than reduce pain, tend to use less medication. And if the cause of your pain can be corrected, you will be able to stop taking your medications.

Physical therapy, biofeedback, relaxation techniques, self-hypnosis, and imagery also may help relieve pain. Other types of pain control include skin stimulation, pressure, vibration, massage, cold or warm compresses, menthol applied to the skin, and transcutaneous electric nerve stimulation. Some of these methods cause nerve endings to become numb in a specific area of the body, providing pain relief without the drowsiness caused by some pain medications. Special procedures that use anesthetics are available for the 10 to 15 percent of patients whose pain therapy is ineffective or causes severe side effects.

You know the most about your pain, such as where it is, how bad it is, what eases it, or what makes it feel worse. Your doctors and nurses rely on you to tell them about your pain. Together, you can decide which methods of relief might be best for you.

Don't hesitate to talk about your pain to your doctor or nurse. You have a right to the best pain control you can get. Relieving your pain means you can continue to do the everyday things that are important to you. A booklet about handling pain, "Questions and Answers about Pain Control: A Guide for People with Cancer and Their Families," is available from the Cancer Information Service (see Chapter 37, "Directory of Additional Resources").

Feelings of Isolation

As cancer progresses, your life is disrupted. Social activities with family, friends, or co-workers become less frequent. Routines change because of treatments, visits to the doctor, or your need to rest.

These changes can lead to feelings of loneliness and isolation, even when you are surrounded by family and friends. One way to lessen these feelings is to live as normally as possible. Continue to do the things you always have done, such as hobbies, reading, walking the dog, or enjoying the company of children. Let your family and friends know that you want to continue with life as it was before. Encourage them, as much as you can, to carry on with their regular routines.

Don't hesitate to ask friends and relatives to visit if you are feeling up to it. They may want to stop by but may be afraid to contact you because they don't know what to say or how to act.

In spite of all your efforts, there will be days when you feel alone because you realize others cannot fully understand or share your experience. Some days you may simply want to be left alone, and that is okay too.

People who live alone or those who do not have family and friends close by may find an illness especially difficult. In these situations, some have found it easier to cope by having volunteers or caregivers visit. For others, the company of a pet often helps.

Talking with other people who have terminal cancer might provide the understanding and companionship you need. Joining a support group, where you can talk with other cancer patients, is another way to ease feelings of isolation.

At times you may need to rely on yourself for encouragement. If this happens, try to focus on the pleasures you can give yourself, such as a leisurely walk, a beautiful bouquet of flowers, or a good book. Draw on your own strength and try to be your own best friend.

Chapter 22

Cerebral Palsy

Jennifer's Story

Jen was born 11 weeks early and weighed only 2½ pounds. The doctors were surprised to see what a strong, wiggly girl she was. But when Jen was just a few days old, she stopped breathing and was put on a ventilator. After 24 hours she was able to breathe on her own again. The doctors did a lot of tests to find out what had happened, but they couldn't find anything wrong. The rest of Jen's time in the hospital was quiet, and after two months she was able to go home. Everyone thought she would be just fine.

At home, Jen's mom noticed that Jen was really sloppy when she drank from her bottle. As the months went by, Jen's mom noticed other things she didn't remember seeing with Jen's older brother. At six months, Jen didn't hold her head up straight. She cried a lot and would go stiff with rage. When Jen went back for her six-month checkup, the doctor was concerned by what he saw and what Jen's mom told him. He suggested that Jen's mom take the little girl to a doctor who could look closely at Jen's development. Jen's mom took her to a developmental specialist who finally put a name to all the little things that hadn't seemed right with Jen—cerebral palsy.

"Cerebral Palsy Fact Sheet FS2," National Information Center for Children and Youth with Disabilities (NICHCY), May 2000.

What Is Cerebral Palsy (CP)?

Cerebral palsy—also known as CP—is a condition caused by injury to the parts of the brain that control our ability to use our muscles and bodies. *Cerebral* means having to do with the brain. *Palsy* means weakness or problems with using the muscles. Often the injury happens before birth, sometimes during delivery, or, like Jen, soon after being born. CP can be mild, moderate, or severe. Mild CP may mean a child is clumsy. Moderate CP may mean the child walks with a limp. He or she may need a special leg brace or a cane. More severe CP can affect all parts of a child's physical abilities. A child with moderate or severe CP may have to use a wheelchair and other special equipment. Sometimes children with CP can also have learning problems, problems with hearing or seeing (called sensory problems), or mental retardation. Usually, the greater the injury to the brain, the more severe the CP. However, CP doesn't get worse over time, and most children with CP have a normal life span.

How Common Is CP?

About 500,000 people in America have some form of CP. Each year 8,000 infants and nearly 1,500 preschool-age children are diagnosed with CP.

What Are the Signs of CP?

There are three main types of CP:

- **Spastic CP** is where there is too much muscle tone or tightness. Movements are stiff, especially in the legs, arms, and/or back. Children with this form of CP move their legs awkwardly, turning in or scissoring their legs as they try to walk. This is the most common form of CP.

- **Athetoid CP** (also called dyskinetic CP) can affect movements of the entire body. Typically, this form of CP involves slow, uncontrolled body movements and low muscle tone that makes it hard for the person to sit straight and walk.

- **Mixed CP** is a combination of the symptoms listed above. A child with mixed CP has both high and low tone muscle. Some muscles are too tight, and others are too loose, creating a mix of stiffness and involuntary movements.

More words used to describe the different types of CP include:

- **Diplegia**—This means only the legs are affected.

- **Hemiplegia**—This means one half of the body (such as the right arm and leg) is affected.

- **Quadriplegia**—This means both arms and legs are affected, sometimes including the facial muscles and torso.

What about Treatment?

With early and ongoing treatment the effects of CP can be reduced. Many children learn how to get their bodies to work for them in other ways. For example, one infant whose CP keeps him from crawling may be able to get around by rolling from place to place. Children younger than three years old can benefit greatly from early intervention services. Early intervention is a system of services to support infants and toddlers with disabilities and their families. For older children, special education and related services are available through the public school to help each child achieve and learn.

Typically, children with CP may need different kinds of therapy, including:

- **Physical therapy (PT),** which helps the child develop stronger muscles such as those in the legs and trunk. Through PT, the child works on skills such as walking, sitting, and keeping his or her balance.

- **Occupational therapy (OT),** which helps the child develop fine motor skills such as dressing, feeding, writing, and other daily living tasks.

- **Speech-language pathology (S/L),** which helps the child develop his or her communication skills. The child may work in particular on speaking, which may be difficult due to problems with muscle tone of the tongue and throat.

The child may also find a variety of special equipment helpful. For example, braces (also called AFOs) may be used to hold the foot in place when the child stands or walks. Custom splints can provide support to help a child use his or her hands. A variety of therapy equipment and adapted toys are available to help children play and have fun while they are working their bodies. Activities such as swimming or horseback riding can help strengthen weaker muscles and relax the tighter ones.

New medical treatments are being developed all the time. Sometimes surgery, Botox injections, or other medications can help lessen the effects of CP, but there is no cure for the condition.

What about School?

A child with CP can face many challenges in school and is likely to need individualized help. Fortunately, states are responsible for meeting the educational needs of children with disabilities.

For children up to age three, services are provided through an early intervention system. Staff work with the child's family to develop what is known as an Individualized Family Services Plan, or IFSP. The IFSP will describe the child's unique needs as well as the services the child will receive to address those needs. The IFSP will also emphasize the unique needs of the family, so that parents and other family members will know how to help their young child with CP. Early intervention services may be provided on a sliding-fee basis, meaning that the costs to the family will depend upon their income.

For school-aged children, including preschoolers, special education and related services will be provided through the school system. School staff will work with the child's parents to develop an Individualized Education Program, or IEP. The IEP is similar to an IFSP in that it describes the child's unique needs and the services that have been designed to meet those needs. Special education and related services, which can include PT, OT, and speech-language pathology, are provided at no cost to parents.

In addition to therapy services and special equipment, children with CP may need what is known as assistive technology. Examples of assistive technology include:

- **Communication devices,** which can range from the simple to the sophisticated. Communication boards, for example, have pictures, symbols, letters, or words attached. The child communicates by pointing to or gazing at the pictures or symbols. Augmentative communication devices are more sophisticated and include voice synthesizers that enable the child to "talk" with others.

- **Computer technology,** which can range from electronic toys with special switches to sophisticated computer programs operated by simple switch pads or keyboard adaptations.

The ability of the brain to find new ways of working after an injury is remarkable. Even so, it can be difficult for parents to imagine what their child's future will be like. Good therapy and handling can help, but the most important "treatment" the child can receive is love and encouragement, with lots of typical childhood experiences, family, and friends. With the right mix of support, equipment, extra time, and accommodations, all children with CP can be successful learners and full participants in life.

Cerebral Palsy as an "Orthopedic Impairment"

The Individuals with Disabilities Education Act (IDEA) guides how early intervention services and special education and related services are provided to children with disabilities. Under IDEA, cerebral palsy is considered an "orthopedic impairment," which is defined as;

". . . a severe orthopedic impairment that adversely affects a child's educational performance. The term includes impairments caused by congenital anomaly (e.g. clubfoot, absence of some member, etc.), impairments caused by disease (e.g., poliomyelitis, bone tuberculosis, etc.), and impairments from other causes (e.g., cerebral palsy, amputations, and fractures or burns that cause contractures)." 34 Code of Federal Regulations Section 300.7(c)(9)

Tips for Parents

- Learn about CP. The more you know, the more you can help yourself and your child. See the list of resources and organizations at the end of this chapter.

- Love and play with your child. Treat your son or daughter as you would a child without disabilities. Take your child places, read together, have fun.

- Learn from professionals and other parents how to meet your child's special needs, but try not to turn your lives into one round of therapy after another.

- Ask for help from family and friends. Caring for a child with CP is hard work. Teach others what to do and give them plenty of opportunities to practice while you take a break.

- Keep informed about new treatments and technologies that may help. New approaches are constantly being worked on and can make a huge difference to the quality of your child's life. However, be careful about unproven new "fads."

- Learn about assistive technology that can help your child. This may include a simple communication board to help your child express needs and desires, or may be as sophisticated as a computer with special software.

- Be patient, keep up your hope for improvement. Your child, like every child, has a whole lifetime to learn and grow.

- Work with professionals in early intervention or in your school to develop an IFSP or an IEP that reflects your child's needs and abilities. Be sure to include related services such as speech-language pathology, physical therapy, and occupational therapy if your child needs these. Don't forget about assistive technology either!

Tips for Teachers

- Learn more about CP. The resources and organizations at the end of this chapter will help you.

- This may seem obvious, but sometimes the "look" of CP can given the mistaken impression that a child who has CP cannot learn as much as others. Focus on the individual child and learn firsthand what needs and capabilities he or she has.

- Tap into the strategies that teachers of students with learning disabilities use for their students. Become knowledgeable about different learning styles. Then you can use the approach best suited for a particular child, based upon that child's learning abilities as well as physical abilities.

- Be inventive. Ask yourself (and others), "How can I adapt this lesson for this child to maximize active, hands-on learning?"

- Learn to love assistive technology. Find experts within and outside your school to help you. Assistive technology can mean the difference between independence for your student or not.

- Always remember, parents are experts, too. Talk candidly with your student's parents. They can tell you a great deal about their daughter or son's special needs and abilities.

- Effective teamwork for the child with CP needs to bring together professionals with diverse backgrounds and expertise. The team must combine the knowledge of its members to plan, implement, and coordinate the child's services.

Resources

Geralis, E. (1998). *Children with cerebral palsy: A parents' guide (2nd ed.).* Bethesda, MD: Woodbine House.

Nolan, C. (1987). *Under the eye of the clock.* New York, NY: St. Martin's Press.

Videos to rent: *My Left Foot Gaby: A True Story.*

Organizations

United Cerebral Palsy Associations, Inc.
1660 L Street NW, Suite 700
Washington DC 20036
Toll-Free Voice/TTY: 800-872-5827
Tel: 202-776-0406
TTY: 202-973-7197; Fax: 202-776-0414
Website: http://www.ucpa.org
E-mail: ucpanatl@ucpa.org

This coalition of associations provide family support, legislative advocacy, public information and education, and training specifically for issues of importance to those who have cerebral palsy. It also publishes newsletters and various brochures and pamphlets. The UCP Research and Educational Foundation supports research to prevent cerebral palsy and develop therapies to improve the quality of life for those affected by this disorder.

Easter Seals—National Office
230 West Monroe Street, Suite 1800
Chicago, IL 60606-4802
Toll-Free: 800-221-6827; Tel: 312-726-6200
TTY: 312-726-4258
Fax: 312-726-1494
Website: http://www.easter-seals.org
E-mail: info@easter-seals.org

Other Websites

- **http://www.ninds.nih.gov**—Site of the National Institute of Neurological Disorders and Stroke at the National Institute of Health.

- **http://www.dreamms.org**—A non-profit information clearing-house on assistive technology.

- **http://www.Lburkhart.com**—Ideas and instructions for adapting toys for use by children with CP.

- **http://www.augcomm.com**—A site dedicated to augmentative/alternative communication device users.

Chapter 23

Multiple Sclerosis

Caring for someone with a chronic illness like MS can be deeply satisfying. Partners, family, and friends can be drawn more closely together when they meet the challenges posed by MS. But caregiving can also be physically and emotionally exhausting, especially for the person who is acting as the primary caregiver. That person is most often a partner or spouse, but can also be a child, parent, or friend.

There is a vast range of caregiving activity, just as there is a vast range of ability and disability among people with MS and even within a given person with MS. Someone giving care to a person who has relatively few functional difficulties may be helping with A, B, or C drug injections and offering support in dealing with the medical team. Someone caring for a person with a more severe level of disability may be responsible for daily activities like toileting, dressing, transferring, and feeding, as well as medical treatments. This chapter provides an overview of the practical and emotional issues that caregivers in all kinds of situations might face. Those caring for someone who is newly diagnosed, or who has little disability may want to concentrate only on those sections relevant to their particular situation.

Throughout this chapter, the terms caregiver and carer are used to refer to the person primarily responsible for providing daily care to the person with MS. It may help to remember that the person giving care and the person receiving it are in this together. They can be

Reprinted with permission, "A Guide for Caregivers," by Tanya Radford, © 2000 National Multiple Sclerosis Society.

thought of as partners; this chapter sometimes refers to them as care-partners. MS doesn't change the fact that important relationships continue to be a two-way street. The person with disabilities may need a great deal of assistance, but the needs and concerns of each care-partner must also be addressed if the relationship is to remain healthy.

Practical Decisions

Most people with MS do not develop such severe disability that they require full-time long-term care. But since there is no way to predict who will develop severe disability, it is wise to make contingency plans. The motto "Hope for the best but plan for the worst" can be a useful philosophy for people with MS. This means investigating the kinds and costs of local long-term options, before a crisis occurs.

Home Care

Even people with severe levels of disability can live at home successfully. There are usually a number of solutions to any problem that arises. For example, someone who cannot transfer from wheelchair to bed or bath can be moved using the proper kind of lift. People with disabilities can be more independent when a home has wide doorways and grab bars. When the caregiver works full-time and the person with MS needs some aid and companionship during the day, adult day care might be an option. Caregiver burnout can be avoided when the care-partner makes use of respite care, friends, and support groups.

Other Care Options

For some people, providing care at home will be impossible. There are different kinds of live-in care facilities, including assisted living facilities, nursing homes, and cooperative care housing. Deciding what kind of facility is best will depend on the level and kind of disability, care needs, and financial resources available.

Caring at Home

Adapting for safety, accessibility, and comfort adaptations to the home can increase safety, accessibility, and comfort for everyone. But before deciding to move or make major home renovations, ask a doctor for a referral to an occupational therapist (OT) for a home visit. OTs can suggest ways to keep the person with MS as independent as possible, ensure safety, and reduce the physical strain on the caregiver. Ramps, widened doorways, and renovations in the kitchen and bath can often solve accessibility problems. Not all changes are major expenses. The National MS Society has information and can give referrals for making some practical low-cost modifications to the home.

Sometimes the best choice involves moving to more accessible housing. Moving to a place that is near public transportation, stores, and other public facilities can give a person with disabilities more choices to be independent. It might also make it easier to hire necessary help.

Flexible Roles

Changes are not confined to doorways or light switches. Carers have to take on more responsibilities. People with severe MS lose independence. The shift of roles can be a source of tremendous anxiety.

Inevitably, the caregiver and the person with MS will have different perspectives about the same issue—whether a necessary adaptation is major or minor, about medication side effects, or how to best schedule hired help. MS affects everyone involved, but it affects everyone differently. It might help to remember this.

Care-partners will need to rethink who does what. List the tasks and responsibilities necessary for the smooth running of the household. These might include:

- Household tasks such as general cleaning, shopping, cooking, laundry, child care, and transportation.

- Care-related tasks such as dressing, bathing, eating, toileting, exercising, transportation, doctor's visits, and taking medication.

- Daily activities such as work, recreation, entertainment, exercise, hobbies, private time, and religious activities.

- Plan to re-evaluate task assignments as needs and circumstances change. And make sure to schedule rewarding personal time for everyone in the household.

Helping with Daily Activities

MS is extremely changeable and unpredictable. People experience attacks and remissions, loss and recovery or partial recovery of abilities. One day a person with MS can dress alone, the next day the person cannot. The caregiver has to take and then give back responsibility for tasks all the time.

If a task seems impossibly difficult or stressful, there is probably an easier way to do it. The medical team can provide tips and techniques for bathing, dressing, toileting, and safe transfers. The National MS Society and other caregivers are also good sources of advice and tips.

Roles and Gender Differences

Women and men who act as caregivers face the same day-to-day responsibilities, frustrations, and satisfactions. However, women caregivers may feel more comfortable than men caregivers, since caregiving has traditionally been viewed as a more feminine role.

Studies have found that many men who are caregivers report difficulty in discussing their problems and are more likely to repress emotional reactions. They find it more difficult to ask for help and many do not use the resources available to carergivers. On the other hand, some men tend to participate more in social and recreational activities that contribute to their overall health and emotional well-being.

Some women are better at expressing their feelings and accessing supportive networks. But women caregivers are more likely to neglect their own health, although they tend to report more physical and emotional ailments than their male counterparts.

When a Child Is a Caregiver

Sometimes children assume major household and personal care responsibilities when the parent has disability due to MS. This is more likely to occur in single-parent households. While it is positive for children to take on household chores and responsibilities, the needs of the children must be carefully balanced with the amount and level of caregiving they are expected to do.

Children are not equipped to handle the stress of being a primary caregiver and should never be responsible for a parent's medical treatments or daily functions such as toileting. Children under 10 can certainly handle some household chores. Young teenagers might be able to handle more responsibility, but they also need to spend some time with their peers. Older teenagers and young adults may be competent carers, but they should not be expected to undertake long-term primary care. After all, they have their own futures to attend to.

When a Parent Is a Caregiver

The return of an adult child to the home can be stressful for both the parents and the adult child. Often, this homecoming reproduces the earlier struggles that occurred before the child became independent. Parents probably have house rules that they want to have respected. But the adult child needs to be treated as an adult, and some house rules may presume the wrong kind of dependence.

As parents age, providing care will become more difficult. In time, one or both parents may become ill and require care themselves. Alternative care plans and living arrangements should be discussed with the adult child well before such a crisis occurs.

Family and Friends

Family and friends can be crucial members in a network of assistance but caregivers often report that it's hard to actually get their help. The first step is to tell friends and family that their help is needed and welcomed. Friends often worry that offering help might seem intrusive, especially when it looks as if things are being handled well.

Keep a list of projects, errands, and services that friends could do. Then, the next time someone offers to help in some way, it will be easy to oblige them. Give people specific, time-limited tasks. Asking a friend or relative to come by on Saturday for 3 hours in the afternoon so the caregiver can run errands is going to be more successful than asking them to stop by when they have a moment.

Hiring Help

People with disabilities need most help with daily care. Unfortunately, this kind of help is generally not covered by insurance plans. Unless one of the care-partners has a long-term care insurance policy with a home care provision, paid care will be limited to what the family can afford.

Professional nurses and therapists are usually referred or assigned by a doctor. However, home care aides and domestic assistants are hired by the care-partners. Hiring capable, reliable, and trustworthy help will be easier if the needs and concerns of the person receiving care are discussed in advance. The person with MS should always be part of the interview process.

Other caregivers, the health care team, and the National MS Society can be of help in locating reliable agencies that screen and refer potential candidates.

Neighborhood teenagers are an underused source of low-cost help. Some schools require community service, and many teenagers would like part-time work. Ask the honors program advisor at the local public high school for names of interested students. Be willing to write recommendation letters and to teach them something about MS and disability. Be prepared to pay at least the minimum wage.

Emotional Support

Handling Stress and Caregiver Burnout

Providing emotional support and physical care to someone with MS is often deeply satisfying, but it is sometimes distressing, and now and then simply overwhelming. The strain of balancing employment, child-rearing, increased responsibilities in the home, and the care of the ill person often leads to feelings of martyrdom, anger, and guilt.

One of the biggest mistakes caregivers make is thinking that they can—and should—handle all caregiving duties alone. Seasoned caregivers and professionals agree that the best way to avoid burnout is to have the practical and emotional support of other people. Sharing problems with others not only relieves stress, but can give new perspectives on problems.

"Why Doesn't Anyone Ask How I Am?"

If the people who give care have one overriding complaint, it is that no one seems to understand what they are going through. Their labor is not particularly visible. It goes on behind closed doors, in bathrooms, and bedrooms.

It is not healthy or reasonable to constantly focus attention on the person with MS. Carers also need to take care of themselves and pay attention to other people as part of their routine. Support groups and religious advisors can help. So can learning to be more assertive.

Take Care of the Caregiver

Many caregivers neglect their own health. They ignore their own ailments and neglect preventative health measures like exercise, diet, and regular medical examinations.

Many caregivers do not get 7 hours of sleep a night. If sleep patterns are regularly disrupted because the person with MS wakes in the night needing help with toileting or physical problems, discuss the problems with a healthcare professional.

Outside Activities

Researchers report that the emotional stress of caring has little to do with the physical condition of the person with MS or the length of time they have been ill. Emotional stress seems more related to how "trapped" caregivers feel in their situation. This, in turn, seems to be closely related to the satisfaction they have in their personal and social relationships, and the amount of time available to pursue their own interests and activities.

Successful caregivers don't give up enjoyable activities. Many organizations have established respite care programs. Family members are often willing—even pleased—to spend time with the person with MS. It may be possible to arrange respite care on a regular basis. Keep a list of people to ask on an occasional basis, as well.

Two-Way Communication

Many emotional stresses are the result of poor communication between care-partners. The caregiver should be able to discuss concerns and fears openly; the person receiving care isn't the only person who needs emotional support. Although collaboration isn't always easy or possible, working out long-term plans and goals together will help both care-partners to feel more secure.

Many care-partners report that the emotional and cognitive symptoms of MS are more distressful than the physical changes. If memory loss, problems with problem solving, mood swings, or depression have become severe and are disrupting daily activities in the household, consult a healthcare professional.

Effective Ways to Acknowledge Feelings

Ignoring a problem will not make it disappear. Anger, grief, and fear soon become guilt, numbness, and resentment. Discussing feelings is important to the health of relationships. Some people find that talking about their concerns happens more easily when they schedule a regular time for conversation. Taking time out to collect feelings before presenting them for discussion will make it easier to speak clearly and calmly.

Handling Unpredictability

Living with MS means expecting the unexpected, making backup plans, and focusing on what can be done rather than what can't. The unpredictability of MS can be very stressful, but it can be managed.

When making plans for outings, always include extra time for travel. Calling ahead to check out bathroom facilities and entranceways is a good idea. Buildings are not always accessible, even when they say they are. Don't make plans too complicated or inflexible. And when plans fall through, have an alternative idea ready. If the planned night out is impossible, order in pizza. A list of backup people who can be contacted for help at short notice is also useful.

Dependency and Isolation

Fear of dependency and isolation are common in the families of the chronically ill. The person with MS is increasingly dependent on the care-partner, and the care-partner is dependent on others for respite and support. Many caregivers feel shame about being dependent on others. As a result, many don't ask for the help that they need. For care-partners who are able to develop a support system—personal and social—anxieties are greatly reduced.

Anger

Anger is a common care-partner emotion. The situation feels—and is—unfair. Hurtful words might be spoken during a difficult task, doors might be slammed during a disagreement, shouting in frustration sometimes replaces conversation. Anger and frustration must be addressed and healthy outlets developed before angry encounters become physically or emotionally abusive.

Avoiding Abuse

Abusive behavior is never acceptable. Circumstances that produce frustration and anger are often unavoidable, but an emotionally damaging or physically aggressive response is not okay. If tensions are mounting, call for a time-out, and call for help.

Physical abuse usually begins in the context of giving or getting personal help—the caregiver might be too rough during dressing or grooming. The person with MS might scratch their care-partner during a transfer. Once anger and frustration reach this level, abuse by either partner may become frequent.

The dangers of physical abuse are obvious, but emotional abuse can also be unhealthy and damaging for either care-partner. Continued humiliation, harsh criticism, or manipulative behaviors can undermine the self-esteem of either partner.

Family and social groups may provide support and counsel. Therapists and marriage counselors can help partners work out problems. The National MS Society can offer local referrals.

The majority of care-partners never experience such levels of distress or become abusive. However, separation, divorce, or a nursing home are healthier options than a corrosive relationship.

Sex and Intimacy

Care-partners who are also spouses or partners usually face changes in their sexual relationship. These changes can have physical or emotional causes. MS can interfere with both sex drive and function. Problems can include decreased vaginal lubrication, numbness or painful sensations, decreased libido, erectile dysfunction, or problems reaching orgasm. MS fatigue can interfere with sexual activity. Spasticity or incontinence problems can negatively affect sexual desire. Most of these symptoms can be managed, so it is a good idea to seek the help of a healthcare professional.

In addition to MS-related functional problems, changes in roles may change the sexual relationship. Caregivers feel that they are performing a parental role, rather than being a lover or spouse, and this can interfere with sexual intimacy.

Sexuality does not have to disappear from the lives of care-partners. Partners might begin by discussing what rewarding sexuality is for them. Many preconceived ideas of what sex should be prevent the satisfaction of actual needs and pleasures. Discussion could lead to the discovery of more imaginative sexual behaviors.

Open and honest communication about sexual needs and pleasures without fear of ridicule or embarrassment is the crucial first step. Counseling by a sex therapist can be helpful in this process.

Support Groups

Support groups can provide an outlet for emotions and can be a source of much needed practical information. All National MS Society chapters have affiliated support groups for people with MS, and many have groups for caregivers, as well. Religious and spiritual communities can also provide support and guidance.

Many caregivers say it is difficult to find a regular time to attend support group meetings. They want to use their limited time for other things. For these people, the benefits of a support group might be obtained through the Internet. There are many useful online caregiver chat groups.

Additional Information

The National Multiple Sclerosis Society
733 Third Avenue
New York, NY 10017
Toll-Free: 800-344-4867
Website: http://www.nationalmssociety.org
E-mail: info@nmss.org

Chapter 24

Parkinson's Disease

Parkinson's disease, a neurological movement disorder that effects approximately one million Americans, has a unique impact on each patient. Some patients experience slowness and tremor, while others complain of problems with posture and balance. Some are severely disabled by the disease while many others are not. Many patients can lead normal lifestyles with proper medical treatments and lifestyle modifications, while others struggle to adapt to physical limitations. Some patients experience more rapid progression of the disease and its symptoms while others do not.

Things I Do to Fight Parkinson's by Richard Chalfon

I am able to take care of myself with few exceptions. I must have someone in the house when I shower, and some mornings I need help getting dressed. I don't drive any more other than to the post office. I fall asleep very quickly. It isn't worth the risk of hurting someone. I have home-care looking after me. They furnish transportation for business, social, and medical appointments. They can do light housework and furnish personal care.

Here is a list of little things that have helped me cope with Parkinson's disease. They are a big help to me.

This chapter contains excerpts from "Good Nutrition in Parkinson's Disease," © 1999 and "PD 'n' Me," © 1997 both reprinted with permission of The American Parkinson Disease Association, Inc., 1250 Hylan Blvd., Suite 4B, Staten Island, NY 10305.

1. Join a support group and be active in it. We have a large one and it's doing a great job.

2. See a mental health counselor on a regular basis.

3. Carry a sharp pocket knife in your pocket or purse. It works well with cutting a tough piece of meat at a restaurant or a banquet.

4. Wear slippery pajamas or nothing at all in bed. One then can slide to turn over or get in and out of bed.

5. Wear clothing that is easy to undo. It can save some embarrassment when nature calls.

6. Have a trapeze on the bed which is a big help in getting in and out of bed and turning over.

7. I have the lifeline system, so I can call for help in an emergency while my wife is at work.

8. Have an electric lift chair. I can't get out of a regular recliner without help. It's also a good place to take a nap in the afternoon.

9. Wear slip-on boots or tennis shoes with velcro fasteners.

10. Use clothes with snaps or zippers. Buttons just don't work anymore.

11. Use an electric toothbrush.

12. Use an electric razor.

13. Have handicap parking for both cars. It works well because of the extra width for opening doors.

14. Have a grab bar in the shower.

15. Use a cane for walking. There are too many uneven spots on the sidewalks. I can trip on a shadow.

16. Put a bath towel over the pillow. As soon as I relax I start drooling.

17. Use a nonslip pad under my plate at mealtime. It keeps the meal from falling on the floor.

18. If you are an amateur photographer, get a new, fully automatic camera, as you could not handle manual settings.

19. Use the telephone a lot. I had trouble with my ears hurting. I would get a spell of shaking and pound my ear with the phone. I now have a speaker phone.

20. Go to the Senior Center in town every morning. There is always a cribbage game going, and I am one of the regulars for that. I can't always shuffle the cards, but the guys are good about doing it for me.

21. Get a pair of reading glasses made for the right distance. I've found it difficult to read because I can't hold a book or newspaper steady. When I put what I was reading on the table, the distance was wrong for my glasses.

These are things I have learned since I got Parkinson's disease. I didn't do them all at once but over the eleven years.

I thought I would have a bad time when I quit driving, because I loved to drive and even worked as a professional driver. It has been no problem. I sure enjoy the roadside scenery.

I have trouble sleeping after two or three hours in the morning, so I use that time for writing. Also, I have thousands of color slides dating as far as 1951. Most of them are from the mountains and our farm. I've been sorting these and have put together some shows for senior citizen groups. I am also about to develop a market for prints from the slides.

We still have our pickup and self-contained camper. We go camping as often as we can get away. We also have an old boat. Fishing is pretty good in this part of Montana.

We belong to the United Church of Christ and try to be active in it.

I am a member of the board of directors for North Central Independent Services. It is a good outfit, which helps disabled or handicapped people get the equipment they need free of charge or at a reduced rate. It is where I got my lift chair. I also work with Easter Seals.

I was kind of hurt when I had to accept help, but with the cost of medication being over $600 per month, we found assistance was mandatory.

I think one of the most important things for Parkinson victims is to keep active physically. There is a man I know who has Parkinson's disease and his family treated him like an invalid. They wouldn't let him walk or go outside when he did walk. He is now in a nursing home completely bedridden. Those of us who became ill about the same time but have kept active are still functioning. My family has been very supportive of me. They are very considerate of my feelings but they don't spoil me, and if I get out of line, they set me straight.

377

Having a good doctor is also very helpful. I write a letter to mine just prior to each visit. I tell him all that has happened and my reaction to my medication. It gives him a chance to study my condition and to plan the treatment for the next four months.

It's not fun having Parkinson's disease, but it need not be the end of the world.

Prevention of Malnutrition: Who Is at Risk?

Preventing malnutrition requires identifying those at risk for inadequate nutrition. There are psychosocial and physical risk factors that predispose to undernutrition (see Table 24.1). If you or the person you are caring for has more than 4 risk factors on this list, careful attention should be given to prevent inadequate nutrition.

What Psychosocial Factors Are Nutritional Risks?

Appetite is reduced by depression and by the loneliness of social isolation. Low income and other social and physical limitations may make it difficult to obtain and prepare nutritious meals.

What Physical Factors in Parkinson's Disease Are Nutritional Risks?

Mobility problems in Parkinson's disease, such as swallowing difficulties and slowness of feeding and chewing, pose nutritional risks. The difficulties with dexterity, balance, and walking may interfere

Table 24.1. Nutritional Risk Factors

Social isolation	Drugs with nutritional interactions
Low income	
Impaired appetite	Increased metabolic requirements (ie, surgery, acute illness)
Depression	
Dementia	Dietary restrictions for weight loss
Poor dentition	
Chewing and swallowing problems	Alcohol/drug abuse
	Acute infection
Immobility and inactivity	

with shopping and meal preparation. Dyskinesia (ie, extra involuntary movements) can impair feeding and eating and, if severe, can increase calorie expenditure by increasing nutritional demands.

Although not specific to Parkinson's disease, other factors that are common in the normal aging population, such as dementia, poor teeth, and other acute and chronic illness, can compound the nutritional risk. It should be emphasized that during an infection or following surgery there are increased nutritional requirements. If a person has borderline nutrition, these increased demands can quickly result in malnutrition.

How Do Anti-Parkinsonian Drugs Affect Nutrition?

Drugs can result in nutritional deficiencies. All anti-parkinsonian drugs (ie, anticholinergics, deprenyl, levodopa-carbidopa, amantadine, pergolide, and bromocriptine) can cause nausea, vomiting, loss of appetite, and constipation. The nausea and loss of appetite usually occur on starting the drug and then subside over time as people become tolerant to these side effects. Other strategies can be used if these symptoms do not improve, but the bottom line is that the person with continuing nausea and loss of appetite should be watched carefully for poor nutritional intake. Many drugs, in addition to anti-parkinsonian drugs, can influence nutrition and should be considered when assessing nutritional risks.

Are There Physical Signs of Undernutrition?

Body weight is probably the best physical indicator of nutritional status. Unexplained weight loss of 10% or more body weight over a short period of time (3 months or less) is a sure sign of undernutrition and should be carefully evaluated. In Parkinson's disease there is a tendency to lose weight; and, therefore, weight should be carefully monitored.

What Should Be Done if a Person Is at Increased Risk of Malnutrition?

Referral to a dietician, who can make a careful assessment and establish a nutritional care plan, should be made. This plan should take into account many of the physical and social factors discussed above. It may require education of family members and referral to appropriate social supports, such as the Meals on Wheels Program.

A Special Diet for Parkinson's Disease

A special diet for Parkinson's disease has evolved out of the knowledge that diet can interfere with the effectiveness of levodopa. Therefore, this section pertains only to those people receiving levodopa who are experiencing fluctuations in their mobility.

Why Are There Interactions between Levodopa and Diet?

First we must understand some special features of levodopa.

1. Levodopa has a very short plasma half-life. This means that levodopa rapidly disappears from the blood. This takes from 60 to 90 minutes. Therefore, the blood levels of the drug bounce up and down. It is easy to imagine that anything that would delay it from entering the blood would also delay how much gets to the brain and, consequently, would affect how well the medication works.

2. Levodopa is not absorbed from the stomach, but from the small bowel. Therefore, anything that delays the emptying of the stomach contents into the small bowel can decrease absorption of the drug.

3. Levodopa is a type of amino acid called a large neutral amino acid (LNAA). To be absorbed, it must attach itself to carrier molecules in the wall of the intestine, which then carry it across the intestinal wall to the blood. This same mechanism is present to move levodopa from blood to brain. Therefore, anything that also uses this carrier system can compete with levodopa and potentially interfere with its ability to get to the brain.

What Factors Interfere with the Absorption of Levodopa?

Since levodopa is not absorbed into the blood stream, the stomach's role is simply to deliver the medication to the place where it is absorbed, which is the small bowel. Because of this, the contents of the stomach, the rate at which they are digested, and the rate at which the stomach empties into the small bowel become very important. Another consideration is that there are enzymes in the stomach lining that play a role in metabolizing the drug. Therefore, the longer the drug stays in the stomach, the more it will be chemically broken down and less of the drug will be available for absorption. There are many dietary factors that affect how rapidly the stomach empties its contents. In regard to the food groups, fat takes the longest to be digested, followed by protein, and then carbohydrates. Dietary fiber also slows the emptying of the stomach. Other factors, such as increased stomach acidity and certain medications (eg, anticholinergics) have been shown to slow the rate of stomach emptying. Experiments are being done to see if decreasing stomach acidity with antacids might improve the absorption of the drug in a few patients. It should also be noted that stomach or bowel diseases, as well as constipation, can affect the rate of absorption.

Research has compared the absorption of levodopa when it is given on an empty stomach versus when it is given with a meal. This clearly demonstrates that, in some people, taking the drug with a meal can dramatically delay the absorption of the drug.

What Is the Recommendation for Timing of Medication?

Sinemet (The same recommendation would apply for Sinemet CR, although it is not thought to be as critical for its absorption.) should be taken 15 to 30 minutes before meals to ensure the most predictable absorption. There are two exceptions to this rule:

1. If this drug produces nausea, the medication should be taken with a light, low-protein snack such as crackers and juice or, if necessary, with a meal. If this does not help, a drug called Domperidone (presently unavailable in the U.S.) can block the nausea side effects and enhance the absorption of the drug.

2. The second exception is if a person experiences too much dyskinesia or involuntary movement after taking the drug. Dyskinesia may be improved by slowing the absorption of the drug by taking it with meals.

What Dietary Factors Affect Levodopa Getting from Blood to Brain?

Once levodopa gets from the stomach to the small bowel, it is absorbed into the blood stream. As mentioned earlier, to get across the intestinal wall, levodopa must be transported by attaching to carrier molecules. This carrier system transports the drug from intestine to the blood stream and from the blood stream to the brain. It can be likened to seats on a train. There are a limited number of seats and when these seats are filled, no more levodopa can be transported. At the level of the intestine, this is not a problem, since the "train" has a large carrying capacity; but at the level of the brain, the "train" is much smaller. Other LNAAs found in the diet use the same carrier system as levodopa. These amino acids are isoleucine, leucine, valine, phenylalanine, tryptophan, and tyrosine. Meals high in protein, and therefore high in LNAAs, can interfere with the ability of levodopa getting into the brain by taking up the seats on the train.

Research has substantiated this idea, suggesting that a low-protein diet can improve the response to levodopa.

Who Should Try the Low-Protein Diet?

Consideration should be given to the severity of the disease. If a person has motor fluctuations that interfere with activities or has noticed that food seems to interfere with how well their medication works, a reduced-protein diet may help these problems.

How Much Protein Should Be Eaten?

People who need to lower the protein in their diet should reduce it to the recommended daily allowance of protein. Most Americans eat far more than this on a daily basis. The RDA for protein is 0.8 g/kg (0.36 g/Ib) body weight.

How Should the Protein Be Distributed Throughout the Day?

Restricting protein to the RDA, compared with the typical American consumption of protein, clearly improves the time a person is mobile throughout the day. Restricting the majority of the protein to the evening meal, compared with evenly distributing it throughout the day, further improves the amount of time a person is mobile. The decision between these two methods of distribution depends on the severity of the disease and the person's life-style needs.

For the person who has moderate motor fluctuations, a diet with protein spread evenly throughout the day will reduce the likelihood of high levels of amino acids and improve the amount of mobile time. For the person with marked motor fluctuations, a diet with protein restricted to the evening meal will allow for an even more predictable response. The drawback to this diet is a less mobile evening. If this is compatible with the life-style of the patient, this diet is best for the person who has marked fluctuations in mobility.

Do Carbohydrates Play a Role in the Parkinsonian Diet?

It has been shown that increased carbohydrates result in increased insulin secretion, which lowers LNAAs circulating in the blood. Therefore, increased carbohydrates plus a decreased protein intake may further enhance the delivery of levodopa to the brain by lowering the competition with other LNAAs. The therapeutic role of carbohydrates in the parkinsonian diet needs further investigation.

What Are the Recommendations for Carbohydrate Use in the Parkinsonian Diet?

If weight is lost when protein is lowered in the diet, carbohydrates should be increased to maintain ideal body weight. The amount should be determined with the help of a dietician. If excessive but predictable dyskinesia results from the increased carbohydrates and lowered dietary protein, it may be helpful to try to evenly distribute carbohydrate intake throughout the day, as well as reduce the dosage of the medication.

Practical Guidelines for a Well-Balanced Diet in Parkinson's Disease

1. Eat a daily diet that has a balance of all food groups. This should include 2 to 3 servings from the meat group, 4 to 5 from fruit and vegetables, 2 to 3 from the milk group, and at least 6 from the bread and cereal group. An average man may need 11 more servings from the bread and cereal group to provide enough calories to maintain weight.

2. On an average, calorie intake should be maintained at 25 to 30 calories per gram of body weight. If dyskinesia is present, additional calories should be added to prevent weight loss. Monitor weight on a weekly basis. Weight loss is the best sign of undernutrition.

3. Fiber and adequate fluids are important in the control of constipation and prevention of bowel disease. Fiber can be found in whole grains, fruits, and vegetables. If necessary, unprocessed bran can be added. To avoid gas, start with 1 teaspoon daily and increase by 1 teaspoon per day to a total of 1 tablespoon twice daily. In addition, adequate amounts of fluid are essential. This should be equivalent to 6 to 8 glasses of water per day.

4. An effort should be made to eat a diet low in saturated fats and low in cholesterol. Cholesterol consumption should be approximately 300 mg per day. If calories are needed in the Parkinson's diet, they are best added in the form of complex carbohydrates and unsaturated fats.

5. The need for vitamin supplements remains controversial. Although most people should be able to get adequate vitamins from a balanced diet, most elderly people with a chronic illness have enough nutritional risk factors to warrant taking a multivitamin. On the other hand, vitamins are drugs, and overuse of some can cause toxicity. High doses of Vitamins C and E used in the hope of slowing the progression of Parkinson's disease have minimal toxicity; however, their true benefit is still unclear.

6. Pyridoxine (B6) does not worsen Parkinson's disease if used in the recommended amount of 2 mg per day. If supplemental vitamins are used, intake should not exceed 5 mg. Pyridoxine-free multivitamins are only needed if a person is taking levodopa rather than Sinemet.

7. Elderly people have many risk factors for decreased calcium intake, which can contribute to osteoporosis and increased risk of broken bones. In Parkinson's disease, decreased calcium intake may occur when protein is restricted in the form of dairy products. Careful attention should be given to ensure daily calcium intake of 1,000 to 1,500 mg.

8. Vitamin D is important in calcium balance. If exposure to sun is inadequate, or chronic use of sunscreen products is necessary, supplements of 200 to 400 IU of Vitamin D should be given daily.

9. Iron is essential in the formation of hemoglobin, which carries oxygen to the cells. If iron supplements are needed, they should be separated from the time levodopa-carbidopa is taken to reduce interference with the effectiveness of the drug.

10. Take levodopa-carbidopa 15 to 20 minutes before meals to ensure more predictable absorption.

11. Avoid high-protein meals.

12. For people on levodopa-carbidopa who are noticing fluctuations in their mobility, protein manipulation may be helpful. The following steps should be followed:

a. Your health care provider should determine if an evenly distributed or restricted protein diet would be best. This is decided by disease severity and life-style needs. Referral is then made to the dietician.

b. The dietician establishes current dietary intakes of calories, protein, and calcium. A nutritional care plan is then established, with appropriate instruction regarding reduction of protein and how it should be distributed throughout the day.

c. Protein should be reduced to meet the recommended daily allowance of 0.8 g/kg (0.36 g/lb) of body weight.

d. If protein is to be evenly distributed, it should be equally divided among three meals. For example, a man who is 170 pounds weighs 77 kilograms and would require 62 grams of protein per day, which is approximately 21 grams per meal.

e. If protein is to be restricted, the protein in breakfast and lunch together should equal approximately 10 grams of high-quality protein. The rest of the protein (ie, 52 g for the 170-lb man) should be eaten from dinner to bedtime.

f. Calorie intake should be calculated to provide adequate calories to prevent weight loss. Decreased calories from protein reduction may need to be replaced by increasing carbohydrates or unsaturated fats.

g. Calcium intake should be monitored to ensure 1,000 to 1,500 mg per day.

h. This diet should be tried for 2 to 4 weeks. The improvement in response to the medication should be evident within a few days. At this time, reevaluation of the benefits should be made by your health care provider. Evaluation of proper use of the diet should be made by the dietician.

Support Group Problems and Solutions by Millie Blome

Bernie and Millie Blome, have been involved with Parkinson's disease since Millie first displayed symptoms in 1969. She was 39 at the time with a five-year old at home and two sons in college. They lived in Florida. Bernie was in the Air Force, headed for Vietnam. Millie moved to Omaha, where there were relatives to help her until Bernie came home in 1971.

Bernie, as a caregiver, and Millie, as a victim, have become widely known for their pioneering work in organizing support groups. Interviewed by the *Transmitter*, they told a story filled with hope for Parkinson's victims and their families.

Transmitter: How many support groups were there in this area when you moved to Omaha?

Bernie: There where no support groups. None in Omaha. None in Nebraska.

Millie: Not a one that we could locate.

Bernie: In those days, people with Parkinson's disease pretty much stayed home by themselves. There were no sources of information (other than their doctors). You couldn't talk to other victims because you didn't know who they were.

Millie: Doctors wouldn't tell you who their patients were because that would have been a breach of privacy.

Bernie: It was very lonely.

Transmitter: What did you do about this situation?

Millie: We decided to contact as many PD victims as possible and organize a support group to serve people in this area.

Bernie: Millie ran ads in the personal columns of the World Herald inviting people with PD to identify themselves.

Millie: We got six names and we got these people together.

Bernie: We called ourselves the "Omaha Area Parkinson's Disease Support Group."

Millie: That was in 1974.

Bernie: We focused on membership.

Millie: We posted signs in hospitals and nursing homes, inviting people to come to our meetings. We weren't always well-received. Some nursing homes wouldn't let us post information.

Bernie: At first we met in homes. Then we met in churches. We met at the Commercial Federal Building at 96th and L.

Millie: We also met at the University of Nebraska Medical Center.

Transmitter: Aside from locating and attracting new members, what was your biggest problem?

Millie: Lack of information.

Bernie: We were able to furnish a social outlet for PD victims right away. But, we had quite a time obtaining reliable technical information. And this information was vital.

Millie: There were many misconceptions about Parkinson's in those days—even amongst those suffering from the disease. The ignorance of the general public was abysmal. People would see you at a restaurant or theater—assume you were drunk.

Bernie: And we had to be very careful not to give medical advice from within the group. We always stressed the importance of checking out information with a neurologist or physician or otherwise qualified individual.

Millie: Later we organized an Information and Referral Center. We sent out books and information about Parkinson's disease.

Transmitter: What happened next?

Millie: We began to get favorable attention from the medical profession.

Bernie: We received valuable help from the APDA.

Millie: We got on mailing lists to receive technical information from various sources.

Transmitter: Were there support groups in other cities at the time?

Bernie: Yes. There was a lot of activity in St. Louis and Kansas City. We learned from them.

Transmitter: What is the support group situation in the Omaha area today?

Bernie: Well, we have the Nebraska Chapter of the APDA. This is an outgrowth of the group we started. The Chapter is a fund-raiser to find the cure and ease the burden of Parkinson's disease.

Millie: There are many other support groups in Omaha and in towns and cities throughout Nebraska and western Iowa, and there are more in the formative stage.

Bernie: There is a special group for young people with Parkinson's disease.

Millie: There are exercise groups and water aerobics classes.

Transmitter: How does a thriving support group help PD victims and their families today?

Bernie: They provide first of all a setting where people with PD—especially those recently diagnosed—can visit with people who've been coping with PD for years. This contact is priceless in terms of building morale and raising shattered hopes.

Millie: A support group provides a source of reliable information about research findings, treatments that work (and some that don't), latest developments. I participated in three research projects trying new drugs and procedures.

Bernie: Everything you learn at a support group isn't confined to medical technology. Take the matter of turning over in bed which some Parkinson's victims find difficult. It was at a support group that we learned to use satin sheets. They make a world of difference. Many ideas are offered that help those with PD cope with the disease.

Millie: Support group get-togethers show caregivers and family members things they can do to assist victims and caregivers.

Bernie: For example, a Parkinson victim often can eat more efficiently with larger utensils and larger plates that don't slip off the table. Using bigger handles on utensils helps.

Millie: And let's hear it for whoever invented Velcro!

Bernie: A telephone head set is a blessing.

Millie: But, most important, the support group offers hope—and Parkinson's disease victims need hope. It is a lonely, depressing disease at best. Having a group of understanding, positive-thinking people to meet with from time to time really helps.

Bernie: We've been active with support groups for a long time now. We really don't know how we could have coped without them.

Transmitter: Thank you, Bernie and Millie. See you at the next support group meeting.

Bernie died in 1996.

American Parkinson Disease Association, Inc. Information and Referral (I&R) Centers

Alabama, Birmingham
University of Alabama at
Birmingham
Tel: 205-934-9100

Arizona Tucson
University of Arizona
Toll-Free: 800-541-4960
Tel: 520-326-5400

Arkansas, Hot Springs
St. Joseph's Regional Health
Center
Toll-Free: 800-407-9295
Tel: 501-318-1690

California, Fountain Valley
Orange Coast Memorial Medical
Center
Tel: 714-378-5062

California, Los Angeles
Cedars-Sinai Health System
Tel: 310-855-7933

California, Los Angeles
(UCLA) Reed Neurological
Research Center
Tel: 310-794-5667

California, San Diego
Information & Referral Center
Tel: 858-273-6763

California, San Francisco
Seton Medical Center
Tel: 650-991-6391

Connecticut, New Haven
Hospital of Saint Raphael
Tel: 203-789-3936

Florida, Jacksonville
Mayo Clinic, Jacksonville
Tel: 904-953-7030

Florida, Pompano Beach
North Broward Medical Center
Toll-Free: 800-825-2732

Florida, St. Petersburg
Columbia Edward White Hospital
Tel: 727-898-2732

Georgia, Atlanta
Emory University School of
Medicine
Tel: 404-728-6552

Idaho, Boise
St. Alphonsus Medical Center
Tel: 208-367-6570

Illinois, Chicago
Glenbrook Hospital
Tel: 847-657-5787

The Arlette Johnson
Young Parkinson Information &
Referral Center
Glenbrook Hospital
Toll-Free: 800-223-9776 (Out of IL)
Tel: 847-657-5787

Louisiana, New Orleans
School of Medicine, LSU
Tel: 504-568-6554

Maryland, Baltimore
Johns Hopkins Outpatient Center
Tel: 410-955-8795

Massachusetts, Boston
Boston University School of
Medicine
Tel: 617-638-8466

Minnesota, Minneapolis
Abbott Northwestern Hospital
Minneapolis Neuroscience Inst.
Toll-Free: 888-302-7762
Tel: 612-863-5850

Missouri, St. Louis
Washington University Medical
Center
Tel: 314-362-3299

Montana, Great Falls
Benefis Health Care
Tel: 406-455-2964

Nebraska, Omaha
Information & Referral Center
Tel: 402-551-9311

Nevada, Las Vegas
University of Nevada School of
Medicine
Tel: 702-464-3132

**Nevada, Reno
V.A. Hospital
Tel: 775-328-1715

New Jersey, New Brunswick
Robert Wood Johnson University Hospital
Tel: 732-745-7520

New Mexico, Albuquerque
Healthsouth Rehabilitation
Hospital
Toll-Free: 800-278-5386

New York, Albany
The Albany Medical College
Tel: 518-452-2749

New York, Far Rockaway
Peninsula Hospital
Tel: 718-734-2876

New York, Manhattan
New York University
Tel: 212-983-1379

New York, Old Westbury
New York College of Osteopathic
Medicine
Tel: 516-626-6114

New York, Smithtown
St. John's Episcopal Hospital
Tel: 516-862-3560

New York, Staten Island
Staten Island University Hospital
Tel: 718-226-6129

North Carolina, Durham
Duke South Hospital
Tel: 919-681-2033

Ohio, Cincinnati
University of Cincinnati Medical
Center
Toll-Free: 800-840-2732
Tel: 513-558-6770

Oklahoma, Tulsa
Hillcrest Medical Center System
Toll-Free: 800-364-4450
Tel: 918-747-3747

Pennsylvania, Philadelphia
Crozer-Chester Medical Center
Tel: 610-447-2911

Pennsylvania, Pittsburgh
Allegheny General Hospital
Tel: 412-441-0100

Rhode Island, Pawtucket
Memorial Hospital of RI
Tel: 401-729-3165

Tennessee, Memphis
Methodist Hospital
Tel: 901-726-8141

Tennessee, Nashville
Centennial Medical Center
Toll-Free: 800-493-2842
Tel: 615-342-4635

Texas, Bryan
St. Joseph Regional
Rehabilitation Center
Tel: 409-821-7523

Texas, Dallas
Presbyterian Hospital of Dallas
Toll-Free: 800-725-2732
Tel: 214-345-4224

Texas, Lubbock
Methodist Hospital
Toll-Free: 800-687-5498

Texas, San Antonio
The University of Texas HSC
Tel: 210-567-6688

Utah, Salt Lake City
University of Utah,
School of Medicine
Tel: 801-585-2354

Vermont, Burlington
University of Vermont
Medical Center
Toll-Free: 888-763-3366
Tel: 802-656-3366

Virginia, Charlottesville
University of Virginia Medical
Center
Tel: 804-982-4482

Washington, Seattle
University of Washington
Tel: 206-543-5369

Wisconsin, Neenah
The Neuroscience Group of
Northeast Wisconsin
Toll-Free: 888-797-2732

Dedicated Centers

*Young Parkinson
**Armed Forces/Veterans

Please contact the nearest I&R Center or the national office for information regarding support groups and chapters. You can also dial the toll-free number 888-400-2732 to contact the I&R Center closest to you.

Chapter 25

Physical Disabilities

One false step on a cellar staircase, an automobile accident, a stroke, and overnight, any of us could end up with disabilities that make us dependent on others for the simplest tasks. We are all vulnerable to the effects of disability, whether it's a matter of caring for an elderly parent devastated by a stroke, supporting a co-worker who has Parkinson's, or hearing about a neighbor's baby born with mental retardation.

As the population ages, more Americans will have illnesses and chronic conditions that limit their ability to carry out ordinary tasks—bathing, rising from a chair, opening a window, and walking to the grocery store. With a current life expectancy of 75 years, newborns, today, can expect to experience an average of 13 years with an activity limitation. Because the 85 plus group is the fastest growing segment of the population, many Americans may live with activity limitations for 20 years or more. Technological and medical advances have made it possible for Americans to live longer but have not been matched by improvements in the delivery of chronic care services. As *Chronic Care in America: A 21st Century Challenge*, a recent report from the Robert Wood Johnson Foundation, sums it up, "There is no effective system to care for those with chronic conditions in the United

---

"Older and Younger People with Disabilities: Improving Chronic Care Throughout the Life Span," Fact Sheet, Administration on Aging (AoA), 1999; and "Persons with Disabilities—Key Messages," National Center for Chronic Disease Prevention and Health Promotion, 1999.

States. As a result, much of the care that is available is fragmented, inappropriate, and difficult to obtain."

One in Six Americans Has a Chronic Condition

According to *Chronic Care in America*, "In 1995, one in six Americans—41 million people—had a chronic condition that inhibited their lives to some degree." Among the conditions counted are arthritis, cancer, heart disease, diabetes, emphysema, Alzheimer's disease, blindness, hearing impairments, mental retardation, mental illness, cerebral palsy, and spinal cord injuries. The report says, "At least 9 million people with disabilities need help either with personal care or home management (40 percent are under age 65)."

Disability rates increase with age. According to the report, in 1994, nearly 40 percent of the elderly not living in institutions—12 million seniors—were limited by chronic conditions. Of these, 3 million (about 10 percent of all elderly) were unable to perform such activities as bathing, shopping, dressing, or eating.

As disheartening as this picture may be, future cohorts of older Americans are expected to have fewer disabilities than past generations. Findings from the National Long-Term Care Surveys regarding the health and disability status of Americans, conducted by Duke University under the auspices of the National Institute on Aging, show that disability rates among older persons are falling, and this trend is expected to continue. The number of older persons with functional problems in 1994 was 7.1 million, rather than the 8.3 million who would have been impaired, if the health of older people had not improved. Nevertheless, the growing number of Americans 85 and older means that there will be a continuing and, indeed, growing need for services and supports.

Lifestyle Changes Prevent Disability

Heart disease accounts for 13 percent of all activity limitations, and injuries cause 13 percent of all disabilities. These two facts, alone, point to the large potential to reduce disabilities by convincing Americans to adopt better nutrition, health, and exercise habits, and to think ahead about building or retrofitting homes to make them safer and more convenient.

Use of assistive devices rises with age, but this is not true of home accessibility features. It is estimated that one million people nationwide need home modifications and without such changes will remain in unsafe environments or end up in institutions. One state, Georgia, has already taken the lead in advocating for the design of homes to accommodate disabilities at all ages, a concept increasingly referred to as "universal design." A bill was introduced in the Georgia legislature to require all new homes to have one entrance without steps, door widths of 32 inches to allow for wheelchairs, bathroom walls reinforced to permit installation of grab bars, and easy-to-reach electrical sockets. In developing this legislation, the Georgia Office on Aging cooperated with disability groups, agencies, and programs, and is working with them on many other projects. Alan Goldman, deputy director of the Georgia Office on Aging, comments, "So many areas overlap when we talk about the long-term care population. The elderly and people with life-long disabilities share so much—the desire to be independent, to have some control over their lives and environments, and to avoid institutionalization."

The frail elderly may have much to learn from younger people with disabilities, including an attitude that refuses to allow society to relegate them to the sidelines and to view them as unfortunate, passive recipients of services. The nationwide network of services to the elderly, led by the U.S. Administration on Aging (AoA), has much to offer the growing numbers of people with life-long disabilities who are living into old age.

Aging and Disability Coalitions Want Shift to Home-Based Care

A National Coalition on Disability and Aging was formed in 1994 and today includes 50 organizations from the disability and aging communities, including the AoA. The Coalition held its first summit on disability and aging before the White House Conference on Aging in 1995.

One of the key objectives of disability and aging coalitions at the federal and state levels is to shift the bias of publicly-funded federal and state programs away from institutional care to home and community-based services. Another is to reverse the cost of medical services to the elderly and to people with developmental disabilities. According to *Chronic Care in America*, the direct costs of medical services for persons with chronic conditions amounted to $425 billion in 1990, and 65 percent of those costs were for hospital care and physician services (39 percent to hospitals and 25 percent to physicians). Home health care expenditures, however, have increased dramatically, rising from $9 to $24 billion between 1989 and 1993, and the number of home health care agencies providing Medicare-reimbursed services doubled between 1979 and 1990. This trend isn't just due to increased use of home health care by elderly people with chronic health problems. It is also due to rules that now send patients home from the hospital "quicker and sicker" to receive services from a home health agency that used to be provided in a hospital.

Services for seniors with chronic conditions, however, are still concentrated in the periods when they need acute care rather than in phases when prevention or rehabilitation services would be beneficial. Costly hospitalizations might be avoided if certain types of services were more affordable and available—transportation to the doctor; installation of railings and ramps; physical therapy to strengthen muscles to prevent falls; education in use of assistive devices; counseling to prevent malnutrition; and provision of home care aides to shop, prepare meals, and assist with personal care.

Physical Activity and Health of Disabled Persons

Nutrition and Physical Activity

- Physical activity need not be strenuous to achieve health benefits.

- Significant health benefits can be obtained with a moderate amount of physical activity, preferably daily. The same moderate amount of activity can be obtained in longer sessions of moderately intense activities (such as 30-40 minutes of wheeling oneself in a wheelchair) or in shorter sessions of more strenuous activities (such as 20 minutes of wheelchair basketball).

- Additional health benefits can be gained through greater amounts of physical activity. People who can maintain a regular routine of physical activity that is of longer duration or of greater intensity are likely to derive greater benefit.

- Previously sedentary people who begin physical activity programs should start with short intervals of physical activity (5-10 minutes) and gradually build up to the desired level of activity.

- People with disabilities should first consult a physician before beginning a program of physical activity to which they are unaccustomed.

- The emphasis on moderate amounts of physical activity makes it possible to vary activities to meet individual needs, preferences, and life circumstances.

Facts

- People with disabilities are less likely to engage in regular moderate physical activity than people without disabilities, yet they have similar needs to promote their health and prevent unnecessary disease.

- Social support from family and friends has been consistently and positively related to regular physical activity.

Benefits of Physical Activity

- Reduces the risk of dying from coronary heart disease and of developing high blood pressure, colon cancer, and diabetes.

- Can help people with chronic, disabling conditions improve their stamina and muscle strength.

- Reduces symptoms of anxiety and depression, improves mood, and promotes general feelings of well-being.

- Helps control joint swelling and pain associated with arthritis.

- Can help reduce blood pressure in some people with hypertension.

What Communities Can Do

- Provide community-based programs to meet the needs of persons with disabilities.

- Ensure that environments and facilities conducive to being physically active are available and accessible to people with disabilities, such as offering safe, accessible, and attractive trails for bicycling, walking, and wheelchair activities.

- Ensure that people with disabilities are involved at all stages of planning and implementing community physical activity programs.

- Provide quality, preferably daily, K-12 accessible physical education classes for children and youths with disabilities.

- Encourage health care providers to talk routinely to their patients with disabilities about incorporating physical activity into their lives.

Family Support Projects

American Association of University Affiliated Programs (AAUAP)—The AAUAP represents the national network of University Affiliated Programs (UAPs) in the United States. The UAPs provide interdisciplinary training for professionals and paraprofessionals and offer programs and services for children with disabilities and their families. Individual UAPs have staff with expertise in a variety of areas and can provide information, technical assistance, and in-service training to agencies, service providers, parent groups, and others. For information on a UAP in your area, write:

American Association of University Affiliated Programs (AAUAP)
8630 Fenton Street, Suite 410
Silver Spring, MD 20910
Tel: 301-588-8252
Fax: 301-588-2842
Website: http://www.aauap.org

The Beach Center on Families and Disability—This center conducts research and training, and disseminates information relevant to families who have members with developmental disabilities or serious emotional disturbances. Write:

The Beach Center on Families and Disability
The University of Kansas
Haworth Hall, Room 3136
1200 Sunnyside Avenue
Lawrence, KS 66045
Tel: 785-864-7600
Fax: 785-864-7605
Website: www.beachcenter.org

Children and Adolescent Service System Programs (CASSP)—CASSPs are federally-funded programs located throughout several states and localities, designed to improve service delivery for children and adolescents with emotional disorders. CASSP provides funding to states for research and training centers and for technical assistance activities. To contact a CASSP in your area, or to obtain a publications list and additional information, write:

National Technical Assistance Center for Children's Mental Health
3307 M Street NW, Suite 401
Washington, DC 20007
Tel: 202-687-5000
Fax: 202-687-1954
Website: http://www.georgetown.edu/research/gucdc/cassp.html
E-mail: gucdc@georgetown.edu

Additional Information

National Center for Chronic Disease Prevention and Health Promotion
Division of Nutrition and Physical Activity
4770 Buford Highway, NE; MS K-46
Atlanta, Georgia 30341-3724
Toll-Free: 888-232-4674
Website: http://www.cdc.gov

The President's Council on Physical Fitness and Sports
200 Independence Avenue, SW
Room 738-H
Washington, DC 20001
Tel: 202-690-9000

National Resource Center on Supportive Housing and Home Modification
University of Southern California
3715 McClintock Avenue
Los Angeles, CA 90089-0191
Tel: 213-740-1364
Fax: 213-740-7069
E-mail: hmap@usc.edu

Offers a *Home Modification Resource Guide* that lists publications, organizations, and web sites on home modification and adaptive equipment. Available for $12. Many publications of this Center are available on Housing Information for seniors and their families.

Adaptive Environments
374 Congress St.
Suite 301
Boston, MA 02210
Tel: 617-695-1225
Fax: 617-482-8099
Website: http://www.adaptenv.org
E-mail: adaptive@adaptenv.org

Offers *A Consumer's Guide to Home Adaptation*, $12.

Center for Universal Design and Accessible Housing Information
North Carolina State University
School of Design
Box 8613
219 Oberlin Road
Raleigh, NC 27695-8613
Toll-Free: 800-647-6777
Tel/TTY: 919-515-3082
Fax: 919-515-3023
E-mail: cud@ncsu.edu

The U.S. Department of Education's National Rehabilitation Information Center
Toll-Free: 800-346-2742.

Provides information to professionals and the public regarding rehabilitation of persons with physical or mental disabilities.

Administration on Aging
U.S. Department of Health and Human Services
330 Independence Avenue, SW
Washington, DC 20201
Tel: 202-619-0724
Fax: 202-260-1012
TDD: 202- 401-7575
Website: http://www.aoa.gov
E-mail: aoainfo@aoa.gov

ARCH National Resource Center for Crisis Nurseries and Respite Care Services
Chapel Hill Training-Outreach Project
800 Eastowne Drive, Suite 105
Chapel Hill, NC 27514
Toll-Free: 800-473-1727
Tel: 919-490-5577

The mission of the ARCH National Resource Center is to provide support to service providers through training, technical assistance, evaluation, and research. The Center provides a central contact point for the identification and dissemination of relevant materials to crisis nurseries and respite care programs. Numerous fact sheets and general resource sheets (including state contact sheets) are available about respite care and crisis nursery care. ARCH also operates the National Respite Locator Service.

National Respite Locator Service
Toll-Free: 800-773-5433

This service helps parents locate respite care services in their area.

Part Four

Care Environments

Chapter 26

Home and Community-Based Care

In 1997 there were approximately two million Americans living in long-term care (LTC) institutions, such as nursing homes or other adult care settings. By comparison, more than 10 million persons of all ages needed some type of assistance with their daily living activities in order to remain in their own homes or in other community-based settings. About 45 percent of persons requiring home and community-based care are between the ages of 18 and 65. Much of the remaining 55 percent are over the age of 65.

What Is Home and Community-Based Care?

The term home and community-based care (HCBC) refers to the full range of services and settings available to both older and disabled people living either in their own homes or in residential care settings. Generally speaking, the basic community services available through an HCBC system are as follows:

- Information and assistance
- Personal care, homemaker, and chore services
- Congregate and home-delivered meals
- Adult day care

This chapter includes "Home and Community-Based Care: Older Americans Month Fact Sheet," 1997 and "Caregivers, Caregiving and Home Care Workers," by June Faris, 1999, from the Administration on Aging (AoA).

- Rehabilitative care

- Transportation assistance

- Home health care

- Caregivers' support, assistance, and respite care

- Housing options, including assisted-living arrangements

- Consumer protection and advocacy

Because older and disabled persons often have multiple and changing health and social service needs, effective HCBC programs can facilitate access to and network among the basic services provided by offering one-stop shopping arrangements, comprehensive assessment, care planning or case management, pre-nursing home admission screening, and linkage to medical care providers.

The national aging network strives to provide a full range of HCBC services and administrative systems to meet the needs of the elderly, disabled persons, and their caregivers in every region and community across the country. The network is headed by the U.S. Administration on Aging (AoA) and comprises 57 State Units on Aging (SUA); more than 661 Area Agencies on Aging (AAA); 222 tribal organizations, representing 300 tribes; and thousands of service providers, senior centers, caregivers and volunteers.

Why Is HCBC Important?

Surveys show that younger and older disabled persons alike and their families prefer to receive services in their own homes and communities, rather than in institutional settings.

All states and localities are concerned about the escalating cost of Medicaid, which paid $45.7 billion for long-term care (LTC) in 1994, representing more than a third of the Medicaid expenditures for the year. States and localities, all of whom have a major financial stake in containing Medicaid costs, are increasingly looking toward HCBC as a possible alternative for reducing the growth of LTC expenditures.

As the aging of the second wave of baby boomers begins to increase the country's population of older Americans, the number of elderly people requiring LTC also will grow. Given the preference of older people to remain at home for as long as possible, the demand for comprehensive HCBC will continue to rise as well. This growing need has major implications with regard to caregiving, employment, and health care policies.

What Is the Aging Network's Involvement in HCBC?

With its legislative mandate under the Older Americans Act to plan, advocate for, coordinate and develop services for the elderly, the network of SUAs and AAAs is in a strategic position to use its long-standing experience and expertise to meet the LTC needs of older persons. As a critical function of administering Older Americans Act funds, many SUAs and AAAs have coordinated and leveraged multiple sources of LTC funds, including the management of the Medicaid Home and Community-based Waiver and Personal Care Option Programs. According to a 1994 AoA report, almost half of the SUAs administer the Medicaid waiver, the most flexible source of funds for HCBC.

Many AAAs, through state allocations of Older Americans Act funds, state and local revenues, Social Services Block Grant funds, and other resources, fund local service providers to deliver basic HCBC services. AAAs also are extensively involved in case management services to ensure older persons are linked to the services they need.

The Eldercare Locator

AoA also supports a nationwide toll-free information and assistance directory for older people and caregivers called the Eldercare Locator, which can provide the name and phone number of the AAA(s) nearest to the person needing assistance. The Eldercare Locator can be reached by dialing toll-free, 1-800-677-1116, Monday through Friday, 9:00 a.m. to 11:00 p.m., Eastern Standard Time. The Eldercare Locator is not an automated, touch-tone information system. Callers speak to a friendly, caring person who can help them. When calling the Eldercare Locator, callers should have the address, zip code, and county of residence for the person needing assistance.

For more information about AoA and the aging network, please contact:

Administration on Aging
U.S. Department of Health and Human Services
330 Independence Avenue, SW
Washington, D.C. 20201
Tel: 202-619-0724
Fax: 202-260-1012
TDD: 202-401-7575
Website: http://www.aoa.gov
E-mail: aoainfo@aoa.gov

As a caregiver, you are one of 12 million Americans who spend all or part of their day assisting 5 million family members or friends who need help to remain at home.

Many caregivers have multiple responsibilities. The great majority of caregivers are women (75 percent)—a quarter of whom care for both older parents and children. Half of all caregivers also work outside the home. It is no wonder then that caregivers—whether they are full or part-time—need respite and support. Otherwise the demands and constraints of caregiving can become overwhelming.

Many working caregivers find that the demands of their job and caregiving responsibilities conflict. When this happens it is important to discuss your needs with your supervisor. Flex-time, job sharing, or rearranging your schedule may help to minimize your stress. Increasingly, companies are also offering resource materials, counseling, and training programs to help caregivers.

You can also encourage your older children to become involved in the care of your family member. Such responsibility, provided it is not over-burdensome, can help young people to become more empathetic, responsible, and self-confident and give you needed support.

Do not hesitate to ask other family members to share in the responsibility of caregiving as well. Your siblings, if they live nearby, have just as much reason as you to assist their aging parent. If you are a caregiving spouse with siblings and/or adult children make your needs known to them. A family conference can often help in sorting out the tasks and schedules that other family members are able to assume. And don't forget neighbors and friends who may be willing to provide transportation, respite care, and help with shopping, household chores, and repair tasks.

The help provided by you, other family members, friends and neighbors may still not be enough to enable an older person to remain independent. In this case you will need to look for other avenues of support. One of the first places you should contact is to your Area Agency on Aging (AAA). If your family member has a limited income, he or she may be eligible for services provided through the AAA including homemaker home health aide services, transportation, home-delivered meals, chore and home repair, as well as legal assistance.

Area Agencies on Aging can direct you to other sources of help for older persons with limited incomes such as subsidized housing, food stamps, Supplemental Security Income, Medicaid, or the Qualified Medicare Beneficiary program which covers the cost of the Part A and B insurance premiums for low-income elderly.

While your Area Agency on Aging may not be able to provide supportive in-home services for older people who have higher incomes, your AAA may be able to make suggestions about how you can find home care workers whom you can hire directly. Your Area Agency also has information on home care agencies and volunteer groups that provide such services as transportation, chore, respite, yard work, and home repair services. In addition to these information and referral services, many AAAs also will provide an assessment of the older person's needs.

AAAs can also direct you to senior center programs which are suitable for older persons who have minor problems with mobility and activities of daily living and to adult day care programs which serve older persons with serious limitations with mobility, dementia, or medical conditions which require daily attention.

In addition to your Area Agency on Aging, good sources for referrals to individual home care workers and home care agencies include the Hospital or Nursing Home Discharge Planner or Social Worker, if your older relative has been hospitalized.

Home Care Workers

If you decide to hire a home care worker, you will need to determine how much help your older relative needs. Will several hours a day be enough, does he or she need help all day until the family returns home, or does your relative live alone and need round the clock care? You also need to decide what type of home care worker your relative needs. Following are descriptions of the types of home care personnel available:

- A Housekeeper or Chore Worker is supervised by the person hiring them and performs basic household tasks and light cleaning.

- A Homemaker or Personal Care Worker is supervised by an agency or you and provides personal care, meal planning, household management, and medication reminders.

- A Companion or Live-In is supervised by an agency or you and provides personal care, light housework, exercise, companionship, and medication reminders.

- A Home Health Aide, Certified Nurse Assistant, or Nurses Aide is supervised by an agency's registered nurse and provides personal care, help with transfers, walking, and exercise; household

409

services that are essential to health care, assistance with medications, reports changes in the patient's condition to the RN or Therapist; and completes appropriate records.

Nonprofit and for profit home care agencies recruit, train, and pay the worker. You pay the agency. Social Service agencies, in addition to home care services, may provide an assessment of the client's needs by a nurse or social worker, and help with the adjustment or coordination of the care plan.

Home Health Care Agencies focus on the medical aspects of care and provide trained health care personnel, such as nurses and physical therapists. Their services may be paid for by Medicare if they are ordered by a physician.

When calling an agency be sure to ask:

1. What type of employee screening is done?

2. Is the employee paid by the agency or the employer?

3. Who supervises the worker?

4. What types of general and specialized training have the workers received?*

5. Whom do you call if the worker does not come?

6. What are the fees and what do they cover?*

7. Is there a sliding fee scale?

8. What are the minimum and maximum hours of service?*

9. Are there service limitations in terms of tasks performed or times of the day when services are furnished?*

*These questions should also be asked if you are hiring the person directly.

Unless your older relative needs care for a limited number of hours each day, the rates charged by private home care agencies for homemaker home health aide services and van services for transportation are often beyond the means of middle income families. There are ways to obtain competent help at lower rates, however.

If an older person is discharged from a hospital and receives skilled health care services at home, such as nursing or physical therapy, they are usually eligible for homemaker-home health aide services from home care agencies paid for under Medicare. When Medicare coverage ends, it is often possible to hire these same aides privately for a half to two-thirds of the cost charged by the home care agency.

Other avenues for finding aides who charge lower fees include churches, senior employment services, and agencies that assist displaced homemakers and others entering the employment market.

If you advertise in the papers for help, screen the applicants carefully. Ask for identification and check their references. Regardless of who cares for your elderly relative, protect their private papers and valuables, make arrangements to pick up the mail yourself, and check the phone bill for unauthorized calls. Stealing and fraud are on the rise among caregivers for the elderly so it is best to "play it safe."

When hiring the worker yourself, be sure that the home care worker has the necessary qualifications and/or training. Ask to see training certificates, particularly if the older person has special medical needs such as insulin injections. If the older person needs to be transferred from a wheelchair make certain that the aide knows how to do this safely. If the prospective aide does not know how to bathe a person in bed or transfer, but seems to be otherwise qualified, they can be trained in these and other necessary procedures.

If your older relative needs a considerable amount of help or round-the-clock care, consider hiring live-in help. In exchange for room and board, these home care aides will usually work for a salary that is far lower than that charged by aides who come in for a few hours, or during the day.

Check with your insurance company about coverage for a full-time home care worker, and contact the appropriate agencies concerning social security taxes, unemployment insurance, and workmen's compensation. If you do not want to deal with these somewhat complicated withholdings from the employee's salary, accountants and companies that specialize in doing payrolls will issue the employee's check with the necessary withholdings.

If public transportation is not available and the older person is not eligible for free or low cost transportation, try to hire someone who drives, since this can save you substantial amounts of money in taxi or commercial van ride fares. If the home care worker is going to drive the family car, be sure to check with your insurance company concerning any limitations on your policy.

Your interview with the prospective home care worker should include a full discussion of the client's needs and limitations; as well as the home care worker's experience in caregiving and her expectations.

Also ask for the names, addresses, and phone numbers of people who have previously employed the home care worker and be certain to contact them.

Once you have hired a home care worker, make sure that the lines of communication are fully open and that both you and the worker have a clear understanding of your responsibilities to the older person and to each other. Explain what you want done and how you would like it done, keeping in mind that the home care worker is there to care for the older person and not the rest of the family. If the home care worker lives in, try to ensure that he or she has living quarters that give you, the older person, and the worker the maximum amount of privacy possible. Be clear about the worker's salary, when he or she will be paid, and about reimbursement for money the worker may spend out of pocket for gas, groceries, etc. If the home care worker has a car, discuss use of the worker's car on the job, insurance coverage for the worker's car, or other travel arrangements.

Be certain to discuss the subject of vacations, holidays, absences, and lateness as well as the amount of time each of you should give if the employment is terminated. If you work and are heavily dependent on the home care worker, emphasize the importance of being informed as soon as possible so that you can make alternative arrangements, if the home care worker is going to be late or absent. You should have a list of home care agencies, neighbors, or family members who can step in should the home care worker be late or absent from work.

Finally, inform the worker about the older person's dietary restrictions, provide a list of contacts in case of an emergency, review security precautions and keys, and discuss the medication requirements of the older person.

Once the home care worker is on the job, periodic and/or ad hoc meetings can be held to discuss any problems the home care worker or the older person may have with the arrangement and to find ways to resolve them. Be positive and open in your approach to resolving difficulties. In most cases, they can be corrected.

However, if, after repeated attempts, you find that major problems are not resolved satisfactorily it may be best to terminate the relationship, and seek another home care worker. During this time, it may be necessary for your older relative to temporarily reside in a long-term care facility or for you to hire a worker through an agency, so it is best to have reserve funds on hand should such an emergency arise.

Another possible avenue of temporary help is respite care. As applied to home care, respite refers to care that provides a needed break for the primary caregiver, ranging from a few hours to days or weeks.

Respite care services can be arranged through your Area Agency on Aging. The service offers assistance with meal preparation, dressing, grooming, feeding, and light housekeeping, and may include some personal care. A four-hour session is usually the minimum, with an 80-hour annual maximum.

While home care may not necessarily be less expensive than nursing home care or assisted living, it offers older people and their families the opportunity to remain at home and together. What is more, it affords a degree of flexibility and choice for the at-risk elderly that few other living arrangements can offer.

Chapter 27

Respite Care

Contents

Section 27.1

Respite Care for Families of Children with Disabilities

"Respite Care," NICHCY *News Digest* #ND12, update June 1996, National Information Center for Children and Youth with Disabilities (NICHCY).

Raising a child with disability or chronic illness poses many challenges. As families meet these challenges, time off can become a necessity for the caretakers. In recent years, the growth of respite care services—short-term specialized childcare—has begun to provide families with some temporary relief.

Social and community support can reduce the stress experienced by families. The support of relatives, friends, service providers, and the community can help families ease the adjustment period.

Over the years, there has been a growing awareness that adjustment to the special needs of a child influences all family members. This awareness has generated interest and has led to the development of support services for families to assist them throughout the lifelong adjustment process. Within the diversity of family support services, respite care consistently has been identified by families as a priority need (Cohen & Warren, 1985).

While respite may be a new word for some people, it is not a new phenomenon; it emerged in the late 1960's with the deinstitutionalization movement. One of the most important principles of this movement was the belief that the best place to care for a child with special needs is in the child's home and community. Families with a child who has a disability or chronic illness know the commitment and intensity of care necessary for their children. The level of dedication and care becomes part of daily life, part of the family routine, but this same commitment can make stress routine too. Parents can become accustomed to having no time for themselves. According to Salisbury and Intagliata (1986), "the need of families for support in general and for respite care in particular has emerged as one of the most important issues to be addressed in the 1980's by policymakers, service providers, and researchers in the field of developmental disabilities," (p. xiii).

Respite care is an essential part of the overall support that families may need to keep their child with a disability or chronic illness at home. United Cerebral Palsy Associations, Inc. (UCPA) defines respite care as "a system of temporary supports for families of developmentally disabled individuals which provides the family with relief. "Temporary" may mean anything from an hour to three months. It may also mean "periodically or on a regular basis. It can be provided in the client's home or in a variety of out-of-home settings," (Warren and Dickman, 1981, p. 3). Respite services are intended to provide assistance to the family, and to prevent "burnout" and family disintegration. Since not all families have the same needs, respite care should always be geared to individual family needs by identifying the type of respite needed and matching the need to the services currently available, or using this information to develop services where none exist. Once identified, it is also important for families to have ready access to that type of respite, in an affordable form.

Family Orientation

Regardless of the type of respite program utilized, the emphasis should be on orienting services toward the entire family. The birth of a child with a disability or the discovery that a child has a disability or chronic illness is obviously a difficult time for the entire family, including siblings, grandparents, and other relatives. Families need to adjust to major changes in their daily lifestyles and in their dreams. Extended family and friends will also need to adjust to these changes. These changes will take planning and time. We are accustomed to typical family life; a child with a significant disability or chronic illness is not typical. Therefore, plans for an untypical lifestyle call for creativity and flexibility. It is also important to bear in mind that the child will change as he or she grows and develops into an individual with his or her own personality and ideas.

Many families will find these changes difficult to handle. Many communities may be limited in their resources or in their interest in meeting the special needs such families present. These combined factors can leave the immediate family with the full-time care of their child and can lead to feelings of isolation from other family members, friends, community activities, religious, and social functions. Even performing the basic necessities of daily life, such as grocery shopping or carpooling, can become difficult to impossible.

It is obvious to anyone who has lived this life that respite care becomes a vital service—a necessity, not a luxury. Parents, of course,

417

are clearly the experts about the need and importance of respite care. Just as families differ, so will the necessity for respite care. Basically, however, all families require some relaxation, diversion, and the security of knowing that their children are safe and happy. The most difficult problem for the family with a child who has a disability is finding the quality of care and expertise the child needs.

As one parent put it, "Families need an uncomplicated, easily accessible means of arranging respite care to suit their wants and needs. When a potential pleasure becomes more trouble than it's worth, then I give it up. I always measure the event against the complications involved in making it happen. Time off is no relaxation if I spend the entire time worrying if the kids are OK. I can't enjoy myself if I think they are unhappy, and certainly I can't relax if I'm not confident about the reliability of the person watching my children. I think many professionals are under the misconception that time away from the cares of rearing a child with a disability is what I need to maintain my sanity. I need much more than time—I need the security that comes from knowing that the person I've left my son with is as capable as I am of providing for his needs. You simply can't relax and enjoy yourself and worry at the same time. It's peace of mind I need—not just time."

Benefits of Respite Care

In addition to providing direct relief, respite has added benefits for families, including:

- **Relaxation.** Respite gives families peace of mind, helps them relax, and renews their humor and their energy;

- **Enjoyment.** Respite allows families to enjoy favorite pastimes and pursue new activities;

- **Stability.** Respite improves the family's ability to cope with daily responsibilities and maintain stability during crisis;

- **Preservation.** Respite helps preserve the family unit and lessens the pressures that might lead to institutionalization, divorce, neglect, or child abuse;

- **Involvement.** Respite allows families to become involved in community activities and to feel less isolated;

- **Time Off.** Respite allows families to take that needed vacation, spend time together, and time alone; and

- **Enrichment.** Respite makes it possible for family members to establish individual identities and enrich their own growth and development.

Often, we hear the question, "Who takes care of the caretakers?" Caretakers can include not only parents, but also brothers and sisters, grandparents, and extended family and friends. Respite gives caretakers the opportunity to have a rest, to take care of personal matters, to enjoy some leisure time, and occasionally to be relieved of the constant need to care for a child with a disability or chronic illness.

The child or youth with disabilities also benefits from respite care, gaining the opportunity to build new relationships and to move toward independence. In many families, it is common for children to attend day care or after-school care, interact with peers and adults outside the family, and stay with a childcare provider while their parents enjoy an evening out. Respite provides these same opportunities for children with special needs.

For older individuals with a disability, respite can assist in building skills needed for independent living. Since the most appropriate living situation for many adults with a disability is in a group home or other supported environment, out-of-home respite care can enable families to test this option, explore community resources and prepare themselves and their family member with a disability for this change.

States and communities are recognizing that respite care also benefits them. On average, the costs for respite services are 65 to 70 percent less than the costs of maintaining people in institutions (Salisbury and Intagliata, 1986). The cost-effectiveness of respite services allows scarce tax dollars to be used for additional community-based services. During the previous decade, over 30 states passed legislation for in-home family support services, including respite care, using either direct services or voucher systems (Agosta and Bradley, 1985).

Federal Level Support

With the 1986 passage of the Children's Justice Act (Public Law 99-401) and its amendment, the Children's with Disabilities Temporary Care Reauthorization Act (P.L. 101-127), respite care has gained support at the Federal level. This legislation authorized funding to states to develop and implement affordable respite care programs and crisis nurseries. Unfortunately, while this Federal funding provides relief for some families, access and affordability continue to be issues for many families in need. As Brill (1994) observes: <u>Families soon discovered that the law fell short of providing national guidelines for respite care.</u> Every state dispensed different versions of the services, and individual agencies devised their own criteria for length of time and funding allotments. (p. 49)

Thus, in spite of the availability of government funding in some areas, many respite care programs must charge for their services. This practice reduces expenses for providers and makes it possible to serve more families. However, charging for respite services can limit their availability to those families who can afford the fees (Cohen and Warren, 1985).

For children and youth with disabilities, their families and communities, and Federal, state, and local governments, the benefits of respite care are enormous. However, the need for maintaining and expanding the levels of available respite services is tremendous.

Respite Care Suggestions for Parents

Parents deciding to leave their child who has special needs in the care of someone else, either in or outside their home, may experience a variety of hesitations. They can have feelings of guilt, anxiety, even a sense of loss of control.

Jeanne Borfitz-Mescon (1988) suggests that a number of fears and concerns are common to parents in this situation: that the child may not get as much attention, or that the care may not be as good; that something may be missed; that the caretaker or staff may not be able to comfort their child, and that he or she might be left crying. The anxiety resulting from these very normal and real concerns or fears can in fact cause parents to believe that respite is just not worth it.

It is important that as a parent you become comfortable with your decision and develop the trust critical to maintaining the peace of mind necessary for relaxation and enjoyment. One way to accomplish this goal is to begin now to think about respite care and whether you, your family, and your child with special needs would benefit from it. The following suggestions may help.

How can you tell if your family could benefit from respite care? Ask yourself the following questions:

1. Is finding temporary care for your child a problem?

2. Is it important that you and your spouse enjoy an evening alone together, or with friends, without the children?

3. If you had appropriate care for your child with special needs, would you use the time for a special activity with your other children?

4. Do you think that you would be a better parent if you had a break now and then?

5. Are you concerned that in the event of a family emergency there is no one with whom you would feel secure about leaving your child?

6. Would you be comfortable going to a trained and reputable respite provider to arrange for care for your child?

If you have answered "Yes" to several of these questions, you and your family could benefit from respite care and should investigate the resources in your community.

Information on Respite Care Services

Many agencies and organizations have information on respite care services. (For a referral, contact the National Respite Locator Service, operated by the ARCH National Resource Center: 800-773-5433). In general, seek groups or professionals who work with children your child's age. For example, if your child is in preschool, contact the school and discuss the need for respite care with the staff. If there is a parent group associated with your school, or if there is a local parent group concerned with children who have needs similar to your child's, ask them. If your child is an adolescent, talk to the staff at his or her school or, again, identify parent groups in your area with needs similar to yours.

The following list presents some of the types of groups you may want to contact in seeking services. Many will be listed in your telephone book. If you experience difficulty locating the organization in your community, often a state contact can be made. For further information and assistance, contact NICHCY, and be sure to ask for a NICHCY State Resource Sheet for your state. Additional resources are listed at the end of this Briefing Paper.

State and Local Government Agencies

- State Department of Mental Retardation
- State Developmental Disabilities Council

- State Program for Children with Special Health Care Needs (formerly Crippled Children's Services)
- Departments of Health and Human Services, or Social Services
- Department of Mental Health
- State and local Departments of Education
- State Protection and Advocacy Agency

State and Local Disability or Support Groups

- The Arc
- United Cerebral Palsy Associations, Inc.
- Autism Society of America
- Brain Injury Association
- Mental Health Association and CASSP
- Spina Bifida Association
- National Easter Seal Society
- Parent Training and Information Center
- Parent-to-Parent * University Affiliated Program(s)
- Community Services Board
- YMCA/YWCA
- Churches
- Recreation Centers

Seeking Respite Care Services in Your Community?

Ask yourself the following questions. The information will be helpful to you when contacting agencies in your local community about respite care (Bradley, 1988).

1. What kind of services do I need? (Long-term, short-term, or both? Why?)

2. Do I prefer services in my home, a cooperative, or in an outside setting? (This will depend on the type of service you need.)

3. Can I donate my time to a cooperative, or is it better for me to obtain help from a respite agency?

4. Does this agency provide the types of service I need?

5. Is there a cost for the service?

6. Am I able to afford this service?

7. If I can't afford the service, are there funds available to assist me?

8. Who is responsible for the direct payment to the provider?

9. How are respite providers selected?

10. Are the providers trained?

11. How many hours of training have they had?

12. Do these providers have training in First Aid and CPR?

13. What other areas are covered in their training?

14. For out-of-home care, does anyone monitor the facility for safety and health measures?

15. Will I be able to have a prior meeting with the care provider?

16. Will I have an opportunity to provide written care instructions to the provider?

17. Will I have an opportunity to assist in training the provider with reference to my son's/daughter's needs?

18. What is the policy that covers emergency situations?

19. Will I have to carry additional insurance to cover the provider while he/she is in my home?

20. Is there a policy which deals with mismatches between providers and the family?

21. Can I request a specific care provider and have the same person with my child each time?

22. Will the respite care provider care for my other children too?

Conclusion

Caring for a child with disabilities or severe health problems can be a full-time job. It is easy to become overwhelmed with the care needs of a child with a disability or chronic illness. Often, families who would not hesitate to call for relief from the constant care of their typical children hesitate to call for relief from the care of their child with a disability or special health care need. That is why respite, as the word implies, is truly an interval of rest. Respite can be your answer to renewed energies and a new perspective. If respite care is not available in your community, make it happen. The best advocate for your family and your child is you. One of the most important goals to strive for is family unity and well-being. It is important to remember that you, too, can have the gift of time that respite care represents.

References

Agosta, J.M., & Bradley, V.J. (Eds.). (1985). "Family care for persons with developmental disabilities: A growing commitment." Boston, MA: Human Services Research Institute.

Borfitz-Mescon, J. (1988). "Parent written care plans: Instructions for the respite setting." *The Exceptional Parent*, 18(3) 20-25.

Bradley, K. (Ed.). (1988). "Issues in respite care." *Kaleidoscope: A spectrum of articles focusing on families*, 1(2) 6.

Brill, J. (1994). "Keys to parenting a child with autism." Hauppauge, NY: Barron's Educational Series.

Cohen, S., & Warren, R.D. (1985). "Respite care: Principles, programs & policies." Austin, TX: Pro-Ed, Inc.

Knitzer, J., & Olson, L. (1982). "Unclaimed children: The failure of public responsibility to children and adolescents in need of mental health services." Washington, DC: Children's Defense Fund.

"Rest a bit: A training program for respite care providers for families of children with emotional problems." (1988). Topeka, KS: Rest a Bit of Family Together, Inc.

Salisbury, C.L., & Intagliata, J. (1986). "Respite care: Support for persons with developmental disabilities and their families." Baltimore, MD: Paul H. Brookes Publishing Co.

Warren, R.D., & Dickman, I.R. (1981). "For this respite, much thanks... Concepts, guidelines and issues in the development of community respite care services." New York, NY: United Cerebral Palsy Associations, Inc.

Family Support Projects

American Association of University Affiliated Programs (AAUAP)—The AAUAP represents the national network of University Affiliated Programs (UAPs) in the United States. The UAPs provide interdisciplinary training for professionals and paraprofessionals and offer programs and services for children with disabilities and their families. Individual UAPs have staff with expertise in a variety of areas and can provide information, technical assistance, and in-service training to agencies, service providers, parent groups, and others. For information on a UAP in your area, write:

American Association of University Affiliated Programs (AAUAP)
8630 Fenton Street, Suite 410
Silver Spring, MD 20910
Tel: 301-588-8252
Fax: 301-588-2842
Website: http://www.aauap.org

The Beach Center on Families and Disability—This center conducts research and training, and disseminates information relevant to families who have members with developmental disabilities or serious emotional disturbances. Write:

The Beach Center on Families and Disability
The University of Kansas
Haworth Hall, Room 3136
1200 Sunnyside Avenue
Lawrence, KS 66045
Tel: 785-864-7600
Fax: 785-864-7605
Website: www.beachcenter.org

Children and Adolescent Service System Programs (CASSP)—CASSPs are federally-funded programs located throughout several states and localities, designed to improve service delivery for children and adolescents with emotional disorders. CASSP provides funding to states for research and training centers and for technical assistance activities. To contact a CASSP in your area, or to obtain a publications list and additional information, write:

National Technical Assistance Center for Children's Mental Health

3307 M Street, NW, Suite 401
Washington, DC 20007
Tel: 202-687-5000
Fax: 202-687-1954
Website: www.georgetown.edu/research/gucdc/cassp.html
E-mail: gucdc@georgetown.edu

Additional Information

ARCH National Resource Center for Crisis Nurseries and Respite Care Services

Chapel Hill Training-Outreach Project
800 Eastowne Drive, Suite 105
Chapel Hill, NC 27514
Toll-Free: 800-473-1727
Tel: 919-490-5577

The mission of the ARCH National Resource Center is to provide support to service providers through training, technical assistance, evaluation, and research. The Center provides a central contact point for the identification and dissemination of relevant materials to crisis nurseries and respite care programs. Numerous fact sheets and general resource sheets (including state contact sheets) are available about respite care and crisis nursery care. ARCH also operates the National Respite Locator Service.

National Respite Locator Service

Toll-Free: 800-773-5433

This service helps parents locate respite care services in their area.

Section 27.2

Respite Care for Adult Patients

Reprinted with permission, "ACP Home Care Guide–Respite Care,"
© 1997 American College of Physicians.

Overview

Understanding the Problem

- What "respite" services are
- Why extra help may be needed
- Who "respite" helpers are

When to Get Professional Help

- Situations indicating that extra help is needed
- What to say when you call for help

What You Can Do to Help

- Make sure you involve the person being cared for in all decisions
- Make sure the extra helpers are both reliable and honest

Possible Obstacles

- "We've never had anyone else help us before."
- "The person I'm caring for doesn't want anyone else here."
- "I feel funny having strangers come into my home."
- "It's too expensive."

Carrying Out and Adjusting Your Plan

- Ask yourself and the person you are caring for how well the plan is working

- If your plan does not work, consider temporarily moving the person you are caring for into a nursing home

Topics with a flag (➤) in front of them are actions you can take or symptoms you can look for.

- The information in this plan fits most situations, but yours may be different.

- If the doctor or nurse tells you to do something other than what is recommended here, follow what they say.

Understanding the Problem

The word respite (pronounced "res-pit") is new to many people. It means "rest." Sometimes, you will see it listed in the telephone book under the ads for local home health care or visiting nurse agencies, which often are called "Respite Care Services." In this type of care, helpers are sent into the home to stay with the care recipient, giving family caregivers and friends a chance to rest.

This type of extra help may be especially needed during the last months or weeks of a patient's life. Only at this time do many caregivers admit they are not sleeping properly, that they are tired, and that they are worn down by emotional tension and stress. Respite helpers can assist by coming in at night and talking to the person, by giving food or drinks to this person, or by helping him or her to move in the bed. Sometimes, respite helpers simply stay with the patient and allow the caregivers time to run errands, visit friends, go to church, and spend some time taking care of themselves. Respite helpers sometimes are trained—families usually want trained helpers to visit rather than having to ask other relatives or friends to help. They want to know that the helpers are skilled in how to give basic nursing care, such as turning someone in bed or giving a weak person a drink.

Most hospice respite workers are women; however, you can ask for a man if that is your preference. For example, an adult man in a wheelchair might want another man to help him with basic needs such as going to the bathroom or washing. It often is best to find this help by asking the hospice social worker or nurse to give you a list of agencies that employ respite workers or the names of reliable self-employed respite workers. It is best not to hire someone out of the newspaper. Instead, ask people who either have used or are using hired respite workers for their recommendations.

Respite workers can be employed by an agency, or they can be self-employed or even volunteers. When they work for an agency, the agency pays them and either bills you or your insurance company, county, or state. Respite workers usually make a bit more than minimum wage. You will have to give the agency more money than this, however, because you must also pay for the time that it takes to supervise and manage their work. The agency bills the county or state if the individual or their families are "eligible," meaning that household incomes are low enough for the government to pick up the cost of extra help at home. If respite workers are self-employed, they bill you directly. Some volunteer respite workers will offer to spend the night, but these volunteers usually are part of a hospice.

Your goals

- Call for help in locating respite workers.

- Make sure the care recipient is involved in all decisions if possible.

- Make sure those providing extra help are both reliable and honest.

When to Get Professional Help

The first question you should ask is whether you need help in locating respite care services. As with most problems, you should plan ahead and not wait for a crisis. The following signs usually point to a home care problem that should be referred to a social worker, nurse, or some other agency, such as your area Agency on Aging, for assistance in finding helpers:

Call a social worker, nurse, or an agency such as your area Agency on Aging for assistance in finding helpers if either of the following is true:

➤ You feel worn out from the extra responsibilities.

Your health and well-being are important. If you are feeling worn out, call and talk the situation over with hospice staff or a health professional who knows about getting help in the home. Many times, a person with advanced cancer or other medical condition is eligible to have a visiting nurse come to the house and find out what your needs are. The nurses also can send out a nurse's aide to help with bathing and bed making. Aides cannot stay longer than 1 to 2 hours, however, and they usually cannot visit in the evening or at night, which is when you may want to rest. If the person you are caring for is not "sick enough" to have visiting nurses call on him or her but is a senior citizen, you can call the local Agency on Aging. They can send a case or social worker to your home to assess the situation and help you find extra help. Sometimes, money from the county or state is available to help pay for respite care workers; other times, you will be asked to pay. Some towns and areas also have volunteers who are experienced in helping people and their families.

➤ **You worry that you will not be able to take on the extra responsibilities or physical labor of helping a weakened person.**

If you are worried about this, start getting extra help early. This has many benefits. Both you and the person will have time to get to know and trust the helpers. You can work out household routines with them before you become stressed, and if the helpers do work out, then you know that you can depend on them should home care grow more difficult in the future. This knowledge can reduce some of your stress or worries about handling future problems.

What You Can Do to Help

There are at least two things you can do at home to find good respite care workers:

- Make sure you involve the person being cared for in all decisions.

- Make sure those providing the extra help are both reliable and honest.

Make sure you involve the person being cared for in all decisions.

Not everyone welcomes extra help right away. Having strangers in the home is a big change. Here are some ideas on how to ease into it:

➤ **Talk over the reasons you want to get extra help. Be honest about your concerns and what you want.**

The person you are caring for may be more willing to accept this situation if you say that you need the extra help to keep giving him or her care at home. This way, the patient realizes that it is very

430

important to you, and that he or she is helping you by accepting the extra helpers.

➤ Set a time limit on how long you will try the extra help to see what it is like.

For example, suggest that the respite helpers visit twice a week for 2 weeks, then talk over how things are working out and decide whether both of you want to continue having the extra help. Maybe a new helper is needed—if so, set a new trial period.

➤ Have the helpers visit for a short time to talk about the tasks they can do and when they can come.

Meeting someone face to face takes away some of the worry about who a new person is. After the first visit, the patient usually will realize that the "stranger" is there to help and will be more willing to get to know what this "visitor" is like.

➤ Make sure those providing the extra help are both reliable and honest.

You want to be sure that extra helpers will not take advantage of the person you are caring for, or of you as a caregiver. Although this problem is rare, it is best to take precautions. Here are some ways to make sure that extra helpers are reliable, honest, and safe:

➤ Get the names of potential helpers from hospice social workers, nurses, or your area Agency on Aging.

Professionals who work with families that are coping with chronic illness are the best people to ask about respite care services. They will explain your options and their costs, and they can recommend workers who they know are "safe" and are good helpers, will show up on time, and will treat everyone in the family with respect. These are people with a good track record. They will not be potential abusers, whether financially, physically, or otherwise.

➤ Avoid getting the names of potential helpers from the newspaper or local flyers and bulletins.

You take an unnecessary risk by hiring someone from of a newspaper or a bulletin board where self-employed people advertise their services. Many times, these people work out just fine. Even so, you increase the chances of getting a worker who is there with bad intentions, such as stealing money or abusing the situation in some way.

> ➤ **Ask someone you know who either has used or is using extra helpers who you should call.**

If people you know are satisfied with the extra help in their homes, ask them for advice on how to find reliable helpers. Maybe you can even use the same helpers. Many respite workers can work more than one job at one time, and volunteers may be willing to do this as well.

> ➤ **Call the American Cancer Society, and ask if it has a volunteer respite program.**

A few Cancer Societies have volunteer respite programs. Home visitors come and relieve caregivers so they can rest, run errands, and take care of their own needs. Some programs have visitors who will stay longer so that caregivers can go to work, though it might take more than one volunteer to cover an 8- or a 10-hour day.

> ➤ **Check at least one reference before using a respite helper who is not employed by an agency or is not a hospice volunteer.**

Possible Obstacles

Here are some obstacles that other caregivers have faced:

1. "We've never had anyone else help us before."

Response: Having helpers in your home takes some getting used to. Even having professionals such as nurses or hospice workers visit is a change. However, you probably will find that you get very close to these people, and that you will look forward to their visits, advice, and conversation. You will grow get close to respite workers and nurse's aides, too. They will spend the most time with the care recipient, and they can share support and love at a difficult period.

2. "The person I'm caring for doesn't want anyone else here."

Response: The person may want to deal with only one or two special people when it comes to bathing, changing the bed, or other personal care tasks. It may take help from more than one or two people to keep the patient at home, however, especially if caregivers are working or have families of their own to look after as well. When this happens, it is important to ask the person to try the extra helpers for your sake.

3. "I feel funny having strangers come into my home."

Response: Getting help at home can feel funny, especially if you have never used it before. You and the care recipient can try it for 2 weeks or so, then decide whether it is working. You probably will find that you like the people who are helping you, and that their help is very important. In fact, you may wonder later how you ever got along without them. This has been the experience of many families who have cared for a person with a chronic illness at home.

4. "It's too expensive."

Response: Lack of money to pay out-of-pocket fees should not stop you. Often, you can get respite help for free from trained volunteers, and in many states, respite help is paid for by the government. Ask a social worker for help. If that fails, ask visiting nurses or hospice workers what kinds of help you can get for free from volunteers or state respite services. Some churches also have respite volunteer programs, and while their volunteers often visit only those families belonging to that church, some do make exceptions and are willing to help. It pays to ask. Of course, if keeping someone at home is just too much, you can choose other options, such as moving the person to a nursing home or a hospice.

Think of other obstacles that could interfere with carrying out your plan.

What additional roadblocks could get in the way of the recommendations in this plan? For example, will the person cooperate? Will other people help? How will you explain your need for help to other people? Do you have the time and energy to carry out the plan?

You need to develop plans for getting around these roadblocks. Use the four COPE ideas (creativity, optimism, planning, and expert information) in developing your plans.

Carrying Out and Adjusting Your Plan

Carrying out your plan.

Many times, people enjoy outsiders visiting and like the extra help. If you do not like the helpers, however, then change helpers. Agencies are accustomed to trying several people before the right one is found. You can check on how well this home care plan is working by asking yourself if having the extra help is worth it. You also can ask the person how he or she feels it is working.

If your plan does not work.

If finding extra help is a problem, review the When to Get Professional Help section of this plan. If the care recipient refuses to try respite care, you may need to find other ways to get the rest that you need, such as moving the patient to a nursing home for a short time. He or she can return when you are rested or if he or she decides that respite help may be better than staying in the nursing home. Decisions like going to a nursing home do not have to be final.

Chapter 28

Hospice Care

Hospice is a concept of care that involves health professionals and volunteers who provide medical, psychological, and spiritual support to terminally ill patients and their loved ones. Hospice stresses quality of life—peace, comfort, and dignity. A principal aim of hospice is to control pain and other symptoms so the patient can remain as alert and comfortable as possible. Hospice services are available to persons who can no longer benefit from curative treatment; the typical hospice patient has a life expectancy of 6 months or less. Hospice programs provide services in various settings: the home, hospice centers, hospitals, or skilled nursing facilities. Patients' families are also an important focus of hospice care, and services are designed to provide them with the assistance and support they need.

There are different types of services available to patients with advanced cancer. In today's changing health care environment, many patients receive their care at home or in a facility such as a clinic or nursing home, rather than in a hospital. Even when hospital care is an option, patients are often able to obtain care at home as a practical and comfortable alternative to hospital care. When you are considering various options, it's helpful to keep in mind that different types of health care service have different goals. Hospice care and home care are two examples.

This chapter includes excerpts from "Advanced Cancer," National Cancer Institute, NIH Publication #98-856, revised September 1998; Fact Sheet 8.6 "Cancer Facts," National Cancer Institute, reviewed 9/3/1999; and excerpts from "Hospices Services," Health Care Financing Administration (HCFA), 1997.

Hospice Care

Hospice care is designed to give supportive care to people in the final phase of a terminal illness and focuses on comfort and a person's quality of life, rather than cure. It is intended for patients who no longer desire or can no longer benefit from treatment aimed at curing their cancer. The goal of hospice is to enable patients to be comfortable and free of pain, so that they live each day as fully as possible. Aggressive methods of pain control may be used. Hospice programs generally are home-based, but they sometimes provide services away from home—in freestanding facilities, in nursing homes, or within hospitals. The philosophy of hospice is to provide support for the patient's emotional, social, and spiritual needs as well as medical symptoms as part of treating the whole person. Hospice caregivers address the needs of the patient and also consider the concerns of those close to the patient.

Hospice programs use a multidisciplinary team approach, including the services of a nurse, doctor, social worker, and clergy in providing care. Additional services provided include drugs to control pain and manage other symptoms; physical, occupational, and speech therapy; medical supplies and equipment; medical social services; dietary and other counseling; continuous home care at times of crisis; and bereavement services. Although hospice care does not aim for cure of the terminal illness, it does treat potentially curable conditions such as pneumonia and bladder infections, with brief hospital stays if necessary. Hospice programs also offer respite care workers, people who are usually trained volunteers, who take over the patient's care so that the family or other primary caregivers can leave the house for a few hours. Volunteer care is part of hospice philosophy.

The first hospice program in the United States began serving patients in 1974; today more than 3,000 hospice programs across the country offer comprehensive hospice care. Most insurance plans include hospice as a covered benefit. The National Hospice Organization promotes and monitors the quality of hospice care.

Home Care

Unlike hospice programs, home care services may include treatment that targets the cancer itself, not just the symptoms of the cancer. Some people prefer to have cancer treatments and care in the familiar setting of a home rather than a hospital. Home care is provided through various for-profit and nonprofit private agencies, public and private hospitals, and public health departments. Members of the health care team visit the patient at home. Home health care professionals can provide cancer treatment, pain medications, nutritional supplements, physical therapy, and many complex nursing and medical care procedures. Like hospice care, home care also can manage pain and relieve or reduce other symptoms.

Home care can be both rewarding and demanding for the patient and caregivers. It often changes relationships and requires addressing new issues and coping with unfamiliar details of the patient's care. To help prepare for these changes, patients and caregivers are encouraged to ask questions and get as much information as possible from the home care team.

Depending on your own needs and concerns and those of your family or others close to you, the home care team may include many or all or of the following professionals: nurses or nurse practitioners, social workers, dietitians, physical therapists, pharmacists, oncologists, radiation therapists, and psychologists or psychiatrists. (Some health team members do not make home visits). In addition, many patients find that they need a home health aide to help with bathing, personal care, or preparation of meals. Your primary care physician will remain in close contact with the team and monitor your care through other team members, phone calls, and office visits.

Most insurance plans cover brief home visits from a nurse and some cover having a home health aide several times a week. Although more frequent visits and other home care services are available, such as 24-hour care or respite care performed by trained volunteers, these services often are not covered by insurance. As always, you need to know exactly what your insurance plan does and does not cover. If you have questions about your insurance coverage, speak to a member of your health care team.

Some Benefits of Hospice and Home Care

Hospice caregivers and home care professionals can help you understand and work through some of the difficult emotional issues that you and your family or others close to you may be experiencing. In this situation, the social worker is an important team member who provides emotional support, assists in planning hospice or home care, and eases the transition between types of care. From the patient's point of view, an advantage to home-based medical services is that family members and friends can be with you and help with your care. As one woman who cared for her mother at home said:

"The times we all were together with Mom, the rest of the family usually sat and talked with her, while I attended to her personal care or coaxed her to eat. [During those times], we quietly seemed to draw strength from each other just by being together."

Insurance Issues

When you are considering different health care services, be sure to check your insurance plan. Insurance coverage may differ depending on the type of care available and its purpose (e.g., comfort versus aggressive treatment). When you call for information about your plan's coverage, it's a good idea to ask for written confirmation of any information you receive by phone. You also may wish to discuss specific options, such as hospice care and home health care, with your nurse, doctor, social worker, or clergy, as well as your insurance company.

Making Treatment Decisions

It is your right to make decisions about your treatment. It is also important for you and those around you to realize that these decisions may change over time. Family, friends, and caregivers may find it hard to accept, but for some patients, trying to cure their cancer is no longer the goal. Quality of life becomes more important. Other patients may want to try every available drug or treatment in the hope that something will be effective. Either way, it is up to you. Many patients turn to family members, friends, or caregivers for advice. But the decision about how much or how little treatment for you to have is yours. Sometimes a patient is unable to make this decision, due to severe illness or change in mental condition. That is why it is important to make your wishes known in advance.

Even though the decisions are yours to make, your family or those close to you should not be left out. Families and loved ones are often the most important source of support for patients at this time. Patients are encouraged to establish a durable power of attorney and a living will so that their wishes are known by family members and the health care team.

Refusal of treatment does not necessarily mean immediate decline and death; however, a decision to refuse treatment should be based on your feelings about life, death, and the benefits and side effects of treatment. If you decide to stop treatment, you can still receive pain medication and treatments to reduce the symptoms of your disease.

This is called palliative care, and its primary focus is helping you remain as comfortable as possible. Remember: You can change your mind and ask to resume more aggressive treatment. If you do, however, be aware that such a decision may raise insurance issues that you will need to explore with your health care plan.

Your doctors will, almost certainly, offer information and advice to help you decide whether or when to stop treatment. Many religious groups have issued statements about the decision to end treatment. You may want to explore the position that your religious group takes on this issue. Contact a member of the clergy or other counselor if you would like more information. In the end, you are the only one who can decide what is best for you.

Additional Information

The National Hospice and Palliative Care Organization (NHO)
1700 Diagonal Road
Arlington, VA 22314
Tel: 703-837-1500
Website: http://www.nhpco.org
E-mail: info@nhpco.org

NHO is dedicated to promoting and maintaining quality care for terminally ill persons and their families, and to making hospice an integral part of the U.S. health care system. The NHO can provide general hospice information and information about hospice services in different areas.

Hospice Association of America (HAA)
228 Seventh St., SE
Washington, D.C. 20003
Tel: 202-546-4759
Fax: 202-547-3540
Website: http://www.nahc.org/HAA/home.html

HAA can provide facts and statistics about hospice programs, and can also supply the publication *Information About Hospice: A Consumer's Guide*. This guide offers information about the advantages and financial aspects of hospice, how to select quality hospice care that is best suited for a patient's needs, and state resources available to patients.

Hospice Education Institute
190 Westbrook Road
Essex, CT 06426-1510
Toll-Free: 800-331-1620
Tel: 860-767-1620
Fax: 860-767-2746
Website: http://www.hospiceworld.org
E-mail: HOSPICEALL@aol.com

Offers information and referrals on various hospice programs around the country and provides regional seminars on hospice care throughout the United States. Comments or suggestions about hospice programs are also welcomed from health professionals and hospice volunteers.

American Cancer Society (ACS)
Toll-Free: 800-ACS-2345
Website: http://www.cancer.org

The ACS offers a variety of services to hospice patients and their families. The ACS has free fact sheets and publications about hospice as well. The address of a local ACS chapter may be obtained by calling their toll-free telephone number.

Hospice Net
401 Bowling Ave, Suite 51
Nashville, TN 37205
Website: http://www.hospicenet.org
E-mail: comments@hospicenet.org

This organization works exclusively through the Internet. It contains more than one hundred articles regarding end-of-life issues and is dedicated to providing information and support to patients, families, and friends facing life-threatening illnesses.

For many people, some hospice expenses are paid by health insurance plans (either group policies offered by employers or individual policies). Information about the types of medical costs covered by a particular policy is available from an employee's personnel office, a hospital or hospice social worker, or an insurance company. Medical costs that are not covered by insurance are sometimes tax deductible.

Medicare

Toll-Free: 800-633-4227
TTY: 877-486-2048
Website: http://www.medicare.gov

Medicare, a health insurance program for the elderly or disabled that is administered by the Health Care Financing Administration (HCFA) of the Federal Government, provides payment for hospice care. When a patient receives services from a Medicare-certified hospice, Medicare hospital insurance pays almost the entire cost, even for some medications that would not be paid for outside a hospice program. The Medicare Hospice Benefit is designed to meet the unique needs of those who have a terminal illness, providing them and their loved ones with special support and services not otherwise covered under Medicare. For information about the location of Medicare-certified hospice programs, people can call their state health department; the telephone number may be found in the state government section of a local telephone directory. The Medicare Hotline can answer general questions about Medicare benefits and coverage; it can also refer people to their regional home health intermediary for information about Medicare-certified hospice programs.

Medicaid

Website for state Medicaid office locations: http://www.hcfa.gov/medicaid/medicaid.htm

Medicaid, a Federal program that is part of HCFA and is administered by each state, is designed for patients who need financial assistance for medical expenses. Information about coverage is available from local state welfare offices, state public health departments, state social services agencies, or the state Medicaid office. In addition, local civic, charitable, or religious organizations also may be able to help patients and their families with hospice expenses.

The hospice service benefit is an optional benefit which States may choose to make available under the Medicaid program. The purpose of the hospice benefit is to provide for the palliation or management of the terminal illness and related conditions. Under Federal guidelines, the hospice benefit is available to individuals who have been certified by a physician to be terminally ill. An individual is considered to be terminally ill if he/she has a medical prognosis that his or her life expectancy is 6 months or less. Individuals who meet these requirements can elect the Medicaid hospice benefit.

In order to receive payment under Medicaid, a hospice must meet the Medicare conditions of participation applicable to hospices and have a valid provider agreement. The provision of care is generally in the home to avoid an institutional setting and to improve the individual's quality of life until he or she dies. However, individuals eligible for Medicaid may reside in a nursing facility (NF) and receive hospice care in that setting.

In order to be covered, a plan of care must be established before services are provided. The following are covered hospice services: nursing care; medical social services; physicians' services; counseling services; home health aide; medical appliances and supplies, including drugs and biologicals; and physical and occupational therapy. In general, the services must be related to the palliation or management of the patient's terminal illness, symptom control, or to enable the individual to maintain activities of daily living and basic functional skills.

Additionally, there are other services that may be provided under the hospice benefit, subject to special coverage requirements. Continuous home care may be provided in a period of crisis. This consists of primarily nursing care to achieve palliation or management of acute medical symptoms. A minimum of 8 hours of care must be provided during a 24-hour day.

National Cancer Institute
Toll-Free: 800-422-6237
Fax on demand (Dial and listen to recorded instructions):
301-402-5874
TTY: 800-332-8615
Website: http://cancer.gov
E-mail: cancermail@icicc.nci.nih.gov (Put the word "help" in the body of the message.)

Chapter 29

Transition from Home to a Residential Facility

There are two kinds of moves to a nursing home: planned and unplanned. In many cases, placement in a nursing home is unplanned and takes place in a crisis. A person is admitted to a hospital for some urgent reason. The doctor says that a nursing home is the best place. The hospital social worker must quickly find a suitable home. In this case, the person's family is caught in a kind of emotional whirlwind. They don't have much time to get their feelings sorted out. There isn't time to think about what they want or need in the nursing home setting.

Placing a person in your care into a nursing home is complex business. An unplanned nursing home placement makes it much harder to do things the way you want and to be clear about your feelings. You have invested a great deal of yourself in providing care to the person. You want to be sure that the home can provide the kind of care you want for the person. You want to know that the new setting will allow you to retain the kind of caregiving role you want with the person. You will also have a great many feelings about placing the person. You may feel grief and loss, anger, sorrow, and a loss of control. After the person is in the home, you may find yourself enjoying the freedom of days not filled with caregiving tasks. You might feel guilt along with this sense of release.

"The Move to the Nursing Home," © Kenneth Hepburn, PhD., Geriatric Research, Education and Clinical Center (GRECC) of the Department of Veterans Affairs Medical Center, Minneapolis, Minnesota, reprinted with permission; and "Nursing Home Checklist," Medicare, Health Care Financing Administration.

At some point, you will decide nursing home placement may be needed for the person in your care. This is the time to begin planning for that move. You need time to select a home that you can afford and that is best for the impaired person and you. For help in making your choice, see the "Nursing Home Checklist" section at the end of this chapter. Then, when the time comes to move the impaired person, you want be ready. Once you have prepared for it, the move will be smoother, whether it is from your home or from the hospital. Once you have chosen a home, sign the person up on the home's admission waiting list. Depending on how long the waiting list is, you can tell roughly how much time you have to get ready for the move.

The rest of this chapter offers suggestions to help you prepare for and make the move. It may help you see problems which may arise, and to plan your role after the move.

Preparing for the Move

There are three major factors in preparing to move a person to a nursing home. You have to make sure that all financial matters are taken care of. You will need to see to the person's medical care. And you will have to decide who will oversee that care.

Financial Arrangements

Ask for a Written Agreement

Ask the home for a detailed written agreement about charges and services. This should be an agreement that is signed by someone in the nursing home with authority to make a contract. The agreement should spell out what the regular monthly fee will be and what services are included. The agreement should also say what regular extra charges you can expect to pay (for hair care, personal laundry service, physical therapy, etc.). Beyond this, you should receive a list of charges for all extra services available in the home.

Make Careful Payment Arrangements

The details of this task will vary depending on how you plan to pay. You may, for instance, need to arrange to transfer Social Security payments to the home. You may need to apply for Medicaid on the patient's behalf. You may want to see a lawyer about setting up a trust account. Or you may need to get agreements from members of the family about sharing in the cost of care. These arrangements should all be in place by the day of the move. The home will expect you to pay in advance for the first month, so you should be prepared to do so.

Attending Physician

Every nursing home patient must have an "attending physician." This is the doctor who will be responsible for the care the person receives in the nursing home. Almost all aspects of nursing home care need an order signed by a doctor. The doctor must order the drugs a person receives and the activities the person takes part in. The doctor must say what physical therapy the person will get. The doctor must write an order that the person may be physically restrained (and for what reason). If the person falls and might need to be taken to an emergency room for X-rays and/or treatment, a doctor's order is needed. Even the kind of special diet a person may eat requires a doctor's order.

At the time of admission, the attending physician provides basic medical information about the patient, including results from a recent physical. The doctor sets up a plan of care, and visits the patient on a regular basis. The visit schedule will vary, but the doctor should see the patient at least once every month or two. The rest of the time, the attending physician can talk with the staff by phone.

As caregiver, you decide who will serve as the attending physician. You may find the following ideas helpful. Find out in advance if the person's current doctor can serve as attending physician at the nursing home. The nursing home may have a policy that all residents must switch to a doctor on staff at the home.

Find out, too, if your current doctor is willing to attend the patient in the nursing home. If the home you have chosen is not nearby, your doctor may not be able to be the attending physician. If you need to choose a new doctor, you may have limited choices. There may be only a few doctors to choose from in the area or on the staff of the home. Try to meet and talk with these doctors. See which one knows the most about dementia patients.

Medical records. If a new doctor will be attending the patient in the nursing home, be sure all medical records are sent to him or her. Ask the impaired person's former doctor to call the new doctor and discuss the case. Your doctor should provide a summary of the patient's care up to this point. You may find you need to follow up with the doctor to be sure this is done.

Consultations on care decisions. Let the new doctor know that you expect to be fully consulted on care decisions and look forward to being helpful. You have a wealth of information about the person. You can be a resource to the attending physician. Be patient, it takes time to learn to work well with a new doctor.

Plan of Care

In almost every nursing home, the care each patient receives is governed by a "plan of care." The plan is based on a clear understanding of what the patient's needs or problems are. The plan sets care or management goals for each of these needs. The plan sets out how the staff will proceed in each of these need or problem areas. It says which departments; nursing, dietary, or social service, for instance will do that part of the work. Generally, the plan of care is set up within the first two or three weeks of a person's stay. The plan is reviewed and revised every three to six months. Many nursing homes invite families to take part in care planning.

Take Part in Setting Up the Care Plan

Plan to take part in setting up the patient's plan of care. You are an expert on the care needs of the impaired person. You know the best techniques for working with this person. Be ready to offer this information to the care planning group. Tell them what you have observed about the person's food preferences, strengths and weaknesses, likes and dislikes, habits, and activities. List for the group the problems you have had and how you handle them. Tell them how you divert the person, how you received him or her, and how you communicate with each other. For example, if the person becomes agitated, how do you calm him or her? How do you tell if the person is in pain or unwell? Do certain gestures signal certain needs, such as the need to go to the toilet?

Put Your Observations in Writing

Prepare for this planning session by putting your observations in writing, if you can. Then they can become a permanent part of the patient's medical record and can be referred to as needed.

Former doctor's detailed plan of care. Ask the patient's former doctor for a detailed plan of care. Even if this doctor will not attend the impaired person at the nursing home, ask him or her to submit a report to the new doctor. The report should detail what kind of care the former doctor, who knows the patient's situation best, would prescribe.

The Day of the Move

Although emotionally hard, the day of the move itself is not as important as it might seem in ensuring the impaired person's adjustment to his or her new home. Your planning and your future efforts to assure the person's well-being matter much more in the long run. Still, the day itself may be charged with very strong feelings.

Keep in mind that these feelings are normal, but try not to let them get in the way of your task. You want to bring the person to the home and leave him or her there in as cheerful a manner as you can. Your task is to minimize any distress the patient may feel. The following ideas may help.

Plan What to Tell or Say to the Person

Think about what you want to tell or say to the person in your care about the move. Let your own knowledge of what the person can understand be your guide. Discuss the move at the person's level and be truthful. This way you will avoid an overly complex explanation. Also you can be at ease with yourself about not deceiving the person. If the person still has powers of memory and thought, you can give more details. Tell him or her about the home and what it will be like. If the person's powers have dwindled, just say that you have chosen a place where he or she will receive good care. In this case, the impaired person will have to adjust to a new home without the information you might like to give in advance. You can still help and reassure, though. Most meaningful will be the emotional tone you use in talking about the new home. If you truly feel good about the home, this feeling will come across.

Bring a Few Favorite Things

If possible, bring a few favorite "things" with the person to his or her new home. Be sure to discuss in advance with the staff any items you wish to bring with the patient. The home may limit the amount and kind of items you can bring. Most nursing homes don't permit large items, sofas or dressers, for instance. Almost every home has a rule barring certain kinds of electrical equipment, electric blankets, and extension cords. Most require that all other electrical items be

447

checked before use in the patient's room. If you want the person to have a radio or TV, and if you can easily do so, bring the items to the home before the day of the move. That way they can be checked and placed in the room before you arrive. Prepare the essential clothes the person will need in the nursing home. Additional clothes can be brought at a later time. Make sure that the person's clothes and personal belongings are marked or labeled clearly with his or her first and last name.

Let the Staff Take Charge

Once you have brought the person to the home, let the staff take charge. They have routines to help a new resident move in and feel at ease. Discuss in advance what they will want you to do. They might want you to remain for a while. They might suggest, based on their experience, that the move will be easier for both you and the person in your care if you plan to leave soon after the person's arrival. You chose this home because you believed the impaired person would receive good care here. Trust that choice. Do what the staff suggests. They will be the caregivers now. You may see that the impaired person is confused, frightened, angry, hurt, or any mix of these. Keep in mind that the staff remembers how hard it is to adjust. They are skilled in helping people through this period.

Foreseeing This as a Hard Day for You

If you foresee that this will be a hard day for you, try to get help. Ask someone else to drive you and the person to the nursing home and to drive you back home afterwards.

Continued Role for You

The amount of contact you have with the person and the care team after placement is your choice. It is subject to many factors. A big factor is distance between your home and the nursing home. Your health and resources enter into this. Events, demands, and interests in the rest of your life will affect your choice. Whatever you choose, your role may be with both the patient and the care team.

Your Role with the Impaired Person

Contact with the person in the nursing home may serve both your needs. You can see for yourself that the person is well cared for. The person can feel your presence even if other communication is no longer possible.

You may also want to invite the person's family and friends to come visit in the new home. Their care and concern for the impaired person doesn't stop with placement. The person can still feel this care. Keep in mind, though, that it may be hard for family and friends to visit the nursing home. They may not be able to handle seeing the person in this setting.

The impaired person's disease will progress and the person's powers will keep on dwindling. If you visit the person once in a while rather than daily you may seem to detect rapid or sudden declines in abilities. This is not because the nursing home placement is speeding up the person's decline, rather, you are now a more distant observer. When you were with the person all the time, you were too involved with your care tasks to notice change. Now that you have "stepped back" the changes may be more noticeable.

Your Role with the Health Care Team

Try for a good working relationship with the nursing home staff. Go about this gently and be tactful. Check with the staff to see if there is anything you can do for them when you visit. You may, for instance, be able to understand what the impaired person is asking for and convey this to the staff. You may be able to coach the staff in how to understand the person better. Keep in mind that nursing home staffs work on a tight schedule. They may not have time to meet with you every time you visit.

Staff members are professionals and should know their jobs. But if you find a problem in the care the person is receiving, bring this up. If the problem cannot be resolved easily, you may need to go to a staff member's supervisor or to the Administrator. If you become very dissatisfied, you may have to think about moving the person to another home. Discuss this step with your lawyer or financial advisor. You may decide to move the person, but you need to think about the costs involved and the strain it will put on you and the person.

Your Life after the Move

What your life will be after the person in your care has moved to a new home depends on many factors. The main thing is to see that you do have a life of your own and a right to live it. Think about some of these ideas as you pick up your own life again.

Rest

Before you become very involved in making plans, take some time to rest and recover. Then you will have the strength you need to make and act on your plans later.

Allow Time to Adjust

Let your feelings come out and work through them. You almost certainly have a lot of feelings stored up. These may be feelings about the person or about the loss of the person. They may be about the disease or about the fairness or unfairness of life. You may have strong feelings about the help you did or did not receive in caring for the person. A lot of grief, sadness, anger, and loneliness can build in caring for a person with a dementing illness. Now that you are no longer providing round-the-clock care, these feelings may hit you quite hard. You may go through a period of grieving, even though the person is still alive. There are resources available to you. Your family and friends, your health care team, counselors, and members of the clergy can help you. The Alzheimer's Disease and Related Disorders Association can help you to locate a group of other caregivers in your situation. Such a group can provide support and practical suggestions.

Take Pride in What You Have Done

Let yourself see how much you did in your caregiving. You took on a task for which you were unprepared, a task you would not have willingly chosen. You dealt with and learned to do things you never imagined you'd have to do. Perhaps you kept providing care long after your strength seemed gone. Sometimes people experience guilt when they place someone in a nursing home. If you feel guilty remember to look at all that you did.

Nursing Home Checklist

Check lists can help you evaluate the nursing homes that you visit. Use a new checklist for each home you visit. Then, compare the lists. This will help you select a nursing home that is a good choice for you or your relative.

Nursing Home Name: _____
Date Visited: _____
Address: _____

Basic Information

1. Medicare Certified:____(yes) ____(no)

2. Medicaid Certified:____(yes) ____(no)

3. Accepting New Patients:____(yes) ____(no)

4. Waiting Period for Admission:____(yes) ____(no)

5. Number of Beds in each category available to you:_____

Useful Tips

- Generally, skilled nursing care is available only for a short period of time after a hospitalization. Basic nursing care is for a much longer period of time. If a facility offers both types of care, learn if residents may transfer between levels of care within the nursing home without having to move from their old room or from the nursing home.

- Nursing homes that only take Medicaid residents might offer longer term but less intensive levels of care. Nursing homes that don't accept Medicaid payment may make a resident move when Medicare or the resident's own money runs out.

- An occupancy rate is the total number of residents currently living in a nursing home divided by the home's total number of beds. Occupancy rates vary by area, depending on the overall number of available nursing home beds.

Nursing Home Information

1. The home and the current administrator are licensed____(yes) ____(no)

2. The home conducts background checks on all staff____(yes) ____(no)

3. The home has Special Services Units____(yes) ____(no)

4. The home has Abuse Prevention Training____(yes) ____(no)

Useful Tips

- **Licensure:** The nursing home and its administrator should be licensed by the State to operate.

- **Background Checks:** Do the nursing home's procedures to screen potential employees for a history of abuse meet your State's requirements? Your State's Ombudsman program might be able to help you with this information.

- **Special Services:** If a nursing home has special service units, learn if there are separate waiting periods or facility guidelines for when residents would be moved on or off the special unit. Some examples are: rehabilitation, Alzheimers, and hospice.

- **Staff Training:** Do the nursing home's training programs educate employees about how to recognize resident abuse and neglect, how to deal with aggressive or difficult residents, and how to deal with the stress of caring for so many needs? Are there clear procedures to identify events or trends that might lead to abuse and neglect, and on how to investigate, report, and resolve your complaints?

- **Loss Prevention:** Are there policies or procedures to safeguard resident possessions?

For Tables 29.1, 29.2, 29.3 and 29.4, give the nursing home a grade from one to five. One is poor, five is best.

Useful Tips

- Good care plans are essential to good care. They should be put together by a team of providers and family and updated as often as necessary.

- Ask the professional staff how the medicine a resident takes can affect what they eat and how often they may want something to drink.

- Visit at meal time. Are residents rushed through meals or do they have time to finish eating and to use the meal as an opportunity to socialize with each other?

- Sometimes the food a home serves is fine, but a resident still won't eat. Nursing home residents may like some control over their diet. Can they select their meals from a menu or select their mealtime?

- If residents need help eating, do care plans specify what type of assistance they will receive?

Table 29.1. Quality of Life

Characteristic	Poor				Best
1. Residents can make choices about their daily routine. Examples are when to go to bed or get up, when to bathe, or when to eat.	1	2	3	4	5
2. The interaction between staff and patient is warm and respectful.	1	2	3	4	5
3. The home is easy to visit for friends and family.	1	2	3	4	5
4. The nursing home meets your cultural, religious, or language needs.	1	2	3	4	5
5. The nursing home smells and looks clean and is well-lighted.	1	2	3	4	5
6. The home maintains comfortable temperatures.	1	2	3	4	5
7. The resident rooms have personal articles and furniture.	1	2	3	4	5
8. The public and resident rooms have comfortable furniture.	1	2	3	4	5
9. The nursing home and its dining room are generally quiet.	1	2	3	4	5
10. Residents may choose from a variety of activities that they like.	1	2	3	4	5
11. The nursing home has outside volunteer groups.	1	2	3	4	5
12. The nursing home has outdoor areas for resident use and helps residents to get outside.	1	2	3	4	5

Total: _____ (Best Possible Score: 60)

Table 29.2. Quality of Care

Characteristic	Poor				Best
1. The facility corrected any Quality of Care deficiencies that were in the State inspection report.	1	2	3	4	5
2. Residents may continue to see their personal physician.	1	2	3	4	5
3. Residents are clean, appropriately dressed, and well groomed.	1	2	3	4	5
4. Nursing Home staff respond quickly to calls for help.	1	2	3	4	5
5. The administrator and staff seem comfortable with each other and with the residents.	1	2	3	4	5
6. Residents have the same care givers on a daily basis.	1	2	3	4	5
7. There are enough staff at night and on weekends or holidays to care for each resident.	1	2	3	4	5
8. The home has an arrangement for emergency situations with a nearby hospital.	1	2	3	4	5
9. The family and residents councils are independent from the nursing home's management.	1	2	3	4	5
10. Care plan meetings are held at times that are easy for residents and their family members to attend.	1	2	3	4	5

Total: _____ (Best Possible Score: 50)

Table 29.3. Nutrition and Hydration

Characteristic	Poor				Best
1. The home corrected any deficiencies in these areas that were on the recent survey.	1	2	3	4	5
2. There are enough staff members to assist each resident who requires help with eating.	1	2	3	4	5
3. The food smells and looks good and is served at proper temperatures.	1	2	3	4	5
4. Residents are offered choices of food at mealtimes.	1	2	3	4	5
5. Residents' weight is routinely monitored.	1	2	3	4	5
6. There are water pitchers and glasses on tables in the rooms.	1	2	3	4	5
7. The staff encourages residents to drink if they are not able to do so on their own.	1	2	3	4	5
8. Nutritious snacks are available during the day and evening.	1	2	3	4	5
9. The dining room environment encourages residents to relax, socialize, and enjoy their food.	1	2	3	4	5

Total: _____ (Best Possible Score: 45)

Table 29.4. Safety

Characteristics	Poor				Best
1. There are handrails in the hallways and grab bars in the bathrooms.	1	2	3	4	5
2. Exits are clearly marked.	1	2	3	4	5
3. Spills and other accidents are cleaned up quickly.	1	2	3	4	5
4. Hallways are free of clutter and well-lighted.	1	2	3	4	5
5. There are enough staff members to help move residents quickly in an emergency.	1	2	3	4	5
6. The nursing home has smoke detectors and sprinklers.	1	2	3	4	5

Total: _____ (Best Possible Score: 30)

Useful Tips Relating to Information in Nursing Home Compare

Nursing Home Compare contains summary information about nursing homes from their last state inspection. It also contains information that was reported by the nursing homes prior to the last State inspection including nursing home and resident characteristics. If you have questions or concerns about the information on a nursing home, you should discuss them during your visit. This section contains useful tips and questions that you may want to ask the nursing home staff, family members, and residents of the nursing home during your visit.

Nursing Home Compare Information on Results of Nursing Home Inspections

- Bring a copy of the Nursing Home Compare inspection results for the nursing home. Ask whether the deficiencies have been corrected.

- Ask to see a copy of the most recent nursing home inspection report.

Nursing Home Compare Information on Resident and Nursing Home Characteristics

1. For the Measure: Residents Who Are Very Dependent in Eating

    - Look at your response to Question 2 in Table 29.3.

    - Observe residents who need help in eating. Are they able to finish their meals or is the food returned to the kitchen uneaten?

2. Residents Who Are Bedfast

    - Ask the Director of Nursing how staff are assigned to care for these residents.

3. Residents with Restricted Joint Motion

    - Ask the Director of Nursing how the nursing home cares for residents with restricted joint motion.

    - Do the residents get help with getting out of chairs and beds when they want to get up?

4. Residents with Restraints

    - Does it appear that there is sufficient staff to assist residents who need help in moving or getting in and out of chairs and bed?

    - Ask the Director of Nursing who is involved in the decisions about restraints.

    - When restraints are used, do the staff remove the restraints on a regular basis to help residents with moving, and with activities of daily living?

    - Do the staff help residents with restraints to get in and out of bed and chairs when they want to get up?

    - Do staff help residents with restraints to move as much as they would like to?

5. Residents with Pressure (Bed) Sores

   • Ask the staff how they identify if a resident is at risk for skin breakdown. Ask them what they do to prevent pressure sores for these residents.

   • Ask the staff about the percentage of their residents that have pressure sores and why.

   • Do you see staff helping residents change their positions in wheelchairs, chairs, and beds?

6. Residents with Urinary Incontinence

   • Does the nursing home smell clean?

   • Ask the staff what steps they take to prevent incontinence for residents who are at risk.

7. Residents with Unplanned Weight Gain or Loss

   • Look at your responses to Questions 2, 3, 4, 5, 8, and 9 in Table 29.3.

8. Residents with Behavioral Symptoms

   • What management and/or medical approaches for behavioral symptoms are being used by the nursing home?

   • How does staff handle residents that have behavioral symptoms such as calling out or yelling?

   • Ask whether residents with behavioral symptoms are checked by a doctor or behavioral specialist.

   • Ask whether staff get special training to help them to provide care to residents with behavioral symptoms.

Nursing Home Compare Information on Nursing Staff

Caring, competent nursing staff who respect each resident and family member are very important in assuring that residents get needed care and enjoy the best possible quality of life. Adequate nursing staff is needed to assess resident needs, plan and give them care, and help them with eating, bathing, and other activities. Some residents (e.g., those who are more dependent in eating or who are bedfast) need more help than other residents depending on their conditions.

The combinations of registered nurses (RNs), licensed practical and vocational nurses (LPNs/LVNs), and certified nursing assistants (CNAs) that nursing homes may have vary depending on the type of care that residents need and the number of residents in the nursing home.

- Look at your responses to Questions 2 and 5 in Table 29.1 and Questions 4, 5, and 10 in Table 29.2. Also look at your responses to Questions 2 and 7 in Table 29.3.

- Are nursing staff members courteous and friendly to residents and to other staff?

- Do nursing staff respond timely to residents calls for assistance such as help getting in and out of bed, dressing, and going to the bathroom?

- Observe meal times. Do all residents who need assistance with eating get help? Do staff give each resident enough time to chew food thoroughly and complete the meal?

- Which nursing staff members are involved in planning the residents individual care? (Are they the same ones who give the care to residents?)

- Ask questions about staff turnover. Is there frequent turnover among certified nursing assistants (CNAs)? What about nurses and supervisors, including the Director of Nursing and the Administrator? If staff changes frequently, ask why.

- While the number of nursing staff is important to good care, also consider other factors, such as education and training. How many registered nurses (RNs) are on the staff, and how many available on each shift? What kind of training do certified nursing assistants (CNAs) receive? How does the nursing home ensure that all staff receive continuing education and keep their knowledge and skills up-to-date?

Part Five

Legal and Financial Information

Chapter 30

Planning for Now and the Future

If you are caring for a family member with Alzheimer's disease or a related disorder, you may feel swamped. The last thing you want to think about is financial planning. But Alzheimer's is a steadily worsening disease. The impaired person will surely lose abilities. One of the most important tasks you may need to assume is the handling of financial matters. In many cases, this may mean taking over these matters for the first time.

The patient's powers often decline slowly, so the person may be able to take part in family affairs for some time. At some point, people suffering from dementing illness will no longer be able to manage legal or financial affairs for themselves or for their families. Making careful plans in advance will ease the stresses of that time when it does come.

You and the impaired person should plan together for the future. Taking over fully for the legal and financial matters of a person will be easier if you know the person's wishes beforehand.

You will need to set goals and determine the best ways to achieve them. For instance, be sure you can afford any extra care needed for the impaired person. You also want to maintain a decent lifestyle and to provide for your family's future. For all these reasons, you want your family's money to yield the best return, both now and for many years to come.

Reprinted with permission, "Working With Financial and Legal Advisors," Parts I and II, © Kenneth Hepburn, Ph.D., Geriatric Research, Education and Clinical Center (GRECC) of the Department of Veterans Affairs Medical Center, Minneapolis, Minnesota.

How Should You Begin?

Start by learning as much as you can about your family's financial situation. This step has two parts: seeking expert help and finding out what resources and obligations exist.

Set Up a Financial Plan

Once you have a plan, you will need to see that each step is carried out. This chapter will give you an outline of the problems involved in taking over the family finances.

Sharing Responsibility

If you share caregiving for an impaired person with other family members, you may need to share the task of financial management. This may simply involve informing others fully of facts and choices made. You may want to share long-term planning decisions or even day-to-day money management chores. In many cases, the primary caregiver of an impaired person is also the person's spouse. If the spouse has little experience managing financial affairs, grown children may be helpful. A grown child who serves as primary caregiver may not wish (or be able) to take on the task of financial management. If this caregiver can take on the added task, he or she needs to keep other family members well informed.

You may want to call a family meeting to deal with these concerns. Then you can discuss all issues, review the expert advice you receive, parcel out extra work, and make choices. For instance, to decide which is the right advice for you, you might obtain suggested plans from two or three sources. Then, with family members putting their heads together, select the ideas which make the most sense. If it doesn't work out to have a family meeting, the caregiver should see that other family members are informed of major decisions. This should be done in writing. This may seem rather formal, but having these things in writing will help avoid conflict and disputes later.

Choosing Competent Help

Even if the impaired person has only a small amount of savings, insurance, or property, you need expert advice. Many financial advisors are willing to assist you with an initial review, often without charge. Such advisors may include bankers and bank trust officers, lawyers, stock brokers, insurance agents, accountants, tax consultants, and certified financial planners. Not all advisors are qualified to give you an overview of your entire financial and legal situation. One primary advisor will consult and work with others to help you plan for your total needs. It is likely that to cover both legal and financial planning, your primary advisor should be a lawyer. The goals of your meeting with an advisor include helping you do the following:

- Organize your records.
- Understand and manage the current financial situation.
- Develop a plan for the future.

The advisor's role is not to choose for you but to help you choose wisely. Nothing is so simple that any one plan will be perfect. More often, each idea will have good and bad points that only you can weigh.

Finding a Good Financial Advisor

To find a good financial advisor, try these suggestions. If you have a family lawyer who knows your situation, start by consulting him or her. Call your local senior citizen's center or other service agencies. Such places often have the names of free volunteer tax preparers or tax advisors. Some can refer you to a lawyer or may even have lawyers for consultation (sometimes for free). Ask friends or family members to suggest a lawyer or other advisor. Ask if they have worked with the person or if this is just hearsay. Ask your banker or someone else you trust to refer you to other good advisors. Call the local Bar Association's "Attorney Referral Service." They can refer you to a lawyer. When you first call, state your needs briefly. Ask about the advisor's experience in dealing with situations like yours. Ask about fees, and ask what the advisor would, in general, suggest you do. If the advisor will not give you this information over the phone or in an initial visit, look elsewhere.

Determining Current Resources and Obligations

You and your advisor need a clear picture of the financial situation. You will need to collect as much information as you can about family assets and income as well as family debts and obligations. This can be harder than it might sound. The impaired person may be of little help. Records have most likely been forgotten, mislaid, or even hidden. Talking about the subject may be upsetting. Also, many people feel financial matters are very private issues. You may feel uneasy about prying into the private affairs of a family member. But someone needs to do so.

Meeting the needs of a person may mean greatly increased medical and living expenses. Living on a fixed income, increasing costs of health care, and inflation must be thought about. Families need to know what resources can be used to meet these costs. Also, someone will need to pay the bills on time.

These added expenses may affect your own financial planning. What if you are the impaired person's spouse? You likely have mingled resources and debts. If you are the person's child, you will likely have to keep separate track of the person's funds and your own. Most of us can list common bills and debts: house mortgages, car loans, other personal loans, or credit card charges, utility bills, insurance premiums, medical bills and taxes, for instance. Financial resources (that is, income and assets) may exist in many forms, however, some of which may be new to you. Normally, creditors will not let you forget any debts owed. But records of assets may be hard to find, especially if the impaired person has been unable to keep good records for some time or has hidden records. Make sure you carefully search the impaired person's home and records to find any trace of resources. Look through the person's mail. Look in other obvious, and not so obvious places. Don't look just in desks, file cabinets, and offices, but also in dresser drawers and containers of all kinds. Search under mattresses, beds, or rugs, and in coat or suit pockets and handbags. Keep in mind that the records could be anywhere: in the attic, in the basement, in the cookie jar, or the medicine cabinet. Check address books for the names of insurance agents, lawyers, accountants, bankers, real estate agents, and other financial advisors. Talk to these people, explain the impaired person's condition and ask if they can tell you about financial dealings they had with the person. You may need a lawyer to help you obtain access to some records.

Look for these items:

- Bank books and statements
- Stock certificates and bonds
- Statements from brokerage firms
- Insurance policies or premium notices for insurance
- Safety deposit boxes
- Personal loans

466

- Disability benefits
- Evidence of foreign bank accounts
- Address books
- Military records pension notices
- Wills
- Trust accounts
- Inheritance records
- Income tax records
- Cemetery plot deeds
- Evidence of real estate property (such as deeds, keys, property tax statements, etc.)
- Other personal property (such as coin or stamp collections, gold, jewelry, autos, antiques, cameras, art pieces, etc.)
- Evidence of other investments (Individual Retirement Accounts or limited partnerships, for example).

Determining Future Resources and Obligations

Find out what resources and income there will be in the future, and estimate future expenses. Don't overlook some ideas that may not have occurred to you before now. Tax credits or deductions and free or low-cost community services, for example, can increase the resources available to you even though these items are not "income." Take into account such "hidden expenses" as inflation and lost insurance coverage. Benefits and income are lost when the impaired person (or caregiver) has to give up a paid job.

Potential Income and Assets

- Income and assets of the impaired person
- VA benefits
- Social Security
- Pensions
- Savings accounts
- Checking accounts
- Real estate investments
- Stocks and bonds

- "Convertible" assets (such as automobiles, jewelry, coin collections, etc.)
- Other income or capital (Individual Retirement Accounts, for example)

Other Sources of Income and Assets

- Impaired person's spouse
- Impaired person's children
- Other relatives

Note: Check state laws about the financial rights and duties of family members.

Insurance Income

- VA coverage
- Health insurance
- Major Medical coverage
- Life insurance
- Medicare
- Medicaid

Note: Be sure to check what such policies cover. Patients with Alzheimer's disease are not always included.

Potential Expenses

To predict future expenses, you need to know what current expenses are averaging. You also need to predict the likely cost of living increases and new expenses. Your advisor should be helpful here. If you don't already know, keep track of the impaired person's monthly living expenses (housing, food, heat, etc.) If you live with the person, keep track of your living expenses too. Some bills are due only once or twice a year (annual water bill, taxes, auto insurance, etc). Average these in. Include savings needs (for a new car, college tuition, retirement, or whatever). Then estimate potential additional expenses of caregiving, using the following questions as a guide.

Remember: Be sure to check out free or low-cost community services which might reduce expenses. For instance, you may find transportation or meal programs, adult day care centers, or counseling services.

Medical Costs

- If you or the impaired person will lose insurance coverage, will you need to purchase extra medical insurance?

- Will the person have more expenses for the services of doctors and nurses?

- Will the impaired person incur extra hospital bills?

- Will the impaired person need more drugs?

- Will you need to purchase special equipment, such as a wheel-chair, to care for the person?

Housing Costs

- If the person will stay at home, will the house have to be modified in any way for safety or ease of use?

- If the impaired person can't stay in the same house, will there be moving costs?

- If the person moves in with you, will you have to make any changes in your own house for either safety or ease of use?

Costs of Hired Help or Services

- Will you need help with housework or yard and home mainte-nance?

- Will you be having meals prepared by someone else, or will you be eating out more often?

- Will you need to use taxis or other transport services?

- Will you need the services of a paid caregiver or day care center when you need a break?

- Will you need daily or weekly nursing help to care for the person?

- Will you or the impaired person have any legal fees or fees for other advisors?

Costs of Miscellaneous Supplies

- Will you need incontinence supplies or other equipment (hand-rails, grab bars, etc.) designed to help in caring for an impaired person?

- Will you need different types of clothing or personal items for the impaired person for safety or ease of use?

Organizing Records

You should keep careful records of expenses of caregiving and of decisions made on the impaired person's behalf. This is to protect you and to avoid confusion later. A lawyer or an accountant can help you set up a simple system. Once you have met with your advisor and arranged the records, prepare a list of documents. The list should say where each document can be found. One copy of the list should be kept at home. Other copies may be given to your financial advisor, lawyer, or close relative.

Your list should include the following items:

- Any "proof of ownership" papers;

- The passbook number and bank branch for all savings and checking accounts;

- The location of all insurance policies (health, disability, life, fraternal, VA, homeowners, automobile, etc.);

- The location of all "vital statistics" documents (marriage, birth, death, citizenship, military, etc.);

- The names, phone numbers and addresses of financial and legal advisors (attorneys, stock brokers, insurance agents, income tax preparers, etc.); and

- A list of all charge accounts.

Taking Over Tactfully

If the impaired person has always controlled the finances in your family, taking charge may be awkward. There is a risk of hurting the person's sense of self-esteem. Also, if the disease has made the person unduly suspicious or paranoid, you may even be accused of trying to steal his or her money. Depending on how impaired the person is, you may be able to go about this slowly. Begin, for instance, by taking over spending decisions and bill paying. Perhaps you will only need to watch over the person's handling of affairs, correcting any mistakes. But you may need to take over fairly abruptly. Either way, the following ideas may help.

- Avoid unnecessary discussion.

- Avoid conflict by avoiding unnecessary discussion. Keep in mind that the person probably finds the whole subject confusing and upsetting. You are quietly but firmly taking care of matters which have just become too hard for the person.

- Review the mail

- Take out bills, checks, bank statements, etc., before the impaired person finds them.

- Direct deposit of income checks.

- Arrange to have all income checks (from pensions, Social Security, etc.) deposited directly into bank accounts you control. *You may want to look into types of accounts that make this easier.

Pocket Money

Make sure the impaired person always has some pocket money. This will help preserve some sense of independence. You will think of other good techniques to help the person and you to make this big change. Support groups are another good source of ideas for coping with problems like these.

Legal and Financial Tools

A financial plan is a major part of taking charge of money matters and legal issues. A financial plan is the way you choose to make the best use of the assets you have. There are a number of legal and financial tools to help you manage these things. The rest of this chapter discusses, in a general way, some of the options that do not require going to court. Not all of these ideas may apply to you right now. Laws and services vary from state to state. You will also need current and detailed advice about how to invest. For all these reasons, you will need to talk to an expert financial advisor.

This chapter covers five tools to help you manage the financial and legal affairs of the impaired person. They can also help assure financial security for yourself and your family:

Wills

Draw up a will, and (if possible) be sure the impaired person has a will. Set up the right kinds of bank accounts for managing day-to-day expenses. Talk about getting a "power of attorney." Explore a "fiduciary," "protective payee," or "representative payee" arrangement. Think about setting up a trust. Wills seem to be the most often overlooked of major legal documents. A will is a document that says how a person wants his or her assets divided after death. Many people never make a will because they have the idea that leaving an estate is for people who have large sums of property or money. This is not true. Anyone who owns any "real properly" (house, land, apartment) or any "personal property" (furniture, bank accounts, jewelry, automobile) has an estate. Even money owed to a person is part of the person's estate. In all these cases, a will should be made. In a marriage, spouses each need a separate will.

Find out if the person in your care has a will. If there is no will, be sure one is drawn up before the person is no longer legally competent. (Your lawyer can tell you how "legal competence" is defined in your state.) A will may be found "invalid" (that is, not binding) if written too late in a person's illness.

Benefits

The benefits of having a properly drawn will include these:

- A will assures that, upon death, a persons estate will be divided according to his or her wishes.

- A will may also provide for the least costly division of the estate.

- A will may reduce delay in the transfer of an estate to heirs.

- A will may save on taxes and other expenses involved in settling the estate.

Without a Will

If people die without making wills, they are said to have died "intestate." Their estates will be split up according to the laws of their home state. The state's way of dividing the estate may not be how you or the impaired person would choose. It might also not be the way that best meets the needs of your family. Here are some ways an estate might be split up if the owner dies intestate:

- If the husband or wife dies, the surviving spouse receives half of the estate and the other half is divided equally among the children.

- Should the husband and wife die at the same time, the entire estate is divided equally among the children. Minor children become wards of the state until guardians and trustees are appointed.

- If a person dies without leaving a surviving spouse or children, the estate goes to any living relatives, excluding any in-laws or their offspring.

- If a person dies without living relatives, the entire estate goes to the state.

Lack of a will may result in increased settlement costs and taxes. It may also cause needless delays in settlement.

How to Write a Will

Each state has its own rules about writing a will and how to assure that a will is valid. Speak to a lawyer about this. In most cases, preparing a will is quite simple. A few hours and as little as $50 to $100 may be all that is needed. A lawyer can help you draw up a will according to your wishes and protect your legal rights. Members of some state Bar Associations offer, as a public service, to prepare simple wills for senior citizens for a small charge. (Check the yellow pages for the number of your local Bar Association and ask if this service is available.)

Many people think they can save a lot of time, trouble, and money by writing their own wills. Such wills are called "holographic" wills. The fact is that only about half of the fifty states accept them as binding. People often lack the legal knowledge and precise knowledge required to ensure that their estate is handled in the manner they want. Also, simple errors, such as failure to include the date or use of a stamped date, may make such a will worthless under the law. All of these problems can lead to bad feelings and very often also result in lawsuits being filed by heirs or others.

If you want to prepare a holographic will, be sure to find out first if it will be binding in your state. Also find out what special rules apply to holographic wills. Check these things with a lawyer.

Keeping a Will Up-to-Date

Review both your own will and the impaired person's will with your lawyer at least every two or three years. Not only may your situation change, but laws (especially tax laws) can change. You should also review the wills right away in the following special situations:

- You or the impaired person must move to a new state.
- Your family situation changes (due to a birth, death, marriage, divorce, etc.).
- The estate changes in size or nature.
- The needs of the heirs change.

Good wills should be seen as a very key part of any family's financial plan. Preparing a will can be hard and can raise a lot of hard feelings. Still, be sure to give this part of your financial planning the time it deserves.

Special Bank Accounts

As the caregiver for an impaired person, you need to think about how to manage day-to-day expenses. A range of simple bank accounts can solve some of these problems. These accounts include personal accounts, joint accounts, and trust accounts. Discuss your choices with a lawyer who can recommend the right account to set up for your family. If there are other adult family members involved, you may also want to discuss all this with them. You can learn about their concerns and ideas and be sure all approve of your final decision. This step can save you family conflicts later. The account balance should be large enough to pay the impaired person's (if need be, the whole family's) normal household expenses for at least a month.

Why Is Such an Account Needed?

The laws of most states "freeze" all the assets of a person who dies. Even assets such as paychecks due may be frozen. This "freeze" lasts until an executor has been named and a list of the deceased person's property has been prepared. This may take two to three weeks or even more. The special cash account is a reserve fund in the event of the person's death. It permits the caregiver to pay the expenses that are part of daily living until the person's estate has been settled.

Joint Bank Accounts

If an impaired person needs help to manage money, think about a "joint bank account." Two or more people may open a joint bank account. Money from this account can be withdrawn by any person named on the account. The joint account is easy to open and use. It leaves you with easy access to funds if the person should die.

If the money in the account belongs to the impaired person, the caregiver should write a letter to the bank stating this. Copies of this letter should be sent to other concerned family members.

If the money is your own, be sure to keep receipts showing how much you have spent on the care of the person. You may want to send copies of this information to certain family members. (If the caregiver is a child of the impaired person, for instance, all other children should receive copies.)

Sometimes the joint account has disadvantages. The main disadvantage is that the impaired person can still withdraw money, even after becoming incompetent. A more remote possibility also exists. If one of the co-signers were to go bankrupt, funds from the account might be withheld from the other co-signer(s) and used to pay debts.

Trust Accounts

You might want to set up a type of simple passbook account called a "trust account." (Note: This is not the same as "setting up a trust.") In this trust account, one person controls funds "in trust for" an impaired person and can sign checks for that person. Funds are protected from a person's faulty judgment, and you have easy access to funds for meeting expenses. There can be a problem with this type of account. You should leave clear guidelines for what to do if you should die before the impaired person.

Power of Attorney

You might think about having the person for whom you provide care give you power of attorney. A "power of attorney" is a written document that permits one person to make certain decisions for another person. This power gives one person the legal right to manage the finances, property, and/or other legal matters of another person.

Note: The person granting the power **must be competent. He or she must fully understand the power of attorney agreement at the time it is written.** If there is any question of the competency of the impaired person in your care, a power of attorney will not be the appropriate way to solve your problem.

475

Simple or Durable Power of Attorney

In some states, a power of attorney may be either "simple" or "durable." A simple power of attorney ends when the person becomes incompetent. A durable power of attorney remains in effect even after the impaired person becomes incompetent.

Not all states permit a durable power of attorney. Where it is allowed, the durable power of attorney is a simpler option than a guardianship. The durable power of attorney permits decisions about care, for instance.

Limited or Broad Power of Attorney

The power of attorney can also be either "limited" or "broad." A "limited" agreement has defined limits. For instance, it could only be used to pay bills, conduct business, or file taxes. A "broad" agreement gives the power to take care of all legal and money matters.

In most states, you are not required to hire a lawyer to complete a power of attorney, but you may save yourself trouble by reviewing things with a lawyer first. A lawyer can help you decide if a power of attorney makes sense in your case. If yes, the lawyer can recommend which type of power of attorney would be best. The lawyer can tell you the right language to give you what you want.

A power of attorney should include the following parts:

- The name of the person granting the power (the impaired person)

- The name of the person to whom power is granted (you or another family member or friend)

- Details of duties and powers being granted

- Details on how long the agreement is to last.

A power of attorney should be signed by both parties before a "notary public." Your bank's staff probably includes a notary. If not, the bank can refer you to one.

The document should be recorded in the County Recorder's office. (This will usually require a small fee.) The procedure will vary from state to state, so ask.

A power of attorney may be cancelled at any time, unless written differently. To cancel, a written and signed statement should be recorded. (Follow the procedure at your County Recorder's office again.)

Fiduciary or Protective/Representative Payee

A "payee" is someone who can receive and use an impaired person's benefits in the best interest of that person. This option is used when a person can no longer manage benefits. Agencies that issue benefits, like the Department of Veterans Affairs and Social Security Administration, can appoint payees.

Agencies use several terms to describe the payee. The person is called a "fiduciary" by the Department of Veterans Affairs. The Social Security Administration uses the term "representative payee." State social services, health, or welfare departments often use the term "protective payee" (or some similar name).

Each state has a different term to describe this arrangement, so be sure to ask. Each agency has its own way of deciding if a payee is needed and how to choose one. An impaired person can request this kind of help. The government agency may require this arrangement. This varies, depending on the agency involved, so be sure to ask.

Trusts

In setting up your financial plan, give thought to the option of a trust. Trusts and a will can work well together to manage and divide financial resources. A trust transfers money or property from one person to another, with certain conditions attached. The trust is managed by a third person. The trust continues until its conditions have been met. (A condition might be that a certain date has arrived, or a certain event has occurred.)

The person creating the trust (the impaired person) is the "trustor." The person who receives the benefit of the trust is the "beneficiary." The beneficiary might be the trustor's child, spouse, grandchild, or anyone else the trustor chooses, including himself or herself. The person who manages the trust is the "trustee." As a caregiver, you could be the trustee. Someone outside your family could also serve as trustee. Banks offer this service.

Trusts are not only for very wealthy people. Still, they are not the right option for persons with very few assets. In that case, a trust-like document may be drawn up with the aid of a lawyer. A lawyer or a banker can tell you which option best meets your needs.

Trusts Are Meant to Achieve the Following Goals

Provide income for beneficiaries. Reduce estate taxes and eliminate some probate fees. Assure that property continues to serve any desired special purpose after the trustor's death. Reduce the trustor's or beneficiary's daily task of money management. VA trust can be written to do many things. The terms could state that the trustee should continue to provide for the care of the trustor (the impaired person) if or when the trustor becomes incompetent. The terms could also state that the trustee should take no action at all unless the trustor becomes incompetent.

Speak to your bank staff or a lawyer about establishing a trust. Going to court is not necessary. The trustor may ask the court to review the operation of the trust. The trust could also allow the beneficiaries to ask for a review by the court. Common kinds of trusts include:

Testamentary Trust—This is a trust created by a will. It takes effect after the trustor's death. Under such a trust, property need not be divided immediately among all heirs. Instead, it can link the division to some event. For instance, the trust may provide that a widow receives the net income from the trust during her lifetime. Then, upon her death, the rest of the funds will be split among any children or other heirs.

Living Trust—People create this kind of trust to help them while they are still alive. It helps them manage their assets. Living trusts can be flexible and controlled by the person. For instance, such a trust can be used to pay the cost of in-home or nursing home care.

Life Insurance Trust—This kind of trust can receive proceeds of life insurance policies. It can make cash available to the administrator of an estate. For instance, this kind of trust can provide income for a family to help meet daily expenses while an estate is being settled.

Chapter 31

Legal Authority

Editor's Note: This document was prepared for residents of North Carolina. Readers need to consult their own state for specific requirements in their state. This chapter is designed to acquaint you with certain legal issues and concerns. It is not designed as a substitute for legal advice, nor does it tell you everything you may need to know about this subject. Future changes in the law cannot be predicted, and statements in this publication are based solely on the laws in force on the date of publication. If you have specific questions on this issue, seek professional advice.

Giving Someone the Power to Act on Your Behalf
Preparing for Possible Future Incompetency

Many people can handle their affairs for most of their lives. Some, however, may need help because of injury, disease, or old age. Unfortunately, many people fail to prepare for the possibility that they may be unable to manage their financial and personal affairs. Preparing for possible future incompetency means giving someone the legal authority to act on your behalf if you are unable to handle your affairs, either temporarily or permanently. Preparing for possible future incompetency involves four basic legal arrangements: joint ownership

Reprinted with permission, "Legal Authority," © North Carolina Cooperative Extension Service, North Carolina State University, Raleigh, North Carolina, 1993.

of personal property, power of attorney, trusts, and guardianship. Some of these arrangements may work better than others. This chapter examines the advantages and disadvantages of each arrangement.

Joint Ownership of Personal Property

Joint ownership of personal property, such as a bank account, gives another person access to some of your funds. If you become incompetent, that person may pay your bills and handle some of your affairs. Although this arrangement is easy and inexpensive to set up, it has limited value and may create additional problems. Some of these problems are discussed later.

You may own a bank account with a spouse, a child, other relative, or trusted friend. You may own an account with one or more persons. Open the account as an "or" account, instead of an "and" account, so either party alone may have access to the funds. For example, open the account as "Mother Smith or Daughter Smith."

Note: Joint ownership of real property (land) is excluded from this discussion. Joint ownership of land is not usually the best way to plan for paying bills during a disabling illness because of the problems in selling, mortgaging, or leasing the land if an owner is not competent.

Potential Problems

If you choose to enter into this type of arrangement, be aware of certain legal and tax consequences. The consequences may depend upon: (1) whether you own the account with or without a right of survivorship; (2) whether your co-owner is your spouse; and (3) whether you are dealing with federal law or state law. The potential problems listed should help you ask questions of your attorney, accountant, or banker before you enter into this type of arrangement.

- Your co-owner may spend the money without your knowledge or permission.

- Your co-owner's creditors may be able to get up to one half of the account (up to one third if there are three owners, etc.), unless you can show that the money in the account is yours. You must keep complete records of your contributions.

- Your co-owner may have to report a share of the income from the account on his or her income tax return.

- You may be making a gift to your co-owner if he or she withdraws your funds for personal use. If your co-owner is not your spouse, you may be liable for gift tax if he or she withdraws more than $10,000 per year for personal use.

- If you own the account without a right of survivorship, your co-owner's share may become part of his or her estate when he or she dies. You may lose all or a portion of those funds, depending upon your right to inherit the funds from your co-owner.

- At the death of your co-owner, part of the account may be used to pay certain debts of your co-owner, such as taxes and the claims of creditors. If you own the account with a right of survivorship, funds in the account will be used to pay these debts only if all other property in your co-owner's estate is spent.

- Your access to the funds may be limited when your co-owner dies. Fifty percent of the funds may be frozen to cover your co-owner's debts and taxes. However, funds in an "absolute right of survivorship" account are not frozen at the death of a co-owner. This type of account is discussed under "Absolute right of survivorship" accounts.

- If you own the account with a right of survivorship and your co-owner dies first, part or all of the account may be included in your co-owner's gross estate for federal estate tax purposes. If your co-owner was not your spouse, the entire account may be included in your co-owner's gross estate. If your co-owner's estate can prove that all or a part of the funds are yours, the amount proven is excluded from your co-owner's gross estate. Your co-owner's personal representative may ask you for records of your contributions to the account. If your co-owner was your spouse, one-half of the value of the account is included in your spouse's gross estate, regardless of how much the spouse contributed to the account.

(Note: The rule for property owned by spouses may be the same as for non-spouses if they owned the property before 1977. This issue is currently open to debate. Application of the non-spouse rule may result in a tax advantage for the surviving spouse. Ask your attorney or accountant for details.)

- If you die first, your co-owner may get all or a portion of the account, regardless of what you have written in your will. If you own the account as joint tenants with right of survivorship, your co-owner may get all of the funds in the account. If you own the account without a right of survivorship, your co-owner may get at least one half of the funds in the account (one-third if there are three owners, one-fourth if there are four owners, etc.).

- If you are incapacitated and your co-owner dies or becomes incapacitated, there may be no one who has legal access to your account to pay your bills and handle your finances.

Alternatives. Because of potential problems, joint ownership of property may not be the best way to plan for possible future incompetency. Consider this method only when you want to make someone a co-owner of your property. If your purpose is simply to give someone access to your bank account, check with your bank for alternatives. A power of attorney and a personal agency account are two alternatives.

Power of attorney. You may give someone a power of attorney to write checks on your account without making that person a co-owner. Your bank may have a special form for this purpose.

Personal agency accounts. On July 1, 1989, personal agency accounts became available in North Carolina. A personal agency account may be a checking account, savings account, time deposit, or any other type of withdrawable account or certificate. Ask your bank if it offers this type of account.

You name an agent (or agents) who may write checks on and make deposits into your account. You may allow your agent to continue writing checks and making deposits even if you become incapacitated. You must specifically choose this option. If you do not choose this option, your agent may not have access to your account if you become incapacitated.

The agent does not have any ownership or survivorship rights in your account. Upon your death, the money remaining in the account is controlled by your will. If you do not have a will, it is inherited by your heirs.

Absolute right of survivorship accounts. On July 1, 1989, joint accounts with an absolute right of survivorship became available in North Carolina. The new account has an advantage over the old right of survivorship account. On the death of a co-owner, the funds in the account are not frozen. The surviving co-owner may withdraw the funds. If the co-owners were not married, the surviving co-owner may need a tax waiver from the Department of Revenue before withdrawing the funds. The deceased co-owner's personal representative may have the right to recover the funds to pay debts. Check with your bank for details on how to open up a new joint account or how to convert an old joint account into a new joint account.

Power of Attorney

A power of attorney is a document in which you give someone the legal authority to act for you. That person is called your attorney-in-fact. You may name your spouse, an adult child, a relative, or trusted friend to be your attorney-in-fact. You should choose someone you trust completely. The actions of your attorney-in-fact authorized by your power of attorney are considered legally to be your actions.

You decide how much or how little authority to give your attorney-in-fact. You may give your attorney-in-fact the authority to deal only with a specific piece of property, or to do one specific act on your behalf. Or, you may give your attorney-in-fact the authority to handle most of your personal and financial matters. The more authority you give your attorney-in-fact, the more likely he or she will be able to handle problems that may arise.

Types of Powers of Attorney

A **durable power of attorney** is effective even though you are incapacitated. If you are planning for possible future incompetency, your power of attorney must be durable. To be durable, a power of attorney must state that it either remains or becomes effective after you become incapacitated, (in North Carolina it must refer to Article 2 of Chapter 32A of the North Carolina General Statutes). If it remains effective after you become incapacitated or if it refers to the statute, it is effective immediately upon signing.

A **regular power of attorney** ends if you become incompetent or incapacitated. Someone may act on your behalf under a regular power of attorney only if you are competent. A regular power of attorney is used for reasons other than planning for incapacity.

Durable Power of Attorney

A durable power of attorney may be effective immediately or only if you become incapacitated. If your power of attorney is effective only if you become incapacitated, you may want to establish a procedure for determining if you are incapacitated. Many lawyers recommend having two doctors' opinions to establish that you are incapacitated. If you do not establish a procedure for making this determination, your power of attorney is effective when your attorney-in-fact swears in an affidavit that you are incapacitated.

Records, inventories, and accountings. If you become incapacitated or mentally incompetent, your attorney-in-fact must keep full and accurate records of anything he or she does on your behalf. Your attorney-in-fact must file inventories and accountings with the clerk of the superior court unless you waive this requirement.

Registration. A durable power of attorney is valid after you become incapacitated only if it is registered in the office of the register of deeds in at least one of the following places:

- in the county named in your power of attorney,
- in the county of your legal residence,
- in a county where you own real property (if you have no legal residence in North Carolina),
- or in the county where your attorney-in-fact lives.

Your durable power of attorney may be registered after you become incapacitated.

If you require your attorney-in-fact to file inventories and accountings, a copy of your durable power of attorney must be filed with the clerk of the superior court within 30 days after filing the power of attorney in the register of deeds office.

The power to make gifts. Your attorney-in-fact may not make gifts of your property unless you have clearly given him or her that power. Giving your attorney-in-fact the power to make gifts may have advantages for you. For example, there may be tax reasons to make gifts of your property. Also, making gifts of your property may help you qualify for certain government benefits to cover the cost of long-term nursing home care. If you are not competent and you have not authorized your attorney-in-fact to make gifts, you may lose these advantages.

Caution: The power to make gifts may have disadvantages for your attorney-in-fact. Ask your lawyer how to minimize or eliminate potential disadvantages. Also, to ensure achieving the desired benefits, no one should make large gifts of property without the advice of an attorney.

The power to make health care decisions. You may want to give someone the specific power to make health care decisions for you if you are unable to make these decisions. This includes the power to consent to your doctor giving, withholding, or stopping any medical treatment, service, or diagnostic procedure. You may give this power to your attorney-in-fact in your durable power of attorney. Or, you may give this power to someone in a separate document, called a health care power of attorney.

The person you give this power to is called your health care agent. Your health care agent should know what you want done if the situation arises. You may want to discuss your medical care preferences with your health care agent and give him or her written suggestions on how you want things done. Your attorney can help you put your suggestions in writing without overly restricting your health care agent's power.

Using a durable power of attorney to recommend a guardian. You may use a durable power of attorney to name the person you would like to be your guardian if you are declared legally incompetent. The court does not have to follow your recommendation, but it usually will accept your choice, unless the person you named is disqualified. You may want to name your choice because a court-appointed guardian may revoke or amend your power of attorney.

To qualify as a guardian for an incompetent adult, the person must be a resident of the state if he or she is appointed to take care of your property. A guardian appointed to take care of you (not your property) may be a nonresident.

What terminates a durable power of attorney? You may revoke your durable power of attorney. If you have not registered your durable power of attorney, it may be terminated in several ways.

- Your death revokes your power of attorney.

- You may provide a method for revoking it in your power of attorney.

- You may destroy the power of attorney if you are competent.

- If you are competent, you may revoke your durable power of attorney by a written document that is signed, notarized, and sent to your attorney-in-fact by certified or registered mail.

Regardless of the method you choose, you should tell your attorney-in-fact that the power of attorney is revoked.

If you have registered your durable power of attorney, the following events will terminate it.

- Your death revokes your power of attorney.

- If you are competent, you may revoke your durable power of attorney by filing a written revocation in the register of deeds office where you filed your power of attorney. You must serve notice of the revocation on your attorney-in-fact (this requires a special procedure).

Also, your power of attorney ends if your attorney-in-fact dies or resigns, and you have not named someone else to take his or her place as your attorney-in-fact. You may arrange to have someone name a substitute attorney-in-fact for you, if necessary.

Paying your attorney-in-fact. In your power of attorney, you may want to set the amount of pay that your attorney-in-fact is entitled to receive or the method for determining the amount of pay. If your power of attorney does not provide for paying your attorney-in-fact, the clerk of court will determine how much to pay your attorney-in-fact. The amount set by the clerk of court may not exceed a fixed percentage of the value of your property.

Trusts

A trust is a legal arrangement in which someone holds and manages property for the benefit of someone else. You transfer money or property to a trustee, and you name yourself or someone else as the beneficiary of the trust.

The trustee holds legal title to the trust property, and the beneficiaries hold equitable title. This means the beneficiaries are the true owners of the trust property. The trustee manages the property for the benefit of the beneficiaries. If you are a beneficiary and you become incapacitated, the trustee has the legal right to continue managing the property for you.

You decide how much power and responsibility to give the trustee. The trustee has a legal duty to act in your best interests and is personally liable for misuse of your property. You may require the trustee to post bond or file regular accountings with the court, or you may waive these requirements.

A trust is a complex legal arrangement that can be set up in many different ways. Different types of trusts have different legal consequences, as well as different income, estate, and gift tax consequences. If you are interested in setting up a trust, you should seek the advice and services of an attorney.

Types of trusts. You may change or terminate a revocable trust. You may not change or terminate an irrevocable trust after you create it. An inter vivos trust, a "living trust," is set up during your lifetime. A testamentary trust is created by will.

Choice of trustee. You may name an experienced financial adviser to manage the trust, or you may name yourself, your spouse, a relative, or a friend. (If you name yourself as sole trustee, you are not preparing for possible future incompetency.) You should choose someone who is knowledgeable and trustworthy and who is available to handle administration of the trust. You may name more than one trustee (co-trustees) to serve at the same time. You may name an alternate trustee (successor trustee) to serve if your first choice cannot or will not serve as trustee.

Naming a corporate trustee, such as a trust company or a trust department in a bank, has some advantages.

- A corporate trustee will not die, get sick, go on vacation, become incapacitated, or move away.

- A corporate trustee has substantial experience in investing and managing money and property.

There are also some possible disadvantages to naming a corporate trustee.

- The services may be impersonal. This depends upon the individuals who work for the corporate trustee.

- Quality of services may vary among corporate trustees. Before choosing a corporate trustee, investigate the quality of the services. Look at the quality of their personnel and the success of their trust division. Try to find out whether their overall investment strategy has produced a profit or loss.

Paying the trustee. You may set the amount of pay the trustee will receive. Professional trustees usually have an established fee schedule. Unless you provide for a different method of payment, the law entitles the trustee to a minimum amount of pay based on a percentage of the trust income and on a percentage of the value of trust property. The clerk of court may pay the trustee more than the minimum amount, as long as the trustee's total annual pay does not exceed the maximum allowed by law.

Guardianship

If you become incapacitated, either temporarily or permanently, your family, friends, business associates, creditors, or the state may need to petition the court to have you declared incompetent and to have a guardian appointed. This is particularly true if you have made no other arrangements for someone to handle your affairs.

Advantages of guardianship. Someone who is closely supervised by the court takes care of you and your property. The law requires your guardian to act in your best interests and to protect your rights.

Disadvantages of guardianship. Guardianship proceedings are open to the public unless you request the court to exclude all persons other than those people directly involved in or testifying at the hearing which is held to determine if you are legally incompetent.

- Guardianship proceedings are expensive. Unless you are indigent, you may have to pay all or a portion of the costs spent to determine if you are incompetent.

- Delays in getting a guardian appointed may cause problems for you and your dependents. An emergency procedure for an appointment of a guardian is available.

- If the court declares you legally incompetent, you lose the right to manage your own affairs until you can prove that you are competent.

How is incompetence determined? Any person, including the state or a local human resource agency, may file a petition with the court for a determination of incompetence.

- You have the right to a lawyer. You may choose your own lawyer, or the court may appoint a lawyer, called a guardian ad litem, to represent you.

- You have the right to request a jury trial. If you do not request a jury trial, you waive this right. The clerk of court may order a jury trial, or the clerk of court may determine if you are competent.

- You may undergo medical, psychological, and social work evaluations.

- A hearing is held, and evidence of your competence or incompetence is presented.

If the clerk or jury finds that you are incompetent, the court declares you incompetent and appoints a guardian or guardians to handle your affairs. You become a ward, and you no longer have the legal right to manage your own affairs. You have the right to appeal from an order declaring you incompetent.

Types of Guardians

A **guardian of the estate** manages your property and business affairs.

A **guardian of the person** performs duties relating to your care, custody, and control. A guardian of the person has the right to approve medical, psychological, legal, or other professional care and treatment.

A **general guardian** takes care of both your property and your person.

Who May Be a Guardian for an Incompetent Person?

The following people or organizations may be appointed as a guardian for an incompetent person.

- A guardian of the estate must be a resident of the state.

- A guardian of the person may be either a resident or nonresident.

- A general guardian must be a resident of the state.

- A corporation authorized by its charter to serve as a guardian may be appointed as guardian.

- A disinterested public agent may be appointed as guardian.

Guardian's Bond

A general guardian and a guardian of the estate usually must post a bond before receiving the ward's property. A guardian of the person does not post a bond, unless he or she is a nonresident of the state.

Conclusion

Preparing for a time when you may be unable to handle your financial and personal affairs involves several choices. What is best for you depends upon your particular needs and circumstances. Professional advice may help you make the best choices for you and your family. Preparing for this time also means taking action before it is too late. If you want to control these decisions, you must make arrangements before you become incompetent. If you fail to make arrangements or if the arrangements you make are inadequate, a court may need to appoint a guardian to manage your affairs. The choice is yours.

—Carol A. Schwab, J.D., LL.M.

Carol A. Schwab is a Member of the North Carolina State Bar, and a Family Resource Management Specialist for the North Carolina Cooperative Extension Service, North Carolina State University, Raleigh, North Carolina.

Chapter 32

Advance Directives: Living Will and Durable Power of Attorney for Health Care

Note: This chapter is not designed as a substitute for legal advice, nor does it tell you everything you may need to know about this subject. Changes in the law cannot be predicted, and statements in this chapter are based solely on the laws in force on the date of publication. If you have specific questions on this issue, seek professional advice.

Patients' Rights

You are entitled to complete information about your illness and how it may impact your life, and you have the right to share or withhold that information from others. You also should be informed about any procedures and treatments that are planned, the benefits and risks, and any alternative treatments that may be available. You may be asked to sign an "informed consent" form, which includes this information. Before you sign such a form, read it carefully and ask your doctor any questions you might have.

The Patient Self-Determination Act

A Federal law, the Patient Self-Determination Act (PSDA), requires all medical care facilities receiving Medicare and Medicaid payments

Reprinted with permission "The Living Will," Carol A. Schwab, J.D., LL.M., © 1993, North Carolina Cooperative Extension Service as publication FCS-364, North Carolina State University, Raleigh, North Carolina, Electronic Publication FCS-364, posted April 1997; and excerpts from "Advanced Cancer," National Cancer Institute, NIH Publication #98-856, September 1998.

to inform patients of their rights and choices in making decisions about the type and extent of their medical care. The PSDA also requires medical care facilities to give patients information about living wills and power of attorney, which are described in this chapter. For more information about the PSDA, contact any hospital or medical care facility in your area.

Advance Directives: The Living Will and Durable Power of Attorney for Health Care

All states allow people to delegate some medical decision-making rights through "advance directives," but state laws differ considerably. The two forms of advance directives are a living will and a durable power of attorney for health care.

A living will is a legal document, which has been properly witnessed by an authority (notary), that allows you to state, in writing, that you do not wish to be kept alive by artificial means or heroic measures. It is a recognized statement of your right to refuse treatment and has been upheld in court. If you decide to prepare a living will, be sure to talk with your doctor, nurse, or lawyer to identify and define terms that may be important to your future medical care, such as "artificial means," "heroic measures," and "code status." You also may want to consider creating a durable power of attorney as a health care proxy (that is, a person who will stand in your place to make medical decisions). This legal document allows you to appoint someone who can make decisions for you about your medical care if you can do so no longer. Choose a person who knows how you feel about specific treatments and who is familiar with any religious considerations that need to be taken into account. And make sure that the term "durable" appears in the power of attorney document you prepare. (A power of attorney can also delegate authority for financial and property management.)

How to Find Out about Your State's Laws

Each state has its own laws concerning living wills and durable powers of attorney, and these laws can vary in important details. It is possible that a living will or power of attorney signed in one state may not be recognized in another. You need to be aware of this possibility if you move to another state or enter a hospital in a state other than the one in which you live. Call Choices in Dying, Inc., a non-profit educational organization, at 1-800-989-WILL to learn how to obtain a copy of the living will used in your state and to learn more about a durable power of attorney for health care (health care proxy). There is a small fee for obtaining the document. You also can contact your state health department for this information.

If you sign a living will or a durable power of attorney, tell everyone close to you that you have these documents and give them copies. Your health care team and lawyer, if you have one, also should be informed and given copies. This information will help ensure that your wishes are carried out.

What Is a Living Will?

A living will is a declaration that you desire to die a natural death. You do not want extraordinary medical treatment, artificial nutrition, or hydration used to keep you alive if there is no reasonable hope of recovery. A living will gives your doctor permission to withhold or withdraw life support systems under certain conditions.

The patient's rights. You have a basic right to control the decisions about your medical care, including the decision to have extraordinary means or artificial nutrition or hydration withheld or withdrawn if your condition is terminal and incurable or if you are in a persistent vegetative state. If you are competent and able to communicate, you may tell your doctor that you do not want extraordinary means, artificial nutrition, or hydration used to keep you alive if there is no reasonable hope of recovery.

What happens if you are not competent or able to communicate this decision? You may decide ahead of time with a living will. If you do not have a living will, someone else may have to decide for you.

A living will is a legal document.

Statutory requirements. You must follow certain requirements to make your living will legally effective.

- You must be at least 18 years old and of sound mind when you sign it.

- Your living will must contain specific statements.

- You must sign your living will in the presence of two qualified witnesses and either a notary public or the clerk of superior court.

493

Required statements. To be valid, your living will must contain two specific statements. Specifics of these statements may vary from state to state. Check with your state for specific requirements.

1. You must declare that you do not want your doctor to use extraordinary means or artificial nutrition or hydration to keep you alive if your condition is terminal and incurable or if you are in a persistent vegetative state (depending upon your instructions).

2. You must state that you know your living will allows your doctor to withhold or stop extraordinary medical treatment, artificial nutrition, or hydration (depending upon your instructions).

Beware of using a living will form provided in a magazine article or distributed by national organizations. These forms may not contain the statements required to make them valid in your state.

Make clear, consistent choices. You must instruct the doctor what you want done if your condition is terminal and incurable or if you are in a persistent vegetative state. You may make these choices in your living will by initialing the appropriate lines. If you make no choices, your living will is meaningless. If you make inconsistent choices, your living will is confusing and may not accomplish what you want. Read the choices carefully before initialing to make sure that your intentions are clear. An attorney can help you fill out the form correctly.

If your condition is terminal and incurable, your living will may instruct your doctor to do the following:

• to withhold or stop extraordinary means only, or

• to withhold or stop both extraordinary means and artificial nutrition or hydration.

If you are in a persistent vegetative state, your living will may instruct your doctor to do the following:

• to withhold or stop extraordinary means only, or

• to withhold or stop both extraordinary means and artificial nutrition or hydration.

The living will must be signed, witnessed, and certified. You must sign your living will in the presence of two witnesses:

- who are not related to you or your spouse;

- who will not inherit property from you, either under your will or under the laws that determine who will get your property if you do not have a will;

- who are not your doctor, your doctor's employees, or the employees of your hospital, nursing home, or group care home; and

- who do not have a claim against you.

Also, a notary public or a clerk or assistant clerk of superior court must certify your living will.

How Does a Valid Living Will Work?

The living will gives your doctor permission to withhold or discontinue life support systems under two conditions. Under the first condition, you must be both terminally and incurably ill. Under the second condition, you must be diagnosed as being in a persistent vegetative state. If two doctors diagnose one of these conditions, your doctor may withhold or discontinue extraordinary medical treatment, artificial nutrition, or hydration as directed by your living will.

Definitions

Artificial nutrition or hydration describes the use of feeding tubes or other invasive means to give someone food or water.

Extraordinary means or medical treatment includes any medical procedure which artificially postpones the moment of death by supporting or replacing a vital bodily function.

You are considered to be in a *persistent vegetative state* if you have had a complete loss of self-aware cognition (you are a vegetable), and you will die soon without the use of extraordinary medical treatment or artificial nutrition or hydration.

How Do You Revoke Your Living Will?

You may revoke your living will by communicating this desire to your doctor. You may use any means available to communicate your intent to revoke. Your mental or physical condition is not considered, so you do not need to be of sound mind. Someone acting on your behalf may also tell your doctor that you want to revoke your living will. Revocation is effective only after your doctor has been notified.

Destroying the original and all copies of your living will may revoke your living will as a practical matter. However, if you have discussed this issue with your doctor, be sure to tell your doctor that you have revoked your living will.

If you sign a new living will, be sure to revoke all prior living wills that may be inconsistent with your new living will.

Where Should You Store Your Living Will?

Keep the original in a place where you or your family members may find it easily. Some lawyers suggest that you sign several copies and have each one witnessed and certified. Then, you may give an original to each of the appropriate people. However, if you change your mind and revoke your living will, make sure that you destroy all the original copies. (Note: North Carolina law allows you to sign more than one original living will because signing a new living will does not revoke a previously signed living will.)

If you have named a health care agent, give him or her a copy of your living will. You may appoint a health care agent with a health care power of attorney or with a general durable power of attorney. Ask your lawyer for details.

Give a copy of your living will to your doctor and any medical facility where you have regular appointments. Give a copy of your living will to your family so they understand your wishes. Also, carry a wallet card stating that you have a living will, where the original is located, and who to contact to get the original.

If you put the original of your living will in a lock box or safe deposit box, make sure someone knows where it is and has access to it. Otherwise, your living will may be found too late.

What Happens if You Do Not Have a Living Will?

If you do not have a living will and you are unable to make your medical decisions, someone else must decide for you. If two doctors diagnose that you are terminally and incurably ill or in a persistent vegetative state, extraordinary means, artificial nutrition, or hydration may be withheld or stopped with the permission of:

- your guardian,
- your health care agent,
- your spouse, or
- the majority of your parents and children.

If you do not have a living will, your family is burdened with the decision. Your family may not be able to agree on what action to take. The lack of decision by your family may lengthen your suffering and increase your medical bills. A living will removes the decision from your family's shoulders and makes the decision yours.

What Is the Effect of Your Living Will if You Move?

Different states have different laws on living wills, so your living will may not be valid in another state. If you move to another state, check with an attorney there to see if you need to sign a new living will.

If you spend a lot of time in other states, you may want to sign a living will for each state. Before signing a living will from another state, ask an attorney if there is any reason why you should not sign a living will from that state. For example, you may not want to sign another state's living will if it revokes all previously signed living wills.

Chapter 33

Medicare, Medicaid, and Medigap

Medicare Is a Health Insurance Program For

- People 65 years of age and older.

- Some people with disabilities, under 65 years of age.

- People with End-Stage Renal Disease (permanent kidney failure requiring dialysis or a transplant).

Medicare Has Two Parts

- Part A (Hospital Insurance). Most people do not have to pay for Part A.

- Part B (Medical Insurance). Most people pay monthly for Part B.

You May Have Choices in How You Get Your Health Care

The Original Medicare Plan—This plan is available everywhere in the United States. It is the way most people get their Medicare Part A and Part B benefits. You may go to any doctor, specialist, or hospital

This chapter includes text from the following Health Care Financing Administration (HCFA) documents: "What is Medicare?" "Who Is Eligible for Medicare?" "Medicare Covered Services," Publication No. HCFA-10116, revised May 1999; "2000 Guide to Health Insurance for People with Medicare." 2000 Publication No. HCFA-02110, Revised March 2000; and "Overview of the Medicaid Program," March 1999.

that accepts Medicare. Medicare pays its share and you pay your share. Some things are not covered, like prescription drugs.

Medicare Managed Care Plans—These are health care choices (like HMOs) in some areas of the country. In most plans, you can only go to doctors, specialists, or hospitals that are part of the plan. Plans must cover all Medicare Part A and B benefits. Some plans cover extras, like prescription drugs. Your out-of-pocket costs may be lower than in the Original Medicare Plan.

Private Fee-for-Service Plans—This is a new Medicare health care choice in some areas of the country. You may go to any doctor, specialist, or hospital. Plans must cover all Medicare Part A and B benefits. Some plans cover extras, like extra days in the hospital. The plan, not Medicare, decides how much you pay.

Medicare Covered Services

Home Health Care

If you meet certain conditions, covered services include intermittent skilled nursing care, physical therapy, speech and language pathology services, home health aide services, durable medical equipment (such as wheelchairs, hospital beds, oxygen, and walkers) and suplies, and other services.
You pay:

- Nothing for Home Health Care services.

- 20% of approved amount for durable medical equipment (such as wheelchairs, hospital beds, oxygen, and walkers). Call your Regional Home Health Intermediary with questions about Home Health Care and conditions of coverage.

Hospice Care

If you meet certain conditions, covered services include pain and symptom relief, and supportive services for the management of a terminal illness. Home care is provided. It also covers necessary inpatient care and a variety of services otherwise not covered by Medicare.
You pay:

- Limited costs for outpatient drugs and inpatient respite care (care given to a hospice patient so that the usual caregiver can rest). Call your Regional Home Health Intermediary about Hospice Care and conditions of coverage.

Who Is Eligible for Medicare?

Generally, you are eligible for Medicare if you or your spouse worked for at least 10 years in Medicare-covered employment and you are 65 years old and a citizen or permanent resident of the United States. You might also qualify for coverage if you are a younger person with a disability or with chronic kidney disease. Here are some simple guidelines. You can get Part A at age 65 without having to pay premiums if:

- You are already receiving retirement benefits from Social Security or the Railroad Retirement Board.

- You are eligible to receive Social Security or Railroad benefits but have not yet filed for them.

- You or your spouse had Medicare-covered government employment.

If you are under 65, you can get Part A without having to pay premiums if:

- You have received Social Security or Railroad Retirement Board disability benefit for 24 months.

- You are a kidney dialysis or kidney transplant patient.

While you do not have to pay a premium for Part A if you meet one of those conditions, you must pay for Part B if you want it. The Part B monthly premium in 2000 was $45.50. It is deducted from your Social Security, Railroad Retirement, or Civil Service Retirement check.

If you have questions about your eligibility for Medicare Part A or Part B, or if you want to apply for Medicare, call the Social Security Administration. You can also get information about buying Part A as well as part B if you do not qualify for premium-free part A.

Social Security Administration
Toll-Free: 800-772-1213
TTY/TDD: 800-325-0778

Overview of the Medicaid Program

Title XIX of the Social Security Act is a program which provides medical assistance for certain individuals and families with low incomes and resources. The program, known as Medicaid, became law in 1965 as a jointly funded cooperative venture between the Federal and State governments to assist States in the provision of adequate medical care to eligible needy persons. Medicaid is the largest program providing medical and health-related services to America's poorest people. Within broad national guidelines which the Federal government provides, each of the States:

1. establishes its own eligibility standards;

2. determines the type, amount, duration, and scope of services;

3. sets the rate of payment for services;

4. and administers its own program.

Thus, the Medicaid program varies considerably from State to State, as well as within each State over time.

Medicaid Eligibility

States have some discretion in determining which groups their Medicaid programs will cover and the financial criteria for Medicaid eligibility. To be eligible for Federal funds, States are required to provide Medicaid coverage for most individuals who receive Federally assisted income maintenance payments, as well as for related groups not receiving cash payments. Some examples of the mandatory Medicaid eligibility groups are:

*   Low income families with children, as described in Section 1931 of the Social Security Act, who meet certain of the eligibility requirements in the State's AFDC plan in effect on July 16, 1996;

*   Supplemental Security Income (SSI) recipients (or in States using more restrictive criteria—aged, blind, and disabled individuals who meet criteria which are more restrictive than those of the SSI program and which were in place in the State's approved Medicaid plan as of January 1, 1972);

*   infants born to Medicaid-eligible pregnant women. Medicaid eligibility must continue throughout the first year of life so long as

502

the infant remains in the mother's household and she remains eligible, or would be eligible if she were still pregnant;

- children under age 6 and pregnant women whose family income is at or below 133 percent of the Federal poverty level. (The minimum mandatory income level for pregnant women and infants in certain States may be higher than 133 percent, if as of certain dates the State had established a higher percentage for covering those groups.) States are required to extend Medicaid eligibility until age 19 to all children born after September 30, 1983(or such earlier date as the State may choose) in families with incomes at or below the Federal poverty level. This phases in coverage, so that by the year 2002, all poor children under age 19 will be covered. Once eligibility is established, pregnant women remain eligible for Medicaid through the end of the calendar month in which the 60th day after the end of the pregnancy falls, regardless of any change in family income. States are not required to have a resource test for these poverty level related groups. However, any resource test imposed can be no more restrictive than that of the AFDC program for infants and children and the SSI program for pregnant women;

- recipients of adoption assistance and foster care under Title IV-E of the Social Security Act;

- certain Medicare beneficiaries (described later); and

- special protected groups who may keep Medicaid for a period of time. Examples are: persons who lose SSI payments due to earnings from work or increased Social Security benefits; and families who are provided 6 to 12 months of Medicaid coverage following loss of eligibility under Section 1931 due to earnings, or 4 months of Medicaid coverage following loss of eligibility under Section 1931 due to an increase in child or spousal support.

States also have the option to provide Medicaid coverage for other "categorically needy" groups. These optional groups share characteristics of the mandatory groups, but the eligibility criteria are somewhat more liberally defined. Examples of the optional groups that States may cover as categorically needy (and for which they will receive Federal matching funds) under the Medicaid program are:

- infants up to age one and pregnant women not covered under the mandatory rules whose family income is below 185 percent

503

of the Federal poverty level (the percentage to be set by each State);

- optional targeted low income children;

- certain aged, blind, or disabled adults who have incomes above those requiring mandatory coverage, but below the Federal poverty level;

- children under age 21 who meet income and resources requirements for AFDC, but who otherwise are not eligible for AFDC;

- institutionalized individuals with income and resources below specified limits;

- persons who would be eligible if institutionalized but are receiving care under home and community-based services waivers;

- recipients of State supplementary payments; and

- TB-infected persons who would be financially eligible for Medicaid at the SSI level (only for TB-related ambulatory services and TB drugs).

Medically Needy Eligibility Groups

The option to have a "medically needy" program allows States to extend Medicaid eligibility to additional qualified persons who may have too much income to qualify under the mandatory or optional categorically needy groups. This option allows them to "spend down" to Medicaid eligibility by incurring medical and/or remedial care expenses to offset their excess income, thereby reducing it to a level below the maximum allowed by that State's Medicaid plan. States may also allow families to establish eligibility as medically needy by paying monthly premiums to the State in an amount equal to the difference between family income (reduced by unpaid expenses, if any, incurred for medical care in previous months) and the income eligibility standard.

Eligibility for the medically needy program does not have to be as extensive as the categorically needy program. However, States which elect to include the medically needy under their plans are required to include certain children under age 18 and pregnant women who, except for income and resources, would be eligible as categorically needy. They may choose to provide coverage to other medically needy persons: aged, blind, and/or disabled persons; certain relatives of children deprived of parental support and care; and certain other financially eligible children up to age 21. In 1995, there were 40 medically needy programs which provided at least some services to recipients.

Amplification on Medicaid Eligibility

Coverage may start retroactive to any or all of the 3 months prior to application, if the individual would have been eligible during the retroactive period. Coverage generally stops at the end of the month in which a person's circumstances change. Most States have additional "State-only" programs to provide medical assistance for specified poor persons who do not qualify for the Medicaid program. No Federal funds are provided for State-only programs.

Medicaid does not provide medical assistance for all poor persons. Even under the broadest provisions of the Federal statute (except for emergency services for certain persons), the Medicaid program does not provide health care services, even for very poor persons, unless they are in one of the groups designated above. Low income is only one test for Medicaid eligibility; assets and resources are also tested against established thresholds. As noted earlier, categorically needy persons who are eligible for Medicaid may or may not also receive cash assistance from the TANF program or from the SSI program. Medically needy persons who would be categorically eligible except for income or assets may become eligible for Medicaid solely because of excessive medical expenses.

States may use more liberal income and resources methodologies to determine Medicaid eligibility for certain AFDC-related and aged, blind, and disabled individuals under sections 1902(r)(2) and 1931 of the Social Security Act. For some groups, the more liberal income methodologies cannot result in the individual's income exceeding the limits prescribed for Federal matching.

Significant changes were made in the Medicare Catastrophic Coverage Act (MCCA) of 1988 which affected Medicaid. Although much of the MCCA was repealed, the portions affecting Medicaid remain in effect. The law also accelerated Medicaid eligibility for some nursing home patients by protecting assets for the institutionalized person's spouse at home at the time of the initial eligibility determination after institutionalization. Before an institutionalized person's monthly income is used to pay for the cost of institutional care, a minimum monthly maintenance needs allowance is deducted from the institutionalized spouse's income to bring the income of the community spouse up to a moderate level.

505

Medicaid/Medicare Relationship

The Medicare program (Title XVIII of the Social Security Act) provides hospital insurance (HI), also known as Part A coverage, and supplementary medical insurance (SMI), also known as Part B coverage. Coverage for HI is automatic for persons aged 65 and older (and for certain disabled persons) who have insured status under Social Security or Railroad Retirement. Coverage for HI may be purchased by individuals who do not have insured status through the payment of monthly Part A premiums. Coverage for SMI also requires payment of monthly premiums.

Medicare beneficiaries who have low income and limited resources may receive help paying for their out-of-pocket medical expenses from their State Medicaid program. There are various benefits available to "dual eligibles" who are entitled to Medicare and are eligible for some type of Medicaid benefit.

For persons who are eligible for full Medicaid coverage, the Medicaid program supplements Medicare coverage by providing services and supplies that are available under their State's Medicaid program. Services that are covered by both programs will be paid first by Medicare and the difference by Medicaid, up to the State's payment limit. Medicaid also covers additional services (e.g., nursing facility care beyond the 100 day limit covered by Medicare, prescription drugs, eyeglasses, and hearing aids).

Limited Medicaid benefits are also available to pay for out-of-pocket Medicare cost-sharing expenses for certain other Medicare beneficiaries. The Medicaid program will assume their Medicare payment liability if they qualify. Qualified Medicare Beneficiaries (QMBs), with resources at or below twice the standard allowed under the SSI program and income at or below 100% of the Federal poverty level (FPL), do not have to pay their monthly Medicare premiums, deductibles, and coinsurance. Specified Low-Income Medicare Beneficiaries (SLMBs), with resources at or below twice the standard allowed under the SSI program and income exceeding the QMB level, but less than 120% of the FPL, do not have to pay the monthly Medicare Part B premiums. Qualifying Individuals (QIs), who are not otherwise eligible for full Medicaid benefits and with resources at or below twice the standard allowed under the SSI program, will get help with all or a small part of their monthly Medicare Part B premiums, depending upon whether their income exceeds the SLMB level, but is less than 135% of the FPL, or their income is at least 135%, but less than 175% of the FPL.

Individuals who were receiving Medicare due to disability, but have lost entitlement to Medicare benefits because they returned to work, may purchase Part A of Medicare. If the individual has income below 200% of the FPL and resources at or below twice the standard allowed under the SSI program, and they are not otherwise eligible for Medicaid benefits, they may qualify to have Medicaid pay their monthly Medicare Part A premiums as Qualified Disabled and Working Individuals (QDWIs).

Home Health Services

Home health services are a mandatory benefit for individuals who are entitled to nursing facility services under the State's Medicaid plan. Services must be provided at a recipient's place of residence, and must be ordered by a physician as part of a plan of care that the physician reviews every sixty days. Home health services must include nursing services, as defined in the State's Nurse Practice Act, that are provided on a part-time or intermittent basis by a home health agency, home health aide services provided by a home health agency, and medical supplies, equipment, and appliances suitable for use in the home. Physical therapy, occupational therapy, speech pathology, and audiology services are optional services that States may choose to provide.

To participate in the Medicaid program, a home health agency must meet the conditions of participation for Medicare.

Physical Therapy, Occupational Therapy, and Services for Individuals with Speech, Hearing and Language Disorders

All of these services are optional Medicaid services States may choose to provide. Physical therapy services are prescribed by a physician or other licensed practitioner of the healing arts within the scope of his or her practice under State law and provided to a recipient by or under the direction of a qualified physical therapist. Included are any necessary supplies and equipment.

Occupational therapy services are prescribed by a physician or other licensed practitioner of the healing arts within the scope of his or her practice under State law and provided to a recipient by or under the direction of a qualified occupational therapist. Included are any necessary supplies and equipment.

Services for individuals with speech, hearing, and language disorders means diagnostic, screening, preventive, or corrective services provided by or under the direction of a speech pathologist or audiologist,

507

for which a patient is referred by a physician or other licensed practitioner of the healing arts within the scope of his or her practice under State law. Included are any necessary supplies and equipment.

Qualifications for providers of physical therapy, occupational therapy, and services for individuals with speech, hearing, and language disorders, are specified in Federal regulations at 42 CFR 440.110(c).

Personal Care Services

Personal care services are an optional Medicaid benefit provided to individuals who are not inpatients or residents of a hospital, nursing facility, intermediate care facility for the mentally retarded, or institution for mental disease. Personal care services must be:

1. authorized for an individual by a physician in accordance with a plan of treatment or (at the State's option) otherwise authorized for the individual in accordance with a service plan approved by the State;

2. provided by a qualified individual who is not a member of the individual's family; and

3. furnished in a home or other location.

Personal care services may include a range of human assistance provided to persons with disabilities and chronic conditions of all ages which enables them to accomplish tasks that they would normally do for themselves if they did not have a disability. Assistance may be in the form of hands-on assistance or cueing so that the person performs the task by him/herself. Such assistance most often relates to performance of activities of daily living (ADLs) and instrumental activities of daily living (IADLs), which includes assistance with daily activities such as eating, bathing, dressing, toileting, transferring, personal hygiene, light housework, medication management, etc. Personal care services can be provided on a continuing basis or on episodic occasions. Skilled services that may be performed only by a health professional are not considered personal care services.

Medicap Insurance

What Is a Medigap Policy and How Does It Work?

A Medigap policy is sold by private insurance companies to fill the "gaps" in Original Medicare Plan coverage. The front of the

Medigap policy must clearly identify it as "Medicare Supplement Insurance." In all but three states (Minnesota, Masschusetts, and Wisconsin), there are 10 standardized Medigap plans called "A" through "J." Each plan has a different set of standard benefits.

Medicare Select is a type of Medigap insurance policy. If you buy a Medicare Select policy, you are buying one of the 10 standardized Medigap plans A through J.

When you buy a Medigap policy you pay a premium to the insurance company. As long as you pay your premium, policies bought after 1990 are automatically renewed each year. This means that your coverage continues year after year as long as you pay your premium. You still must pay your monthly Medicare Part B premium.

Medigap Policy Coverage

Each standardized Medigap policy must cover basic (core) benefits. Medigap policies pay most, if not all, of the Original Medicare Plan coinsurance amounts. These policies may also cover the Original Medicare Plan deductibles. Some of the policies cover extra benefits to fill more of the gaps in your coverage, like prescription drugs.

Medigap policies do not cover:

- Long-term care
- Vision or dental care
- Hearing aids
- Private-duty nursing
- Unlimited prescription drugs

Considerations before buying a Medigap policy

- How much am I spending on health care?
- What are my health care dollars spent on?
- Which Medigap benefits do I need?
- How much can I afford to spend on premiums?
- What will my future health care costs be? Remember, you may need more health care as you get older.

Information on Medigap Policies in Your State

You can get information about Medigap policies in your state by calling:

- Your State Insurance Department to find out what Medigap policies are available in your state and which companies sell them; or

- Your State Health Insurance Assistance Program to get free counseling to help you decide which policy is best for you.

You can also use a computer to find information on and compare Medigap policies offered in your state. Look on the Internet at www.medicare.gov and click on "Medigap Compare." This website has information on:

- Which Medigap policies are sold in your state.

- How to shop for a Medigap policy.

- What the policies must cover.

- How insurance companies decide what to charge you for a Medigap policy premium.

- Your Medigap rights and protections.

If you don't have a computer, your local library or senior center may be able to help you look at this information.

Watch Out for Illegal Insurance Practices

It is illegal for anyone to:

- Sell you a second Medigap policy when they know that you already have one, unless you tell the insurance company in writing that you plan to cancel your existing Medigap policy.

- Sell you a Medigap policy if they know you have Medicaid except in certain situations.

- Sell you a Medigap policy if they know you are enrolled in a Medicare managed care plan with a Medicare + Choice contract or Private Fee-for-Service plan.

- Claim that a Medigap policy is part of the Medicare program or any other federal program.

- Use the mail to advertise Medigap policies that are not approved for sale in your state.

- Misuse the names, letters, symbols, or emblems of the U.S. Department of Health and Human Services (DHHS), Social Security Administration (SSA), Health Care Financing Administration (HCFA), or any of their various programs like Medicare.

You should report any suspected violations of the laws on marketing insurance policies to your State Insurance Department.

If you believe that a federal law has been violated, you may call 1-800-MEDICARE (1-800-633-4227, TTY/TDD: 1-877-486-2048 for the hearing and speech impaired). In most cases, however, your State Insurance Department can help you with insurance-related problems.

Chapter 34

Long Term Care Insurance and Other Insurance Choices

Other Kinds of Health Insurance

There are several kinds of health coverage, besides Medigap, that pay for some of your health care costs not covered by Medicare. They include:

- Employee or retiree coverage from an employer or union: Call your benefit administrator to find out if you have or can get health care coverage based on your or your spouse's past or current employment. Since this kind of health insurance coverage is not a Medigap policy, the rules that apply to Medigap policies do not apply.

- COBRA Coverage (Consolidated Omnibus Budget Reconciliation Act of 1985): This law requires an employer to let you and your dependents stay covered under the employer's group health plan for a certain length of time after losing your job, having your work hours reduced, or after your spouse's death,or a divorce. However, you may have to pay both your share and the employer's share of the premium.

- The PACE Program (Programs of All-Inclusive Care for the Elderly): This program combines both inpatient and outpatient medical and long-term care services for eligible persons. To be

Excerpts from "2000 Guide to Health Insurance for People with Medicare," Health Care Financing Administration (HCFA), Publication No. HCFA-02110.

eligible, you must be at least 55 years old, live in the service area of a PACE program, and be certified as eligible for nursing home care by the appropriate state agency. The goal of PACE is to keep you independent, and living in your community as long as possible, and to provide quality care at low cost.

Caution: If you drop your employer or union group health coverage, you may not be able to get it back. For more information, call your benefit administrator.

Note: When you have retiree coverage from an employer or union, they have control over this insurance. They may change the benefits or premiums, and can also cancel the insurance if they choose.

- *Federally Qualified Health Centers (FQHCs)*: These are special health centers, like a community health center, tribal health clinic, migrant health service, and health center for the homeless, that can give you routine health care at a lower cost.

- *Medicaid*: This is a joint federal and state program that helps pay medical costs for some people with low incomes and limited resources. Medicaid programs vary from state to state, but most health care costs are covered if you qualify for both Medicare and Medicaid. If you cannot afford to pay your Medicare premiums and other health care costs, you may be able to get help from your state.

- *Hospital Indemnity Insurance*: This kind of insurance pays a certain cash amount for each day you are in the hospital up to a certain number of days. It is not designed to fill gaps in your Medicare coverage.

- *Specified Disease Insurance*: This kind of insurance pays benefits for only a single disease, such as cancer, or for a group of diseases. It is not designed to fill gaps in your Medicare coverage.

- *Long-Term Care Insurance*: This kind of insurance policy may cover medical and non-medical care to help you with your daily needs, such as bathing, dressing, using the bathroom, and eating. Generally, Medicare does not pay for long-term care. This type of insurance may help fill some gaps in the coverage that you and/or your spouse may need in the future.

Other Private Health Insurance Options

The following types of policies are generally limited in scope and are not substitutes for Medigap insurance or comprehensive health coverage. Benefits under these policies are not designed to fill gaps in your Medicare coverage.

What Is Hospital Indemnity Insurance?

Hospital indemnity insurance pays a fixed cash amount for each day you are in the hospital up to a certain number of days. Some policies may have added benefits such as surgical benefits or skilled nursing home confinement benefits. Some policies have a maximum number of days or a maximum payment amount.

What Is Specified Disease Insurance?

Specified disease insurance, which is only available in some states, pays benefits for only one disease, such as cancer, or for a group of specified diseases. The value of this coverage depends on the chance you will get the specific disease or diseases covered. Benefits are usually limited to a fixed amount for each type of treatment.

Remember, Medicare and any Medigap policy you have will very likely cover costs from any specified diseases you may have.

What Is Long-Term Care?

Long-term care is different from traditional medical care. Someone with a long physical illness, or a disability, or a memory or thought problem (such as Alzheimer's disease) often needs long-term care. Long-term care is made up of many different services to help people with chronic conditions overcome limitations that keep them from being independent. Long-term care may include help with activities of daily living, home health care, respite care, adult day care, care in a nursing home, and care in an assisted living facility. Long-term care may also include case management services, which will evaluate your needs and coordinate and monitor the delivery of long-term care services.

Does Medicare Cover Long-Term Care?

No. Generally, Medicare only covers medically necessary care under Part A (Hospital Insurance) and Part B (Medical Insurance). You

515

must meet certain conditions for Medicare to cover skilled nursing facility home health, and hospice care.

What Is Long-Term Care Insurance?

Long-term care insurance is one way you may pay for long-term care. This type of insurance will pay for some or all of your long-term care. Long-term care insurance is a relatively new type of insurance. It was introduced in the 1980s as nursing home insurance. It has changed a lot and now often covers much more than nursing home care.

If you are shopping for long-term care insurance, find out which types of long-term care services the different policies cover. For more information about long-term care insurance, get a copy of *A Shopper's Guide to Long-Term Care Insurance* from either your State Insurance Department or the National Association of Insurance Commissioners, 120 W. 12th Street, Suite 1100, Kansas City, MO 64105-1925.

Who Sells Long-Term Care Insurance?

Private insurance companies sell long-term care insurance policies. You can buy them from an insurance agent or through the mail. Or, you can buy a group policy through an employer or through membership in an association. You can also get long-term care benefits through a life insurance policy. Insurance companies must be licensed in your state to sell long-term care insurance. Be certain that you are dealing with a company that you know. If you decide to buy long-term care insurance, be sure that the company and the agent, if one is involved, is licensed in your state. If you are not sure, call your State Insurance Department.

How Can I Find Out about Nursing Homes in My Area?

You can now get important information about the nursing homes in your area by using a computer to look on the Internet at www.medicare.gov. Click on "Nursing Home Compare" to see where nursing homes are located in your area, how big they are, what types of residents they have, and whether or not the nursing home accepts Medicare or Medicaid. With "Nursing Home Compare," you can also see nursing home inspection reports that can tell you if any problems were found during the inspection. If you don't have a computer, your local library or senior center may be able to help you look at this information.

Chapter 35

Viatical Settlements

If you have a terminal illness—or if you are caring for someone who is terminally ill—chances are you're giving a great deal of thought to time and money. You may be thinking about life insurance, too. It's in that context that you may hear the phrases "accelerated benefits" and "viatical settlements."

Accelerated benefits sometimes are called "living benefits." They are the proceeds of life insurance policies that are paid by the insurer to policy holders before they die. Occasionally, these benefits are included in policies when they are sold, but usually, they are offered as riders or attachments to new or existing policies.

Viatical settlements involve the sale of a life insurance policy. If you have a terminal illness, you may consider selling your insurance policy to a viatical settlement company for a lump sum cash payment. In a viatical settlement transaction, people with terminal illnesses assign their life insurance policies to viatical settlement companies in exchange for a percentage of the policy's face value. The viatical settlement company, in turn, may sell the policy to a third-party investor. The viatical settlement company or the investor becomes the beneficiary to the policy, pays the premiums, and collects the face value of the policy after the original policyholder dies.

Decisions affecting life insurance benefits can have a profound financial and emotional impact on dependents, friends, and caregivers.

"Viatical Settlements," Federal Trade Commission, May 1998.

Before you make any major changes regarding your policy, talk to your friends and family as well as to someone whose advice and expertise you can count on—a lawyer, an accountant, or a financial planner.

Investigating Your Options

Many options exist for people with terminal illnesses when financial needs are critical. For example, you may consider a loan from someone such as the original beneficiary of your life insurance policy. Or, if you've already ruled out less expensive alternatives to raise cash, you might sell your life insurance policy through a viatical settlement.

Many life insurance policies in force nationwide now include an accelerated benefits provision. Companies offer anywhere from 25 to 100 percent of the death benefit as early payment, but policyholders can collect these payments only under very specific circumstances. The amount and the method of payment vary with the policy.

If you own a life insurance policy, call your state Insurance Commissioner or your company's Claims Department to find out about alternatives. Ask whether your life insurance policy allows for accelerated benefits or loans, and how much it will cost. Some insurers add accelerated benefits to life insurance policies for an additional premium, usually computed as a percentage of the base premium. Others offer the benefits at no extra premium, but charge the policyholder for the option if and when it is used. In most cases, the insurance company will reduce the benefits advanced to the policyholder before death to compensate for the interest it will lose on its early payout. There also may be a service charge.

In addition, you may consider selling your life insurance policy to a viatical settlement company, a private enterprise that offers a terminally ill person a percentage of the policy's face value. It is not considered an insurance company.

The viatical settlement company becomes the sole beneficiary of the policy in consideration for delivering a cash payment to the policyholder and paying the premiums. When the policyholder dies, the viatical settlement company collects the face value of the policy.

Viatical settlements are complex legal and financial transactions. They require time and attention from physicians, life insurance companies, lawyers, and accountants or financial planners. The entire transfer process can take up to four months to complete.

Eligibility for Viatical Settlements

Each viatical settlement company sets its own rules for determining which life insurance policies it will buy. For example, most viatical companies will require that:

- you've owned your policy for at least two years;

- your current beneficiary sign a release or a waiver;

- you are terminally ill, some companies require a life expectancy of two years or less, while others may buy your policy even if your life expectancy is four years;

- you sign a release allowing the viatical settlement provider access to your medical records.

Most companies will require that the company issuing your life insurance policy be financially sound. If your life insurance policy is provided by your employer, purchasers will want to know if it can be converted into an individual policy or otherwise be guaranteed to remain in force before it can be assigned.

Financial Implications

Because the decision to sell your life insurance policy is a very complex matter, you should consult a tax advisor before doing so. Generally, if you sell your policy to a viatical settlement company, the proceeds are tax-free if you have a life expectancy of less than two years. However, you still may owe state tax, although a number of states, including New York and California have made these settlements tax-free.

Collecting accelerated benefits or making a viatical settlement also may affect your eligibility for public assistance programs based on financial need, such as Medicaid. The federal government does not require policyholders either to choose accelerated benefits or cash in their policies before qualifying for Medicaid benefits. But once the policyholder cashes in the policy and receives a payment, the money may be counted as income for Medicaid purposes and may affect eligibility.

In 1997, Congress changed the tax code so that proceeds from accelerated benefits and viatical settlements are tax-exempt. Under the law, proceeds from accelerated benefits and viatical settlements are tax-exempt as long as your life expectancy is less than two years and the viatical settlement company is licensed—if you live in a state that requires licensing. If your state does not require viatical settlement companies to be licensed, state law will still require that these companies meet other standards and make certain other disclosures.

Most states have declared that payments of accelerated benefits or viatical settlements are exempt from state taxes. However, some states do not give these payments tax-free status. Because of the complexity of the situation, seek professional tax advice from a lawyer, an accountant, or a financial planner.

Guidelines for Consumers

The daily physical and emotional demands of a terminal illness can be overwhelming, and financial burdens can seem insurmountable. If you are considering making a viatical settlement on your life insurance policy—or if you are helping someone with this decision— these consumer guidelines should help you avoid costly mistakes and make the choice that's right.

- Contact two or three viatical settlement companies to make sure offers are competitive, and be aware of prevailing discount rates. A viatical settlement company may pay 80 percent of the face value of a policy to a person whose life expectancy is six months or less.

- Check with your state insurance department to see if viatical settlement companies or brokers must be licensed. If so, check the status of the companies with whom you are considering doing business.

- Don't fall for high pressure tactics. You don't have to accept an offer, and you can change your mind. Some states require a 15-day cooling off period before any viatical settlement transaction is complete.

- Verify that the investor or the company has the money for your payout readily available. Large companies may have cash on hand; smaller ones may have uneven cash flows or may be "shopping" the policy to third parties.

- Insist that the company set up an escrow account with a reputable, independent financial institution before the company sends the offer papers for your signature. An escrow account will let you be sure that the funds are available to cover the offer.

- Insist on a timely payment. Once the insurance company has made the necessary changes, you should get your money within two to three business days from the escrow agent. No more than a few months should go by from the initial contact with the company to the closing. Check with your state Attorney General's office or department of insurance to see if there are complaints against the company before you do business.

- Ask the company about possible tax consequences and implications for public assistance benefits. Some states require viatical settlement companies to make these disclosures and tell you about other options that may be available from your life insurance company.

- Ask about privacy. Some companies may not protect a policyholder's privacy when they act as brokers for payouts from potential investors.

- Contact a lawyer to check on the possible probate and estate considerations. If you make a viatical settlement, there will be no life insurance benefits for the person you originally designated as beneficiary.

For More Information

Any decision that affects your life insurance benefits can affect the people who care for and about you. Before you make a decision, talk to your friends and family as well as to someone whose advice and expertise you can count on—a lawyer, an accountant, or a financial planner. You also may want to contact the following organizations for more information.

American Council on Life Insurance
1001 Pennsylvania Avenue, N.W.
Washington, DC 20004-2599
Tel: (202) 624-2000
Website: http://www.acli.com

National Association of Insurance Commissioners
2301 McGee, Suite 800
Kansas City, MO 64108-2604
Tel: 816-842-3600
Website: http://www.naic.org

National Association of People with AIDS
1413 K Street, N.W., 7th Floor
Washington, DC 20005
Tel: 202-898-0414
Fax: 202-898-0435
Website: http://www.napwa.org
E-mail: napwa@napwa.org

National Viatical Association
1030 15ᵗʰ Street, Suite 870
Washington, DC 20005
Toll-Free: 800-741-9465
Tel: 202-347-7361
Fax: 202-393-0336
Website: http://
www.nationalviatical.org
E-mail: nva@rgminc.com

North American Securities Administrators Association
10 G Street N.E., Suite 710
Washington, D.C. 20002
Tel: 202-737-0900
Fax: 202-783-3571
Fax-on-Demand: 888-84-NASAA
Website: http://www.nasaa.org

Viatical and Life Settlement Association of America
2025 M Street, N.W., Suite 800
Washington, DC 20036
Tel: 202-367-1136
Fax: 202-367-2136
Website: http://www.viatical.org
E-mail: VLSSA@dc.sba.com

Your State Attorney General
Office of Consumer Protection
Your State Capital

Your State Insurance Commissioner
Department of Insurance
Your State Capital

Federal Trade Commission
CRC-240
Washington, DC 20580
Toll-Free: 877-382-4357
Tel: 202-326-2000
Website: http://www.ftc.gov

The FTC works for the consumer to prevent fraudulent, deceptive, and unfair business practices in the marketplace and to provide information to help consumers spot, stop, and avoid them. Contact them to file a complaint or to get free information on any of 150 consumer topics. The FTC enters Internet, telemarketing, and other fraud-related complaints into Consumer Sentinel—a secure, online database available to hundreds of civil and criminal law enforcement agencies worldwide.

Part Six

Additional Help and Information

Chapter 36

Glossary

A

Activities of Daily Living (ADL). A term used to describe basic tasks that are a part of most people's regular day, such as bathing, dressing, moving around the house, and eating.

Administration on Aging (AoA). The principal agency in the federal government responsible for the administration of the provisions of the Older Americans Act. It advocates at the federal level for the needs, concerns, and interests of older citizens throughout the nation.

Adult Care Homes. A custodial level of care provided in a licensed residence for aged or disabled adults who require some personal care and supervision. Three types of licensed adult care facilities are: family care homes, homes for the aged and disabled, and group homes for developmentally disabled adults.

Adult Day Care. The provision of group care and supervision of adults who may be physically or mentally disabled in a place other than their usual residence on a less than 24-hour basis. Services are designed to support the adult's personal independence, as well as their physical, social, and emotional well-being.

Reprinted with permission, "Glossary of Terms on Aging," © 2000 Land-of-Sky Regional Council, Area Agency on Aging.

Adult Day Health Care. A community-based day care program that provides health, social and recreational care, along with rehabilitative services. Staffing is by trained paraprofessionals and is under the supervision of a registered nurse. The program is ideal for the elderly or physically impaired adult who needs assistance in a protective setting during the day.

Adult Foster Care. A community living alternative serving primarily the elderly in family-like settings that provide assistance with activities of daily living. Programs receive major financial support from state and local governments.

Alzheimer's Disease. A progressive, degenerative disease that attacks the brain and results in impaired memory, thinking, and behavior.

American Association of Retired Persons (AARP). The nation's leading membership organization for people age 50 and older. Emphasis is placed on utilizing the lifetime experiences and leadership skills available in the mature adult population for improving local communities. The national AARP advocates for senior's rights and interests, promoting research, financial services, pharmaceutical services, travel discounts, and insurance programs for this age group.

Athetoid Cerebral Palsy (also called dyskinetic CP). Can affect movements of the entire body. Typically, this form of CP involves slow, uncontrolled body movements and low muscle tone that makes it hard for the person to sit straight and walk.

Area Agency on Aging (AAA). Area Agencies on Aging (AAA) plan, coordinate, and advocate for the development of a comprehensive service delivery system to meet the needs of older people in a specific geographic area. The AAAs provide training and technical support to county agencies that offer services to older adults.

Artificial Nutrition or Hydration. Describes the use of feeding tubes or other invasive means to give someone food or water.

C

Care Management. This service provides professional assistance to older adults and their families by identifying, accessing, and coordinating services that are necessary to enable the older adult to remain in the least restructured environment.

Certificate of Need (CON). A competitive application process by which providers acquire new institutional health care services (i.e., nursing home beds, hospital beds, rehabilitative beds, etc.) in accordance with the State Medical Facilities Plan. This serves as a quality assurance process for the state to manage quantity and costs of medical services. This varies from state to state.

Chore Services. See In-Home Aide Services

Cognitive Impairment. A term that refers to damage or loss of intellectual or mental functioning. The act or process of "knowing," including awareness or judgment, is impaired. Alzheimer's disease is the most common cause of cognitive impairment among older adults.

Community Alternatives Program (CAP). A Medicaid waiver program that provides community-based services to disabled adults, mentally retarded adults, and children who meet the medical requirements for nursing home level care. CAP services may include traditional Medicaid home health services (nursing, physical therapy, home health aide, etc.), as well as services not generally available under Medicaid (home delivered meals, respite care, chore services, etc.).

Congregate Living. A living arrangement in which two or more unrelated individuals reside in a house or apartment.

Congregate Meals. A nutrition program that provides meals in a group setting that often promotes socialization among the participants. The site for meals can be in churches, schools, senior centers, or recreational centers.

Continuing Care Facility (CCF). A facility that offers a continuum of care—from independent living, assisted-living, or domiciliary care, to nursing home care. Individuals are offered an independent living lifestyle with the security of knowing supportive and health care services are available if needed.

Congregate Nutrition. The provision of a hot meal in a group setting. This meal is to meet 1/3 of the USDA daily nutrition requirement.

Council on Aging (COA). A private, nonprofit organization or public agency that serves as a county focal point on aging and traditionally provides supportive services to older adults (located in some, but not all counties). Sometimes these are advisory boards to the county board of commissioners.

D

Demographics of Aging. The characteristics of the current older population in terms of numbers, proportionate size, attributes, and geographic distribution. Attributes could include gender, age, and race/ethnicity. A study of the demographics of aging also typically looks at projected changes in these areas and seeks to explain why they are occurring and what their probable effect will be.

Department of Health and Human Services. Umbrella agency for all human resource programs.

Department of Social Services (DSS). County agency provider services are available for older and disabled adults through departments of social services. Adult Placement Services, Individual and Family Adjustment, Foster Care Services for Adults, Protective Services for Adults, and at least one level of in-home aide service, are usually provided by county departments.

Direct Services. Activities used to support maintain, or improve an individual's condition or circumstance. Such basic services for high-risk older adults include: in-home aide services; nursing services; transportation for required care; assistance with durable medical equipment and medical supplies; adult day care or attendant care; home-delivered meals; and physical, speech, and occupational therapy.

Division of Aging (DOA). The State agency responsible for planning, administering, coordinating, and evaluating the activities, programs, and services developed under the Older Americans Act, as well as for advocacy and development of other programs for older adults.

Durable Medical Equipment. Equipment often prescribed by a doctor to serve a medical purpose. Example: wheelchairs, bedside commodes, and hospital beds. Insurance considers payment on rental or purchase of this equipment.

Durable Power of Attorney. Effective even though you are incapacitated. If you are planning for possible future incompetency, your power of attorney must be durable. To be durable, a power of attorney must state that it either remains or becomes effective after you become incapacitated.

E

Emergency Assistance Crisis Intervention Program. Immediate financial help for fuel, food, utilities, medications, clothing, and rent provided for individuals and families in crisis situations. These services are often handled through local public agencies, churches, private organizations, or the Salvation Army.

Employment/Training Adjustment Services. Basic counseling and referral services, leading to training, educational opportunities, and/or paid employment for blind or visually impaired individuals.

Extraordinary Means. Includes any medical procedure which artificially postpones the moment of death by supporting or replacing a vital bodily function.

F

Family Care Home. A licensed adult care home that provides residential care for two to six adults who require some supervision, along with room and board, to assure their safety and comfort.

Food Stamps. A program to assist eligible households with the purchase of food through the use of coupons.

Foster Care Services for Adults. Assistance to aging, blind, or disabled individuals and other adults in need of finding suitable licensed substitute homes when they are unable to remain in their own homes or when such service is needed to enable adults to move out of institutional care. Services include assessment of the individual and/or his/her family for the need of an initial or continued placement; arranging for appropriate services to support the social, emotional, and physical well-being of the individual during the placement; counseling to help the individual attain and maintain an adequate psychosocial adjustment; and casework services to support and strengthen the individual's relationship with his own family.

Foster Grandparent Program. Low-income older persons receive a stipend to help special needs children for about 20 hours per week.

H

Health Promotion. Activities to maintain and improve the health and well-being of older adults. Health promotion focus areas may include, but are not limited to, exercise/physical fitness, nutrition/diet, drug management, accident prevention/injury control, smoking cessation, immunization, dental health, vision care, foot care, and environmental health.

Health Screening. General medical testing, screening, and referral for the purpose of promoting the early detection and prevention of health problems of older persons.

High-Risk Older Adults. Those who experience multiple functional impairments in activities of daily living (ADLs) that jeopardize their independence and control over the quality of their lives. Individuals at high risk often need multiple health and social service interventions to substitute for lost functions and to maintain and rehabilitate other areas of functioning.

Home and Community Care Block Grant (HCCBG). Federal and state funds administered by the Division of Aging (DOA), includes the Older Americans Act (OAA), Social Services Block Grant (SSBG), and State funds.

Home Delivered Meals. A nutrition program that utilizes volunteers to deliver at least one hot nutritious meal per day (usually 5 days a week) to homebound adults.

Home Health Services. Health care prescribed by a physician and given in the home to an older adult in need of medical care. Allowable services are skilled nursing services, therapy services (physical therapy, occupational therapy, and speech therapy), medical social services, and health promotion services.

Homemaker Services. See In-Home Aide Services

Hospice Care. A service provided for terminally ill patients and their families. This agency provides medical, nursing, and supportive services to meet the needs of families and patients in the last six months of the patient's life.

I

ICF-MR. Intermediate care facilities for the mentally retarded.

In-Home Aide Services. The in-home aide services are also known as Chore, Homemaker, Homemaker-Home Health Aide, Respite, and

Personal Care Services. These are paraprofessional services that assist children and adults, their families, or both, with essential home management tasks, personal care tasks, supervision, or all of the above. Their purpose is to allow these individuals to function effectively in their own homes for as long as possible. The four levels of care are:

- Level I—Home Management: In-Home Aide Services at this level are intended to provide support to those needing assistance with basic home management tasks, such as housekeeping, cooking, shopping, and bill paying. Personal care tasks may not be performed at this level.

- Level II—Home Management/Personal Care: In-Home Aide Services at this level are intended to provide support to persons/families who predominately require assistance with basic personal care (bathing, shaving, toileting, and personal hygiene), and home management tasks.

- Level III—Home Management: In-Home Aide Services at this level are intended to provide intensive education and support to persons/families in carrying out home management tasks and improving family functioning skills.

- Level III—Personal Care: In-Home Aide Services at this level are intended to provide substantial activities of daily living (ADL) support to individuals/families who require assistance with health and personal care tasks. Provision of these tasks involves extensive "hands-on" care and potential assistance with a wide range of health related conditions.

- Level IV—Home Management: In-Home Aide Services at this level are intended to provide a wide range of educational and supportive services to persons/families who are in crisis or who require long-term assistance with complex home management tasks and family functioning skills. Provision of the service involves quick and creative response to individual/family crisis situations identified by the case manager; it also focuses on conducting appropriate learning sessions with small groups of persons from different families who have similar needs.

Informational Referral and Case Assistance (I&R). Provision of information about services available and efforts to assist individuals in identifying the types of assistance needed, placing individuals in contact with appropriate services and follow-up activities to determine whether services were received and met the identified needs.

Institutional Respite Care. Provides needed relief to primary caregivers of individuals who cannot be left alone because of mental and physical problems.

Instrumental Activities of Daily Living (IADL). Basic tasks that may not be a part of people's regular day, but are essential to living independently, such as paying bills, shopping, and using the telephone.

Intermediate-Level Care. A level of care in a nursing facility that provides 24-hour assistance, with a minimum of eight hours of coverage daily by a licensed nurse but no requirement for 24-hour skilled nursing services.

L

Legal Services. A service to provide older people with information on their legal rights, legal advice, legal benefits, entitlements and/or appeals when referral to a human service agency or a pro bono (for free) service is inappropriate; also includes preventive measures such as community education.

Life Insurance Trust. This kind of trust can receive proceeds of life insurance policies. It can make cash available to the administrator of an estate. For instance, this kind of trust can provide income for a family to help meet daily expenses while an estate is being settled.

Living Trust. People create this kind of trust to help them while they are still alive. It helps them manage their assets. Living trusts can be flexible and controlled by the person. For instance, such a trust can be used to pay the cost of in-home or nursing home care.

Living Will. This is a declaration that you desire to die a natural death. You do not want extraordinary medical treatment, artificial nutrition, or hydration used to keep you alive if there is no reasonable hope of recovery. A living will gives your doctor permission to withhold or withdraw life support systems under certain conditions.

Long-Term Care Ombudsman. A professional who serves as an advocate for long term-care residents. Advocacy includes educating individuals about their rights and complex rules or regulations governing the long-term care system. An Ombudsman can be requested to investigate concerns and serve as a mediator for conflict resolution should a resident encounter difficulty exercising rights.

Low-Income Emergency Assistance (LIEAP). Provides funds to help low income families cope with cost increases in heating and provides emergency assistance to those families who are experiencing a heating related crisis. LIEAP funding is 100% federal.

M

Medicaid (Title XIX). A Federal- and State-funded health care program for income eligible persons. Administered by the state, the program provides medical care for qualifying recipients. Applications for Medicaid can usually be made through the local department of Social Services.

Medicare. A Federal health insurance program for persons aged 65 and over who are eligible for Social Security or Railroad Retirement benefits and for some people who are disabled regardless of age. There are two parts: Part A is hospital insurance which is automatic, for those eligible, and Part B covers the physician and other services. Part B is voluntary and requires a monthly premium.

Mixed Cerebral Palsy. A combination of symptoms, a child with mixed CP has both high and low tone muscle. Some muscles are too tight, and others are too loose, creating a mix of stiffness and involuntary movements.

N

Nursing Homes. Skilled nursing and intermediate-care facilities.

O

Occupational Therapist. Occupational therapists assist in rehabilitation through the design and implementation of individualized programs to improve or restore functions impaired by illness or injury.

Occupational Therapy (OT). Helps the individual develop fine motor skills such as dressing, feeding, writing, and other daily living tasks.

Older Americans Act (OAA). Federal legislation established in 1965 providing broad policy objectives designed to meet the needs of older persons. The key philosophy of the program has been to help maintain and support older persons in their homes and communities and to avoid unnecessary or premature institutionalization.

Outreach. Agency activities to increase the public awareness of services to older persons and to provide information on services available to older adults.

P

Personal Care. See In-Home Aide Services

Persistent Vegetative State. If you have had a complete loss of self-aware cognition (you are a vegetable), and you will die soon without the use of extraordinary medical treatment or artificial nutrition or hydration.

Personal Emergency Alarm Response. A service that uses telephone lines to alert a central monitoring facility (often a hospital emergency room) of an emergency in the household. This service is predominantly used by older adults who live alone and are at risk of medical emergencies (Example: Lifeline).

Physical Therapy (PT). Helps the individual develop stronger muscles such as those in the legs and trunk. PT skills include walking, sitting, and keeping his or her balance.

Poverty Level. An income guideline established federally to define individuals who are economically disadvantaged.

Power of Attorney. Someone may act on your behalf under a regular power of attorney only if you are competent. This ends if you become incompetent or incapacitated. A regular power of attorney is used for reasons other than planning for incapacity.

Primary Adjustment Services. Services are provided to enable eligible blind or visually impaired individuals to attain and/or maintain the highest level of functioning possible, to promote their well-being, and to prevent or reduce dependency. This is achieved through a focused regimen of counseling and casework assistance to individuals and their families.

Protective Services for Adults. Services provided to correct or prevent further abuse, neglect, exploitation, or hazardous living conditions of individuals 18 years of age or older, or lawfully emancipated minors who are unable to manage their own resources, carry out the activities of daily living or protect their own interests. Services include: evaluation of reports of the need of individuals for protective services; planning and counseling with such individuals and their relatives or caretakers to identify, remedy and/or prevent problems which result in abuse, neglect, or exploitation; assisting in arranging for appropriate alternative living arrangements in the community or in an institution; and arranging for the provision of medical, legal, and other services as needed and appropriate. Also included is assistance in arranging for protective placement, guardianship, or commitment when needed as part of the protective services plan, and the provision of medical and psychological diagnostic studies, and evaluations where needed to substantiate and assess the circumstances of abuse or neglect.

Q

Qualified Medicare Beneficiary/Medicare-Aid (QMB). Assistance for those who do not qualify for Medicaid, but whose income is very low (pays Medicare Part B premiums/deductibles for A and B, etc).

R

Refugee Assistance. Support services to help refugees with resettlement, job training, and employment. Refugee Assistance is 100% federally funded.

Respite. Provides needed relief to primary caregivers of individuals who cannot be left alone because of mental or physical problems.

Retired and Senior Volunteer Program. Encourages volunteerism among retired and senior adults 55 years of age and older.

Retirement Community. A housing complex designed for older adults. Many of the retirement communities allow monthly rental, while others require purchase of the unit. Persons living in retirement communities are generally able to care for themselves; however, assistance from home care agencies is allowed by some communities. Activities and socialization are provided.

S

Screening. Assessment activities performed by a team of at least two persons, a social worker, and a nurse to determine a person's current functional abilities and resources in six areas: physical health, mental health, social support, activities of daily living, environmental conditions, and financial situation. Screening must include a home visit by at least one member of the screening team. (once the assessment is completed, activities related to developing and implementing a client service plan becomes part of case management.)

Senior Center. A multipurpose center designed with the older adult in mind. Scheduled activities, crafts, and programs provide social stimulation and interaction among participants.

Senior Companion Program. Provides a stipend to low income older adults to provide in home services to the elderly to help them live independently.

Senior Community Service Employment Program (Title V). Provides federally subsidized part-time community service employment for about 20 people.

Senior Health Insurance Information Program (SHIIP). Volunteers assist older adults with information about all types of insurance issues.

Social Services Block Grant (SSBG). Federal, state, and local fund block grants providing a variety of services for children and adults. Examples—Adult Protective Services (APS), Placement, Guardianship, In-Home Aide Services, and transportation.

Spastic Cerebral Palsy. A condition where there is too much muscle tone or tightness. Movements are stiff, especially in the legs, arms, and/or back. Children with this form of CP move their legs awkwardly, turning in or scissoring their legs as they try to walk. This is the most common form of CP.

Speech-Language Pathology (S/L). Helps the individual develop his or her communication skills.

State/County Special Assistance for Adults (S/CSA). Provides a cash supplement to eligible persons in adult care homes or, at county option, to certain disabled persons in private living arrangements who do not meet Supplemental Security Income (SSI) Medicaid eligibility standards. This is a state/county supported program (50% state funded and 50% county funded) with no federal funds involved. It is not available in all states.

Special Assistance for the Blind. Provides special financial assistance to blind individuals in need of domiciliary care. Funding is 50% state and 50% county paid to an individual or institution.

State Senior Center Outreach/Development. A service designed for the expansion of senior center activities to unserved or underserved areas. Development of new centers is allowable if county commissioners commit to the ongoing support of that center.

Supplemental Security Income (SSI). Additional monthly income for seniors whose Social Security is below a given level.

Support Groups. Usually made up of caregivers, family members, and friends of a person experiencing an illness such as Alzheimer's disease, cancer, Parkinson's, etc. People are brought together by a common concern, situation, or experience. A professional sometimes facilitates group discussion and sharing of experiences and feelings. Educational programs are also common among support groups.

T

Testamentary Trust. This is a trust created by a will. It takes effect after the trustor's death. Under such a trust, property need not be divided immediately among all heirs. Instead, it can link the division to some event. For instance, the trust may provide that a widow receives the net income from the trust during her lifetime. Then, upon her death, the rest of the funds will be split among any children or other heirs.

Title III Older Americans Act. Supports a wide array of community-based and in-home services that permit older adults aged 60 years and older to remain in their homes and avoid premature institutionalization. The Act is targeted to older persons with the greatest economic or social needs with particular attention to low-income minorities. Funding under the Older Americans Act supports: In-home meals to at-risk older adults (generally a noon day meal is provided at least five days a week); in-home aide or health care services; congregate nutrition programs; housing and home improvement; adult day care; information and case assistance; senior companion programs; health screening; care management; senior center operations; mental health counseling; institutional respite care; transportation; and volunteer program development.

Title XIX Medical Transportation. Provides transportation for medical services to authorized Medicaid recipients. Title XIX Medical Transportation funding is 33.48% county and 66.52% federal.

V

Vocational Rehabilitation. Supported by both Federal and State moneys, allocated for the specific purpose of vocational services. Services may include: diagnostic procedures, surgery and treatment, prosthetic devices, hospital convalescent, training material, maintenance, occupational expenses, interpreter services, transportation.

Volunteer Program Development. The development and operation of a systematic program for volunteer participation. The objective is to involve volunteers of all ages in providing services to older adults in their community. Older adults are also encouraged to volunteer.

Chapter 37

Directory of Additional Resources

Government Agencies

The Administration on Aging offers several services including: National Association of Area Agencies on Aging, Inc; National Association of State Units on Aging; National Institute on Aging (NIA) Information Center; and Eldercare Locator. Contact information for each service is listed.

Administration on Aging
U.S. Department of Health and Human Services
330 Independence Avenue, SW
Washington, DC 20201
Eldercare Locator Toll-Free:
800-677-1116, Monday-Friday, 9 a.m. to 8 p.m. ET
Tel: 202-619-0724
Fax: 202-260-1012
TDD: 202-401-7575
Website: http://www.aoa.gov
E-mail: aoainfo@aoa.gov

National Association of Area Agencies on Aging, Inc.
927 15th Street, N.W., 6th Floor
Washington, DC 20005
Tel: 202-296-8130
Fax: 202-296-8134
Website: http://www.n4a.org

This chapter contains information from the National Aging Information Center of the Administration on Aging.

National Association of State Units on Aging (NASUA)
1225 I Street, NW, Suite 725
Washington, DC, 20005
Tel: 202-898-2578
Fax: 202-898-2583
Website: http://www.nasua.org
E-mail: staff@nasua.org

National Institute on Aging (NIA) Information Center
P.O. Box 8057
Gaithersburg, MD 20898-8057
Toll-Free: 800-222-2225
TTY: 800-222-4225
Website: http://www.nih.gov/nia

Federal Trade Commission
CRC-240
Washington, DC 20580
Toll-Free: 877-382-4357
Tel: 202-326-2000
Website: http://www.ftc.gov

Medicare Hotline
Health Care Financing Administration
U.S. Department of Health and Human Services
Toll-Free: 800-638-6833
TTY: 877-486-2048
Website: http://www.medicare.gov

National Center for Chronic Disease Prevention and Health Promotion
Division of Nutrition and Physical Activity
Mail Stop K-46
4770 Buford Highway, NE
Atlanta, Georgia 30341-3724
Toll-Free: 888-232-4674
Website: http://www.cdc.gov

National Center for Injury Prevention and Control
Division of Unintentional Injury Prevention
Mailstop K-59
4770 Buford Highway NE
Atlanta, GA 30341-3724
Tel: 770-488-4656
Fax: 770-488-1665
Website: http://www.cdc.gov/ncipc/osp/data.htm

The President's Council on Physical Fitness and Sports
200 Independence Avenue
Room 738-H
Washington, DC 20004
Tel: 202-690-9000

Worklife Enrichment & Studies Team
Center for Employee Services
Social Security Administration
G122A West High Rise Building
6401 Security Boulevard
Baltimore, MD 21235
Tel: 410-965-0479

State Agencies on Aging

National Association of State Units on Aging (NASUA)
1225 I Street, NW, Suite 725
Washington, DC, 20005
Tel: 202-898-2578
Fax: 202-898-2583
Website: http://www.nausa.org
E-mail: staff@nasua.org

Alabama: Region IV

Alabama Department of Senior Services
RSA Plaza, Suite 470
770 Washington Avenue
Montgomery, AL 36130-1851
Tel: 334-242-5743
Fax: 334-242 5594
Website: http://
www.adss.state.al.us

Alaska: Region X

Alaska Commission on Aging
Division of Senior Services
Department of Administration
Juneau, AK 99811-0209
Tel: 907-465-3250
Fax: 907-465-4716
Website: http://alaskaaging.org

Arizona: Region IX

Aging and Adult Administration
Department of Economic Security
1789 West Jefferson St., #950A
Phoenix, AZ 85007
Tel: 602-542-4446
Fax: 602-542-6575
Website: http://de.state.az.us

Arkansas: Region VI

Division Aging and Adult Services
Arkansas Dept of Human Services
P.O. Box 1437, Slot 1412
1417 Donaghey Plaza South
Little Rock, AR 72203-1437
Tel: 501-682-2441
Fax: 501-682-8155
Website: http://
www.accessarkansas.org

California: Region IX

California Department of Aging
1600 K Street
Sacramento, CA 95814
Tel: 916-322-3887
Toll-Free Senior Services:
800-510-2020
Fax: 916-324-4989
Website: http://
www.aging.state.ca.us
E-mail:
ohidalgo@aging.state.ca.us

Colorado: Region VIII

Aging and Adult Services
Department of Social Services
1575 Sherman St., Ground Floor
Denver, CO 80203
Tel: 303-620-4147; 303-866-2800
Fax: 303-620-4191; 303-866-2696
Website: http://
www.cdhs.state.co.us/oss/aas

541

Connecticut: Region I

Division of Elderly Services
25 Sigourney Street, 10th Floor
Hartford, CT 06106-5033
Tel: 860-424-5277
Fax: 860-424-4966
Website: http://dss.state.ct.us/
dss.htm

Delaware: Region III

Delaware Division of Services for Aging and Adults with Physical Disabilities
Department of Health and
Social Services
1901 North DuPont Highway
1st Floor Annex
New Castle, DE 19720
Tel: 302-577-4791
Fax: 302-577-4793
E-mail: dsaapdinfo@state.ed.us

District of Columbia: Region III

District of Columbia Office on Aging
One Judiciary Square, 9th Floor
Suite 900-S
441 Fourth Street, NW
Washington, DC 20001
Tel: 202-724-5622
Fax: 202-724-4979
Website: http://www.dcoa.dc.gov

Florida: Region IV

Department of Elder Affairs
Suite 315
4040 Esplanade Way
Tallahassee, FL 32399-7000
Tel: 850-414-2000
Fax: 850-414-2004
Website: http://fcn.state.fl.us/ddea

Georgia: Region IV

Division of Aging Services
Department of Human Resources
2 Peachtree St. N.W., 36th Floor
Atlanta, GA 30303-3176
Tel: 404-657-5258
Fax: 404-657-5285
Website: http://
www.dhr.state.ga.us

Guam: Region IX

Division of Senior Citizens
Department of Public Health &
Social Services
P.O. Box 2816
Agana, Guam 96910
Tel: 671-475-0263
Fax: 671-477-2930
Website: http://admin.gov.gu/
pubhealth

Hawaii: Region IX

Executive Office on Aging
No. 1 Capitol District
250 South Hotel Street, Room 109
Honolulu, HI 96813-2831
Tel: 808-586-0100
Fax: 808-586-0185
Website: http://www.state.hi.us/
health/eoa

Idaho: Region X

Idaho Commission on Aging
P.O. Box 83720
Boise, ID 83720-0007
Tel: 208-334-3833
Fax: 208-334-3033
Web: http://www.idahoaging.com

Illinois: Region V

Illinois Department on Aging
421 East Capitol Ave., Suite 100
Springfield, IL 62701-1789
Tel: 217-785-3356
Chicago Office Tel: 312-814-2630
Fax: 217-785-4477
Web: http://www.state.il.us/aging

Indiana: Region V

Bureau of Aging and In-Home Services
Division of Disability, Aging and
Rehabilitative Services
Family and Social Services Adm.
402 W. Washington Street, #W454
P.O. Box 7083
Indianapolis, IN 46207-7083
Tel: 317-232-7020
Fax: 317-232-7867
Web: http://www.in.gov/ai/social

Iowa: Region VII

Iowa Dept. of Elder Affairs
Clemens Building, 3rd Floor
200 Tenth Street
Des Moines, IA 50309-3609
Tel: 515-242-3333
Fax: 515-242-3300
Web: http://www.state.ia.us/
elderaffairs

Kansas: Region VII

Department on Aging
New England Building
503 S. Kansas Ave.
Topeka, KS 66603-3404
Tel: 785-296-4986
Fax: 785-296-0256
Website: http://www.k4s.org

Kentucky: Region IV

Office of Aging Services
Commonwealth of Kentucky
275 East Main Street
Frankfort, KY 40621
Tel: 502-564-6930
Fax: 502-564-4595
Website: http://
www.chs.state.ky.us/aging

Louisiana: Region VI

Governor's Office of Elderly Affairs
P.O. Box 80374
Baton Rouge, LA 70898-0374
Tel: 225-342-7100
Fax: 225-342-7133
Web: http://www.gov.state.la.us/
depts/elderly.htm

Maine: Region I

Bureau of Elder and Adult Services
Department of Human Services
#1 State House Station
35 Anthony Avenue
Augusta, ME 04333
Tel: 207-624-5335
Fax: 207-624-5361
Website: http://www.me.state.us/
dhs/beas

Maryland: Region III

Maryland Dept. of Aging
State Office Building, Rm. 1007
301 West Preston Street
Baltimore, MD 21201-2374
Tel: 410-767-1100
Fax: 410-333-7943
Website: http://
www.mdoa.state.md.us

Massachusetts: Region I

**Massachusetts Executive
Office of Elder Affairs**
One Ashburton Place, 5th Floor
Boston, MA 02108
Tel: 617-727-7750
Fax: 617-727-9368
Website: http://
www.state.ma.us/elder

Michigan: Region V

**Michigan Office of Services
to the Aging**
Ottawa Building, 3rd Floor
611 W. Ottawa
Lansing, MI 48933
Tel: 517-373-8230
Fax: 517-373-4092
Website: http://www.miseniors.net

Minnesota: Region V

Minnesota Board on Aging
444 Lafayette Road
St. Paul, MN 55155-3843
Toll-Free: 800-882-6262
Tel: 651-296-1531
Fax: 651-297-7855
TTY: 800-627-3529
Website: http://www.mnaging.org

Mississippi: Region IV

**Division of Aging and Adult
Services**
750 N. State Street
Jackson, MS 39202
Tel: 601-359-4900
Fax: 601-359-4370
Website: http://
www.mdhs.state.ms.us

Missouri: Region VII

Division on Aging
Department of Social Services
221 West High Street
P.O. Box 1527
Jefferson City, MO 65102-1337
Tel: 573-751-3082
Fax: 573-751-8687
Website: http://
www.dss.state.mo.us

Montana: Region VIII

**Senior and Long Term Care
Division**
Department of Public Health &
Human Services
111 Sanders, Room 210
P.O. Box 4210
Helena, MT 59604
Aging (Toll Free) Hotline: 800-
332-2272
Tel: 406-444-4077
Fax: 406-444-7743
Website: http://
www.dphhs.state.mt.us/sltc

Nebraska: Region VII

Department of Health and Human Services
Division on Aging
1343 M Street
P.O. Box 95044
Lincoln, NE 68509-5044
Tel: 402-471-2307
Fax: 402-471-4619
Website: http://
www.hhs.state.ne.us/
ags.agsindex.htm

Nevada: Region IX

Nevada Division for Aging Services
Department of Human Resources
State Mail Room Complex
3416 Goni Road, Building D 132
Carson City, NV 89706
Tel: 775-687-4210
Fax: 775-687-4264
Website: http://aging.state.nv.us

New Hampshire: Region I

Elderly and Adult Services Division
129 Pleasant Street
Concord, NH 03301
Tel: 603-271-4680
Fax: 603-271-4643

New Jersey: Region II

Department of Health and Senior Services
New Jersey Division of Senior Affairs
P.O. Box 807
Trenton, NJ 08625-0807
Toll-Free: 800-792-8820
Tel: 609-588-3141
Fax: 609-588-3601
Website: http://www.state.nj.us/
health

New Mexico: Region VI

State Agency on Aging
228 East Palace Avenue
Santa Fe, NM 87501
Tel: 505-827-7640
Fax: 505-827-7649
Website: http://
www.nmaging.state.nm.us

New York: Region II

New York State Office for the Aging
2 Empire State Plaza
Albany, NY 12223-1251
Toll-Free: 800-342-9871
Tel: 518-474-5731
Fax: 518-474-0608
Website: http://
www.aging.state.ny.us

North Carolina: Region IV

Department of Health and Human Services
Division of Aging
2101 Mail Service Center
Raleigh, NC 27699-2101
Tel: 919-733-3983
Fax: 919-733-0443
Website: http://
www.dhhs.state.nc.us/aging

North Dakota: Region VIII

Department of Human Services
Aging Services Division
600 South 2nd Street, Suite 1C
Bismarck, ND 58504
Tel: 701-328-8910
Fax: 701-328-8989
E-mail: sosena@state.nd.us

North Mariana Islands: Region IX

CNMI Office on Aging
P.O. Box 2178
Commonwealth of the Northern
Mariana Islands
Saipan, MP 96950
Tel: 670-233-1320/1321
Fax: 670-233-1327/0369

Ohio: Region V

Ohio Department of Aging
50 West Broad Street, 9th Floor
Columbus, OH 43215-5928
Tel: 614-466-5500
Fax: 614-466-5741
Website: http://www.state.oh.us/age

Oklahoma: Region VI

Aging Services Division
Department of Human Services
P.O. Box 25352
312 N.E. 28th Street
Oklahoma City, OK 73105
Tel: 405-521-2281 or 405-521-2327
Fax: 405-521-2086
Website: http://www.okdhs.org

Oregon: Region X

Senior and Disabled Services Division
500 Summer Street, N.E., E02
Salem, OR 97301-1073
Toll Free: 800-282-8096 (V/TTY)
Tel: 503-945-5811
Fax: 503-373-7823
Website: http://
www.sdsd.hr.state.or.us
E-mail: sdsd.info@state.or.us

Palau: Region X

State Agency on Aging
Republic of Palau
Koror, PW 96940
Tel: 9-10-288-011-680-488-2736
Fax: 9-10-288-680-488-1662

Pennsylvania: Region III

Pennsylvania Department of Aging
Commonwealth of Pennsylvania
555 Walnut Street, 5th floor
Harrisburg, PA 17101-1919
Tel: 717-783-1550
Fax: 717-772-6842
Website: http://
www.aging.state.pa.us

Puerto Rico: Region II

Commonwealth of Puerto Rico
Governor's Office of Elderly Affairs
Call Box 50063
Old San Juan Station, PR 00902
Tel: 787-721-5710; 787-721-4560; 787-721-6121
Fax: 787-721-6510
E-mail:
administrator@ogave.prstar.net

Rhode Island: Region I

Department of Elderly Affairs
160 Pine Street
Providence, RI 02903-3708
Tel: 401-222-2858
TDD: 401-222-2880
Fax: 401-222-3389
Website: http://www.dea.state.ri.us

American Samoa: Region IX

Territorial Adm. on Aging
Government of American Samoa
Pago Pago, American Samoa 96799
Tel: 011-684-633-2207
Fax: 011-684-633-2533

South Carolina: Region IV

Office of Senior and Long Term Care Services
Department of Health and Human Services
P.O. Box 8206
Columbia, SC 29202-8206
Tel: 803-898-2501
Fax: 803-898-4515
Website: http://www.dhhs.state.sc.us

South Dakota: Region VIII

Office of Adult Services and Aging
Richard F. Kneip Building
700 Governors Drive
Pierre, SD 57501-2291
Tel: 605-773-3656
Fax: 605-773-6834
Website: http://www.state.sd.us/asa

Tennessee: Region IV

Commission on Aging
Andrew Jackson Bldg., 9th Floor
500 Deaderick Street,
Nashville, Tennessee 37243-0860
Tel: 615-741-2056
Fax: 615-741-3309
Website: http://www.state.tn.us/comaging

Texas: Region VI

Texas Department on Aging
4900 North Lamar, 4th Floor
Austin, TX 78751-2316
Tel: 512-424-6840
Fax: 512-424-6890
Website: http://www.tdoa.state.tx.us

Utah: Region VIII

Division of Aging & Adult Services
Box 45500
120 North 200 West, Room 401
Salt Lake City, UT 84103
Tel: 801-538-3910
Fax: 801-538-4395
Website: http://www.hsdaas.state.ut.us

Vermont: Region I

Vermont Department of Aging and Disabilities
Waterbury Complex
103 South Main Street
Waterbury, VT 05671-2303
Tel: 802-241-2400
Voice/TTY: 802-241-2186
Fax: 802-241-2325
Website: http://
www.dad.state.vt.us

Virginia: Region III

Virginia Department for the Aging
1600 Forest Avenue, Suite 102
Richmond, VA 23229
Tel: 800-552-3402
Fax: 804-662-9354
Website: http://
www.aging.state.va.us

Virgin Islands: Region II

Senior Citizen Affairs
Virgin Islands Department of
Human Services
Knud Hansen Complex
Building A
1303 Hospital Ground
Charlotte Amalie, VI 00802
Tel: 340-774-0930
Fax: 340-774-3466
Website: http://
www.gov.vi.human

Washington: Region X

Aging and Adult Services Administration
Department of Social & Health
Services
P.O. Box 45050
Olympia, WA 98504-5050
Toll-Free: 800-422-3263
Tel: 360-725-2300
TTY: 800-737-7931
Fax: 360-438-8633
Website: http://www.dshs.wa.gov
E-mail: askdshs@dshs.wa.gov

West Virginia: Region III

West Virginia Bureau of Senior Services
1900 Kanawha Boulevard, East
Holly Grove, Building 10
Charleston, WV 25305
Tel: 304-558-3317
Fax: 304-558-0004
Website: http://www.state.wv.us/
seniorservices

Wisconsin: Region V

Bureau of Aging and Long Term Care Resources
Department of Health and
Family Services
1 Wilson Street
Madison, WI 53707
Tel: 608-266-2536
Fax: 608-267-3203
Website: http://
www.dhfs.state.wi.us/aging

Wyoming: Region VIII

Aging Division
6101 Yellowstone Road
Room 259-B
Cheyenne, WY 82002
Tel: 307-777-7986
Fax: 307-777-5340
Website: http://
wdhfs.state.wy.us/aging/
index.html

Private Organizations

Adaptive Environments
374 Congress St., Suite 301
Boston, MA 02210
Tel: 617-695-1225
Fax: 617-482-8099
Website: http://
www.adaptenv.org
E-mail: adaptive@adaptenv.org

American Association of Retired Persons
601 E Street, N.W.
Washington, DC 20049
Toll-Free: 800-424-3410
Tel: 202-434-2277
Website: http://www.aarp.org
E-mail: member@aarp.org

American Business Collaboration for Quality Dependent Care
200 Talcott Avenue West
Watertown, MA 02472
Toll-Free: 800-447-0543
Website: http://
www.abcdependentcare.com

Bay Area Emergency Care Consortium
Managing Director or Director
Caregivers on Call: 800-225-1200

Center for Universal Design and Accessible Housing Information
North Carolina State University
School of Design
Box 8613
219 Oberlin Road
Raleigh, NC 27695-8613
Toll-Free: 800-647-6777
Tel/TTY: 919-515-3082
Fax: 919-515-3023
E-mail: cud@ncsu.edu

Children of Aging Parents (CAPS)
1609 Woodbourne Rd, Suite 302A
Levittown, PA 19057
Toll-Free: 800-227-7294
Tel: 215-945-6900
Website: http://
www.caps4caregivers.org

Easter Seals—National Office
230 West Monroe Street
Suite 1800
Chicago, IL 60606-4802
Toll-Free: 800-221-6827
Tel: 312-726-6200
TTY: 312-726-4258
Fax: 312-726-1494
Website: http://www.easter-seals.org
E-mail: info@easter-seals.org

Family Caregiver Alliance
690 Market Street, Suite 600
San Francisco, CA 94104
Toll-Free in California: 800-445-8106
Tel: 415-434-3388
Fax: 415-434-3508
Website: http://www.caregiver.org
E-mail: info@caregiver.org

National Academy of Elder Law Attorneys, Inc.
1604 North Country Club Road
Tucson, AZ 85716
Tel: 520-881-4005
Fax: 520-325-7925
Website: http://www.naela.com

National Alliance for Caregiving
4720 Montgomery Lane
Bethesda, MD 20814
Tel: 301-718-8444

National Association for Home Care
228 Seventh Street, SE
Washington, DC 20003
Tel: 202-547-7424
Fax: 202-547-3540
Website: http://www.nahc.org

National Meals on Wheels Association of America
1414 Prince Street, Suite 202
Alexandria, VA 22314
Toll-Free: 800-999-6262
Tel: 703-548-5558
Fax: 703-548-8024
Website: http://www.mealsonwheelsassn.org

The American Health Care Association
1201 L St., NW
Washington, DC 20005-4014
Tel: 202-842-4444
Fax: 202-842-3860
Website: http://www.ahca.org

Brain Injury

Brain Injury Association (formerly the National Head Injury Foundation)
105 North Alfred Street
Alexandria, VA 22314
Toll-Free: 800-444-6443
Tel: 703-236-6000
Website: http://www.biausa.org
E-mail: FamilyHelpline@biausa.org

Emergency Medical Services for Children–National Resource Center
111 Michigan Avenue N.W.
Washington, DC 20010-2970
Tel: 202-884-4927

Epilepsy Foundation–National Office
4351 Garden City Drive
Suite 500
Landover, MD 20785
Toll-Free: 800-332-1000
Tel: 301-459-3700
TTY: 800-332-2070
Website: http://www.efa.org
E-mail: postmaster@efa.org

Family Caregiver Alliance
690 Market Street, Suite 600
San Francisco, CA 94104
Tel: 415-434-3388
Website: http://www.caregiver.org

Family Voices
P.O. Box 769
Algodones, NM 87001
Tel: 505-867-2368
Website: http://www.familyvoices.org
E-mail: kidshealth@familyvoices.org

Head Injury Hotline
212 Pioneer Building
Seattle, WA 98104-2221
Tel: 206-621-8558
Website: http://www.headinjury.com
E-mail: brain@headinjury.com

National Information Center for Children and Youth with Disabilities
P.O. Box 1492
Washington, DC 20013
Toll-Free (Voice/TTY): 800-695-0285
Fax: 202-884-8441
Website: http://www.nichcy.org
E-mail: nichcy@aed.org

Cerebral Palsy

United Cerebral Palsy Associations, Inc.
1660 L Street NW, Suite 700
Washington DC 20036
Toll-Free Voice/TTY: 800-872-5827
Tel: 202-776-0406
TTY: 202-973-7197
Fax: 202-776-0414
Website: http://www.ucpa.org
E-mail: ucpanatl@ucpa.org

Easter Seals—National Office
230 West Monroe Street
Suite 1800
Chicago, IL 60606-4802
Toll-Free: 800-221-6827
Tel: 312-726-6200
TTY: 312-726-4258
Fax: 312-726-1494
Website: http://www.easter-seals.org
E-mail: info@easter-seals.org

Elder Abuse

National Center on Elder Abuse
1225 I Street, NW Suite 725
Washington, DC 20005
Tel: 202-898-2586
Website: http://www.elderabusecenter.org

Grandparent Resources

Grandparent Information Center—AARP
601 E. Street, N.W.,
Washington, DC 20049
Toll-Free: 800-424-3410
Website: http://www.aarp.org
E-mail: gic@aarp.org

The Brookdale Foundation
126 East 56th Street, 10th Floor
New York, NY 10022
Website: http://www.ewol.com/brookdale
E-mail: bkdlfdn@aol.com

Child Welfare League of America (CWLA)
440 First St. NW
Washington, DC 20001
Tel: 202-638-2952
Fax: 202-638-4004
Website: http://www.cwla.org

Creative Grandparenting, Inc.
100 W. 10th Street, Suite 1007
Wilmington, DE 19801
Tel: 302-656-2122
Fax: 302-656-2123

The Foundation for Grandparenting
108 Farnham Rd.
Ojai, CA 93023
Website: http://
www.grandparenting.org
E-mail:
gpfound@grandparenting.org

Generations United
122 C St. NW, Suite 820
Washington, DC 20001
Tel: 202-638-1263
Fax: 202-638-7555
Website http://www.gu.org

GrandsPlace
154 Cottage Rd.
Enfield, CT 06082
Tel: 860-763-5789
Website: http://
www.grandsplace.com

The National Foster Parent Association
P.O. Box 81
Alpha, OH 45301
Toll-Free: 800-557-5238
Fax: 937-431-9377
Website: http://www.nfpainc.org

National Coalition of Grandparents
137 Larkin Street
Madison, WI 53705
Tel: 608-238-8751

National Committee to Preserve Social Security and Medicare
10 G St., NE, Suite 600
Washington, DC 20002
Toll-Free: 800-966-1935
Fax: 202-216-0447

R.O.C.K.I.N.G., Inc
P.O. Box 96
Niles, MI 49102
Tel: 616-683-9038

Hospice

The National Hospice and Palliative Care Organization (NHO)
1700 Diagonal Road
Arlington, VA 22314
Tel: 703-837-1500
Website: http://www.nhpco.org
E-mail: info@nhpco.org

Hospice Association of America (HAA)
228 Seventh St., SE
Washington, D.C. 20003
Tel: 202-546-4759
Fax: 202-547-3540
Website: http://www.nahc.org/
HAA/home.html

Hospice Education Institute
190 Westbrook Road
Essex, CT 06426-1510
Toll-Free: 800-331-1620
Tel: 860-767-1620
Fax: 860-767-2746
Website: http://
www.hospiceworld.org
E-mail: HOSPICEALL@aol.com

American Cancer Society (ACS)
Toll-Free: 800-ACS-2345
Website: http://www.cancer.org

Hospice Net
401 Bowling Ave, Suite 51
Nashville, TN 37205
Website: http://
www.hospicenet.org
E-mail:
comments@hospicenet.org

Medicare
Toll-Free: 800-633-4227
TTY: 877-486-2048
Website: http://
www.medicare.gov

National Cancer Institute
Toll-Free: 800-422-6237
Fax on demand (Dial and listen
to recorded instructions):
301-402-5874
TTY: 800-332-8615
Website: http://cancer.gov
E-mail:
cancermail@icicc.nci.nih.gov
(Put the word "help" in the body
of the message.)

Independent Living Resources

Listed are some companies that feature products, equipment, and clothing designed to make self-care skills easier.

Adaptability
P.O. Box 513
Colchester, CT 06415
Toll-Free: 800-243-9232

After Therapy Catalog
North Coast Medical
18305 Sutter Blvd.
Morgan Hill, CA 95037-2845
Toll-Free: 800-821-9319
Tel: 408-776-5000

American Walker
4683 Schneider Dr.
Oregon, WI 53575
Tel: 608-835-9255

Bell Atlantic Center for Customers with Disabilities
280 Locke Drive, 4th Floor
Marlboro, MA 01752
Toll-Free: 800-974-6006
Fax: 508-624-7645
Web: http://www.bellatlantic.com
E-mail: baccd@bellatlantic.com

Bruce Medical Supply
411 Waverly Oaks Rd.
Suite 154
Waltham, MA 02454
Toll-Free: 800-225-8446
Fax: 781-894-9519
Website: http://
www.brucemedical.com

Comfort House
189 -V Frelinghuysen Avenue
Newark, NJ 07114-1595
Toll-Free: 800-359-7701
Website: http://
www.comforthouse.com

Dr. Leonard's Health Care Catalog
100 Nixon Lane
Edison, NJ 08818
Toll-Free: 800-785-0880
Fax: 732-572-2118
Website: http://
www.drleonards.com

Dressing Tips and Clothing Resources for Making Life Easier [book available from:]
The Best 25 Catalogues
Resources for Making Life Easier
933 Chapel Hill Road
Madison, WI 53711
Website: http://
www.makinglifeeasier.com
E-mail:
help@makinglifeeasier.com

Metro Medical Equipment
12985 Wayne Road
Livonia, MI 48150
Toll-Free: 800-877-7285
Fax: 734-522-9380

Durable Medical Equipment (over 3500) Plate Guards, Aids for Daily Living
Yes I Can
35325 Date Palm Drive
Suite 131
Cathedral City, CA 92234
Toll-Free: 800-366-4226
Tel: 760-321-1717

Sammons Preston
P.O. Box 5071
Bolingbrook, IL 60440-5071
Toll-Free: 800-323-5547
Fax: 800-547-4333
Website: http://
www.SammonsPreston.com

Fashion Ease
1541 60th Street
Brooklyn, NY 11219
Toll-Free: 800-221-8929
Tel: 718-871-8188
Fax: 718-436-2067
Website: http://
www.fashionease.com

Independent Living Aids Inc.
200 Robbins Lane
Jericho, NY 11753-2341
Toll-Free: 800-537-2118
Fax: 516-937-3906
Website: http://
www.independentliving.com

J C Penny's Special Needs Catalog
P.O. Box 2021
Milwaukee, WI 53201

Patients Transfer Systems
Beatrice M. Brantman, Inc.
207 E. Westminster
Lake Forest, IL 60045
Toll-Free: 800-232-7987
Fax: 847-615-8894

Personal Pager
The Greatest of Ease Company
2443 Fillmore Street, #345
San Francisco, CA 94115

Sears Health Care Catalog
Sears Roebuck and Company
P.O. Box 804203
Chicago, IL 60680-4203
Toll-Free: 800-326-1750

The Speedo Aquatic Exercise System
7911 Haskell Avenue
Van Nuys, CA 91409
Toll-Free: 800-547-8770

The Do Able Renewable Home
Consumer Affairs Program Dept.
American Association of Retired Persons (AARP)
Toll-Free: 800-424-3410

Voice Amplifiers

Rand Voice Amplifier
Park Surgical Company, Inc.
5001 New Utrecht Avenue
Brooklyn, NY 11219
Toll-Free: 800-633-7878
Tel: 718-436-9200
Fax: 718-854-2431
Website: http://www.parksurgical.com

Luminaud Inc.
8688 Tyler Blvd.
Mentor, OH 44060-4348
Toll-Free: 800-255-3408
Fax: 440-255-2250
Website: http://www.luminaud.com

Anchor Audio, Inc.
3415 Lomita Blvd.
Torrance, CA 90505
Toll-Free: 800-262-4671
Tel: 310-784-2300
Fax: 310-784-0066
Website: http://www.anchoraudio.com

Walkers

Noble Motion Inc.
P.O. Box 1520
Pittsburgh, PA 15206
Toll-Free: 800-234-9255
Fax: 412-363-7189
Website: http://
www.wheels4walking.com

Wander Prevention Systems

WanderGuard
Toll-Free: 800-235-8085

Hand-Held Showerhead with an On-Off or Pause Control

Access with Ease
Toll-Free: 800-531-9479

Alsons
Toll-Free: 800-421-0001

Jaclo
Toll-Free: 800-852-3906
Tel: 908-789-7008

M.O.M.S.
Toll-Free: 800-232-7443

Sears Home Health Care Catalogue
Toll-Free: 800-326-1750

Door Alarms

The Safety Zone
Toll-Free: 800-999-3030

WanderGuard
Toll-Free: 800-235-8085

Secure Care Products
Toll-Free: 800-451-7917
Tel: 603-223-0745

Grab Bars

DSI
Tel: 818-782-6793

Franklin Brass Co.
Toll-Free: 800-829-0089

Häfele
Toll-Free: 800-423-3531

Maxi Aid
Toll-Free: 800-522-6294

Anti-Scalding Devices

Accent on Living
Toll-Free: 800-787-8444

Insurance

Any decision that affects your life insurance benefits can affect the people who care for and about you. Before you make a decision, talk to your friends and family as well as to someone whose advice and expertise you can count on—a lawyer, an accountant, or a financial planner. You also may want to contact the following organizations for more information.

American Council on Life Insurance
1001 Pennsylvania Avenue, N.W.
Washington, DC 20004-2599
Toll-Free: 800-589-2254
Tel: 202-624-2000
Website: http://www.acli.com

National Association of Insurance Commissioners
2301 McGee, Suite 800
Kansas City, MO 64108-2604
Tel: 816-842-3600
Website: http://www.naic.org

National Association of People with AIDS
1413 K Street, N.W., 7th Floor
Washington, DC 20005
Tel: 202-898-0414
Fax: 202-898-0435
Website: http://www.napwa.org
E-mail: napwa@napwa.org

National Viatical Association
1030 15th Street, Suite 870
Washington, DC 20005
Toll-Free: 800-741-9465
Tel: 202-347-7361
Fax: 202-393-0336
Website: http://
www.nationalviatical.org
E-mail: nva@rgminc.com

North American Securities Administrators Association
10 G Street N.E., Suite 710
Washington, D.C. 20002
Tel: 202-737-0900
Fax: 202-783-3571
Fax-on-Demand: 888-84-NASAA
Website: http://www.nasaa.org

Viatical and Life Settlement Association of America
2025 M Street, N.W., Suite 800
Washington, DC 20036
Tel: 202-367-1136
Fax: 202-367-2136
Website: http://www.viatical.org
E-mail: VLSSA@dc.sba.com

Your State Attorney General
Office of Consumer Protection
Your State Capital

Your State Insurance Commissioner
Department of Insurance
Your State Capital

Multiple Sclerosis

The National Multiple Sclerosis Society
733 Third Avenue
New York, NY 10017
Toll-Free: 800-344-4867
Website: http://
www.nationalmssociety.org
E-mail: info@nmss.org

Respite Family Support Projects

American Association of University Affiliated Programs (AAUAP)
8630 Fenton Street, Suite 410
Silver Spring, MD 20910
Tel: 301-588-8252
Fax: 301-588-2842
Website: http://www.aauap.org

The Beach Center on Families and Disability
The University of Kansas
1200 Sunnyside Avenue
3111 Haworth Hall
Lawrence, KS 66045
Tel: 785-864-7600
Fax: 785-864-7605
Website: http://
www.beachcenter.org

National Technical Assistance Center for Children's Mental Health
3307 M Street, NW, Suite 401
Washington, DC 20007
Tel: 202-687-5000
Fax: 202-687-1954
Website: http://
www.georgetown.edu/research/
gucdc/cassp.html
E-mail: gucdc@georgetown.edu

ARCH National Resource Center for Crisis Nurseries and Respite Care Services
Chapel Hill Training-Outreach Project
800 Eastowne Drive, Suite 105
Chapel Hill, NC 27514
Toll-Free: 800-473-1727
Tel: 919-490-5577

National Resource Center on Supportive Housing and Home Modification
Univ. of Southern California
3715 McClintock Avenue
Los Angeles, CA 90089-0191
Tel: 213-740-1364
Fax: 213-740-7069
E-mail: hmap@usc.edu

Parkinson Disease

American Parkinson Disease Association, Inc. Information and Referral (I&R) Centers

Alabama, Birmingham
University of Alabama at Birmingham
Tel: 205-934-9100

Arizona Tucson
University of Arizona
Toll-Free: 800-541-4960
Tel: 520-326-5400

Arkansas, Hot Springs
St. Joseph's Regional Health Center
Toll-Free: 800-407-9295
Tel: 501-318-1690

California, Fountain Valley
Orange Coast Memorial Medical Center
Tel: 714-378-5062

California, Los Angeles
Cedars-Sinai Health System
Tel: 310-855-7933

California, Los Angeles
(UCLA) Reed Neurological Research Center
Tel: 310-794-5667

California, San Diego
Information & Referral Center
Tel: 858-273-6763

California, San Francisco
Seton Medical Center
Tel: 650-991-6391

Connecticut, New Haven
Hospital of Saint Raphael
Tel: 203-789-3936

Florida, Jacksonville
Mayo Clinic, Jacksonville
Tel: 904-953-7030

Florida, Pompano Beach
North Broward Medical Center
Toll-Free: 800-825-2732

Florida, St. Petersburg
Columbia Edward White Hospital
Tel: 727-898-2732

Georgia, Atlanta
Emory University School of
Medicine
Tel: 404-728-6552

Idaho, Boise
St. Alphonsus Medical Center
Tel: 208-367-6570

Illinois, Chicago
Glenbrook Hospital
Tel: 847-657-5787

***The Arlette Johnson**
Young Parkinson Information &
Referral Center
Glenbrook Hospital
Toll-Free: 800-223-9776 (Out of IL)
Tel: 847-657-5787

Louisiana, New Orleans
School of Medicine, LSU
Tel: 504-568-6554

Maryland, Baltimore
Johns Hopkins Outpatient Center
Tel: 410-955-8795

Massachusetts, Boston
Boston University School of
Medicine
Tel: 617-638-8466

Minnesota, Minneapolis
Abbott Northwestern Hospital
Minneapolis Neuroscience Inst.
Toll-Free: 888-302-7762
Tel: 612-863-5850

Missouri, St. Louis
Washington University Medical
Center
Tel: 314-362-3299

Montana, Great Falls
Benefis Health Care
Tel: 406-455-2964

Nebraska, Omaha
Information & Referral Center
Tel: 402-551-9311

Nevada, Las Vegas
University of Nevada School of
Medicine
Tel: 702-464-3132

****Nevada, Reno**
V.A. Hospital
Tel: 775-328-1715

New Jersey, New Brunswick
Robert Wood Johnson
University Hospital
Tel: 732-745-7520

New Mexico, Albuquerque
Healthsouth Rehabilitation
Hospital
Toll-Free: 800-278-5386

New York, Albany
The Albany Medical College
Tel: 518-452-2749

New York, Far Rockaway
Peninsula Hospital
Tel: 718-734-2876

New York, Manhattan
New York University
Tel: 212-983-1379

New York, Old Westbury
New York College of Osteopathic
Medicine
Tel: 516-626-6114

New York, Smithtown
St. John's Episcopal Hospital
Tel: 516-862-3560

New York, Staten Island
Staten Island University Hospital
Tel: 718-226-6129

North Carolina, Durham
Duke South Hospital
Tel: 919-681-2033

Ohio, Cincinnati
University of Cincinnati Medical
Center
Toll-Free: 800-840-2732
Tel: 513-558-6770

Oklahoma, Tulsa
Hillcrest Medical Center System
Toll-Free: 800-364-4450
Tel: 918-747-3747

Pennsylvania, Philadelphia
Crozer-Chester Medical Center
Tel: 610-447-2911

Pennsylvania, Pittsburgh
Allegheny General Hospital
Tel: 412-441-0100

Rhode Island, Pawtucket
Memorial Hospital of RI
Tel: 401-729-3165

Tennessee, Memphis
Methodist Hospital
Tel: 901-726-8141

Tennessee, Nashville
Centennial Medical Center
Toll-Free: 800-493-2842
Tel: 615-342-4635

Texas, Bryan
St. Joseph Regional
Rehabilitation Center
Tel: 409-821-7523

Texas, Dallas
Presbyterian Hospital of Dallas
Toll-Free: 800-725-2732
Tel: 214-345-4224

Texas, Lubbock
Methodist Hospital
Toll-Free: 800-687-5498

Texas, San Antonio
The University of Texas HSC
Tel: 210-567-6688

Utah, Salt Lake City
University of Utah,
School of Medicine
Tel: 801-585-2354

Vermont, Burlington
University of Vermont
Medical Center
Toll-Free: 888-763-3366
Tel: 802-656-3366

Virginia, Charlottesville
University of Virginia Medical
Center
Tel: 804-982-4482

Washington, Seattle
University of Washington
Tel: 206-543-5369

Wisconsin, Neenah
The Neuroscience Group of
Northeast Wisconsin
Toll-Free: 888-797-2732

Dedicated Centers
*Young Parkinson
**Armed Forces/Veterans

Please contact the nearest
I&R Center or the national office for information regarding
support groups and chapters.
You can also dial the toll-free
number 888-400-2732 to contact
the I&R Center closest to you.

Transportation

American Automobile
Association
1000 AAA Drive
Heathrow, FL 32746-5063
Tel: 407-444-7000
Fax: 202-444-4247
Website: http://www.aaa.com

AAA Foundation for Traffic
Safety
1440 New York Avenue, N.W.,
Suite 201
Washington, DC 20005
Tel: 202-638-5944
Fax: 202-638-5943
Website: http://www.aaafts.org

Internet Resources

Caregiving by family members is the primary source of support in our society for individuals of all ages with physical, mental, and chronic health care conditions. Changing trends in family size, low unemployment, employment of women, and the increasing longevity of individuals due to better health care—have increased public policy attention to this traditionally very private and personal service. Thousands of Internet sites now have information relevant to parents, children of parents, spouses, and others suddenly thrust into the role of caring for a loved one. Caregiver web sites listed here include non-profit membership groups and commercial sites selling information products and services. Viewers are encouraged to find caregiver resources on the web pages of state, area, and local government, and service agencies. If you cannot find the information you seek, call the toll-free National Eldercare Locator at 800-677-1116 to find the telephone number of your local information and referral service.

Administration on Aging

Because We Care—A Guide for People Who Care
Website: http://www.aoa.gov/wecare

Information about Services in Your Community
Website: http://www.aoa.gov/elderpage/locator.html

Information for Older Persons and Their Families
Website: http://www.aoa.gov/elderpage.html

Resource Directory for Older Persons
Website: http://www.aoa.gov/aoa/resource.html

Administration on Aging Fact Sheets
Website: http://www.aoa.gov/factsheets

National Institute on Aging Fact Sheets
Website: http://www.aoa.gov/elderpage.html

ElderAction
Website: http://www.aoa.gov/elderpage.html

Other Federal Government Sites Access

America for Seniors
Website: http://www.seniors.gov/

Healthfinder—a gateway consumer health information web site
Website: http://www.healthfinder.gov

Medicare
Website: http://www.medicare.gov/publications/overview.asp

National Institute of Neurological Disorders and Stroke
Website: http://www.ninds.nih.gov

National Caregiver Organizations

Alliance for Aging Independently
Website: http://agingindependently.org

The Center for Family Caregivers
Website: http://www.familycaregivers.org

National Family Caregivers Association
Website: http://www.nfcacares.org

National Alliance for Caregiving
Website: http://www.caregiving.org

Family Caregiving Alliance
Website: http://
www.caregiver.org

Well Spouse Foundation
Website: http://
www.wellspouse.org

Other Sites

American Association of Homes and Services for the Aging
Website: http://www.aahsa.org

Augmentative/Alternative Communication Device Users
Website: http://
www.augcomm.com

Caregiver Issues
Website: http://health-center.com/senior/caregiver

Caregiver Survival Resources
Website: http://
www.caregiver911.com

CaregiversWorld
Website: http://
www.caregiversworld.com

CaregiverZone
Website: http://
www.caregiverzone.com

CareThere.com
Website: http://
www.carethere.com

Elder Web
Website: http://
www.elderweb.com

Empowering Caregivers
Website: http://www.care-givers.com

Family Caregiver America
Website: http://
www.familycareamerica.com

Health Caregiver.com
Website: http://
www.healthycaregiver.com

Ideas and Instructions for Adapting Toys for Children with Cerebral Palsy
Website: http://
www.lburkhart.com

Non-Profit Information Clearinghouse on Assistive Technology
Website: http://
www.dreamms.org

Support Group.com
Website: http://www.support-group.com

Today's Caregivers Magazine
Website: http://
www.caregiver.com

Index

Index

Page numbers followed by 'n' indicate a footnote. Page numbers in *italics* indicate a table or illustration.

A

571

O

Health Reference Series

COMPLETE CATALOG

AIDS Sourcebook, 1st Edition

Basic Information about AIDS and HIV Infection, Featuring Historical and Statistical Data, Current Research, Prevention, and Other Special Topics of Interest for Persons Living with AIDS

Along with Source Listings for Further Assistance

Edited by Karen Bellenir and Peter D. Dresser. 831 pages. 1995. 0-7808-0031-1. $78.

"One strength of this book is its practical emphasis. The intended audience is the lay reader . . . useful as an educational tool for health care providers who work with AIDS patients. Recommended for public libraries as well as hospital or academic libraries that collect consumer materials."
— *Bulletin of the Medical Library Association, Jan '96*

"This is the most comprehensive volume of its kind on an important medical topic. Highly recommended for all libraries."   — *Reference Book Review, '96*

"Very useful reference for all libraries."
— *Choice, Association of College and Research Libraries, Oct '95*

"There is a wealth of information here that can provide much educational assistance. It is a must book for all libraries and should be on the desk of each and every congressional leader. Highly recommended."
— *AIDS Book Review Journal, Aug '95*

"Recommended for most collections."
— *Library Journal, Jul '95*

∎

AIDS Sourcebook, 2nd Edition

Basic Consumer Health Information about Acquired Immune Deficiency Syndrome (AIDS) and Human Immunodeficiency Virus (HIV) Infection, Featuring Updated Statistical Data, Reports on Recent Research and Prevention Initiatives, and Other Special Topics of Interest for Persons Living with AIDS, Including New Antiretroviral Treatment Options, Strategies for Combating Opportunistic Infections, Information about Clinical Trials, and More

Along with a Glossary of Important Terms and Resource Listings for Further Help and Information

Edited by Karen Bellenir. 751 pages. 1999. 0-7808-0225-X. $78.

"Highly recommended."
— *American Reference Books Annual, 2000*

"Excellent sourcebook. This continues to be a highly recommended book. There is no other book that provides as much information as this book provides."
— *AIDS Book Review Journal, Dec-Jan 2000*

"Recommended reference source."
— *Booklist, American Library Association, Dec '99*

"A solid text for college-level health libraries."
— *The Bookwatch, Aug '99*

Cited in *Reference Sources for Small and Medium-Sized Libraries, American Library Association, 1999*

∎

Alcoholism Sourcebook

Basic Consumer Health Information about the Physical and Mental Consequences of Alcohol Abuse, Including Liver Disease, Pancreatitis, Wernicke-Korsakoff Syndrome (Alcoholic Dementia), Fetal Alcohol Syndrome, Heart Disease, Kidney Disorders, Gastrointestinal Problems, and Immune System Compromise and Featuring Facts about Addiction, Detoxification, Alcohol Withdrawal, Recovery, and the Maintenance of Sobriety

Along with a Glossary and Directories of Resources for Further Help and Information

Edited by Karen Bellenir. 613 pages. 2000. 0-7808-0325-6. $78.

"This book is an excellent choice for public and academic libraries."
— *American Reference Books Annual, 2001*

"Recommended reference source."
— *Booklist, American Library Association, Dec '00*

"Presents a wealth of information on alcohol use and abuse and its effects on the body and mind, treatment, and prevention."   — *SciTech Book News, Dec '00*

"Important new health guide which packs in the latest consumer information about the problems of alcoholism."   — *Reviewer's Bookwatch, Nov '00*

SEE ALSO Drug Abuse Sourcebook, Substance Abuse Sourcebook

∎

Allergies Sourcebook, 1st Edition

Basic Information about Major Forms and Mechanisms of Common Allergic Reactions, Sensitivities, and Intolerances, Including Anaphylaxis, Asthma, Hives and Other Dermatologic Symptoms, Rhinitis, and Sinusitis

Along with Their Usual Triggers Like Animal Fur, Chemicals, Drugs, Dust, Foods, Insects, Latex, Pollen, and Poison Ivy, Oak, and Sumac; Plus Information on Prevention, Identification, and Treatment

Edited by Allan R. Cook. 611 pages. 1997. 0-7808-0036-2. $78.

Allergies Sourcebook, 2nd Edition

Basic Consumer Health Information about Allergic Disorders, Triggers, Reactions, and Related Symptoms, Including Anaphylaxis, Rhinitis, Sinusitis, Asthma, Dermatitis, Conjunctivitis, and Multiple Chemical Sensitivity

Along with Tips on Diagnosis, Prevention, and Treatment, Statistical Data, a Glossary, and a Directory of Sources for Further Help and Information

Edited by Annemarie S. Muth. 600 pages. 2001. 0-7808-0376-0. $78.

Alternative Medicine Sourcebook

Basic Consumer Health Information about Alternatives to Conventional Medicine, Including Acupressure, Acupuncture, Aromatherapy, Ayurveda, Bioelectromagnetics, Environmental Medicine, Essence Therapy, Food and Nutrition Therapy, Herbal Therapy, Homeopathy, Imaging, Massage, Naturopathy, Reflexology, Relaxation and Meditation, Sound Therapy, Vitamin and Mineral Therapy, and Yoga, and More

Edited by Allan R. Cook. 737 pages. 1999. 0-7808-0200-4. $78.

"Recommended reference source."
—Booklist, American Library Association, Feb '00

"A great addition to the reference collection of every type of library." —American Reference Books Annual, 2000

Alzheimer's, Stroke & 29 Other Neurological Disorders Sourcebook, 1st Edition

Basic Information for the Layperson on 31 Diseases or Disorders Affecting the Brain and Nervous System, First Describing the Illness, Then Listing Symptoms, Diagnostic Methods, and Treatment Options, and Including Statistics on Incidences and Causes

Edited by Frank E. Bair. 579 pages. 1993. 1-55888-748-2. $78.

"Nontechnical reference book that provides reader-friendly information."
—Family Caregiver Alliance Update, Winter '96

"Should be included in any library's patient education section." —American Reference Books Annual, 1994

"Written in an approachable and accessible style. Recommended for patient education and consumer health collections in health science center and public libraries." —Academic Library Book Review, Dec '93

"It is very handy to have information on more than thirty neurological disorders under one cover, and there is no recent source like it." —Reference Quarterly, American Library Association, Fall '93

SEE ALSO Brain Disorders Sourcebook

Alzheimer's Disease Sourcebook, 2nd Edition

Basic Consumer Health Information about Alzheimer's Disease, Related Disorders, and Other Dementias, Including Multi-Infarct Dementia, AIDS-Related Dementia, Alcoholic Dementia, Huntington's Disease, Delirium, and Confusional States

Along with Reports Detailing Current Research Efforts in Prevention and Treatment, Long-Term Care Issues, and Listings of Sources for Additional Help and Information

Edited by Karen Bellenir. 524 pages. 1999. 0-7808-0223-3. $78.

"Provides a wealth of useful information not otherwise available in one place. This resource is recommended for all types of libraries."
—American Reference Books Annual, 2000

"Recommended reference source."
—Booklist, American Library Association, Oct '99

Arthritis Sourcebook

Basic Consumer Health Information about Specific Forms of Arthritis and Related Disorders, Including Rheumatoid Arthritis, Osteoarthritis, Gout, Polymyalgia Rheumatica, Psoriatic Arthritis, Spondyloarthropathies, Juvenile Rheumatoid Arthritis, and Juvenile Ankylosing Spondylitis

Along with Information about Medical, Surgical, and Alternative Treatment Options, and Including Strategies for Coping with Pain, Fatigue, and Stress

Edited by Allan R. Cook. 550 pages. 1998. 0-7808-0201-2. $78.

". . . accessible to the layperson."
—Reference and Research Book News, Feb '99

Asthma Sourcebook

Basic Consumer Health Information about Asthma, Including Symptoms, Traditional and Nontraditional Remedies, Treatment Advances, Quality-of-Life Aids, Medical Research Updates, and the Role of Allergies, Exercise, Age, the Environment, and Genetics in the Development of Asthma

Along with Statistical Data, a Glossary, and Directories of Support Groups, and Other Resources for Further Information

Edited by Annemarie S. Muth. 628 pages. 2000. 0-7808-0381-7. $78.

"This informative text is recommended for consumer health collections in public, secondary school, and community college libraries and the libraries of universities with a large undergraduate population."
—American Reference Books Annual, 2001

"Highly recommended." —The Bookwatch, Jan '01

Back & Neck Disorders Sourcebook

Basic Information about Disorders and Injuries of the Spinal Cord and Vertebrae, Including Facts on Chiropractic Treatment, Surgical Interventions, Paralysis, and Rehabilitation

Along with Advice for Preventing Back Trouble

Edited by Karen Bellenir. 548 pages. 1997. 0-7808-0202-0. $78.

"The strength of this work is its basic, easy-to-read format. Recommended."
> — *Reference and User Services Quarterly, American Library Association, Winter '97*

■

Blood & Circulatory Disorders Sourcebook

Basic Information about Blood and Its Components, Anemias, Leukemias, Bleeding Disorders, and Circulatory Disorders, Including Aplastic Anemia, Thalassemia, Sickle-Cell Disease, Hemochromatosis, Hemophilia, Von Willebrand Disease, and Vascular Diseases

Along with a Special Section on Blood Transfusions and Blood Supply Safety, a Glossary, and Source Listings for Further Help and Information

Edited by Karen Bellenir and Linda M. Shin. 554 pages. 1998. 0-7808-0203-9. $78.

"Recommended reference source."
> —*Booklist, American Library Association, Feb '99*

"An important reference sourcebook written in simple language for everyday, non-technical users. "
> —*Reviewer's Bookwatch, Jan '99*

■

Brain Disorders Sourcebook

Basic Consumer Health Information about Strokes, Epilepsy, Amyotrophic Lateral Sclerosis (ALS/Lou Gehrig's Disease), Parkinson's Disease, Brain Tumors, Cerebral Palsy, Headache, Tourette Syndrome, and More

Along with Statistical Data, Treatment and Rehabilitation Options, Coping Strategies, Reports on Current Research Initiatives, a Glossary, and Resource Listings for Additional Help and Information

Edited by Karen Bellenir. 481 pages. 1999. 0-7808-0229-2. $78.

"Belongs on the shelves of any library with a consumer health collection." —*E-Streams, Mar '00*

"Recommended reference source."
> — *Booklist, American Library Association, Oct '99*

SEE ALSO *Alzheimer's, Stroke & 29 Other Neurological Disorders Sourcebook, 1st Edition*

Breast Cancer Sourcebook

Basic Consumer Health Information about Breast Cancer, Including Diagnostic Methods, Treatment Options, Alternative Therapies, Self-Help Information, Related Health Concerns, Statistical and Demographic Data, and Facts for Men with Breast Cancer

Along with Reports on Current Research Initiatives, a Glossary of Related Medical Terms, and a Directory of Sources for Further Help and Information

Edited by Edward J. Prucha and Karen Bellenir. 600 pages. 2001. 0-7808-0244-6. $78.

SEE ALSO *Cancer Sourcebook for Women, 1st and 2nd Editions, Women's Health Concerns Sourcebook*

■

Breastfeeding Sourcebook

Basic Consumer Health Information about the Benefits of Breastmilk, Preparing to Breastfeed, Breastfeeding as a Baby Grows, Nutrition, and More, Including Information on Special Situations and Concerns, Such as Mastitis, Illness, Medications, Allergies, Multiple Births, Prematurity, Special Needs, and Adoption

Along with a Glossary and Resources for Additional Help and Information

Edited by Jenni Lynn Colson. 350 pages. 2001. 0-7808-0332-9. $48.

SEE ALSO *Pregnancy & Birth Sourcebook*

■

Burns Sourcebook

Basic Consumer Health Information about Various Types of Burns and Scalds, Including Flame, Heat, Cold, Electrical, Chemical, and Sun Burns

Along with Information on Short-Term and Long-Term Treatments, Tissue Reconstruction, Plastic Surgery, Prevention Suggestions, and First Aid

Edited by Allan R. Cook. 604 pages. 1999. 0-7808-0204-7. $78.

"This key reference guide is an invaluable addition to all health care and public libraries in confronting this ongoing health issue."
> —*American Reference Books Annual, 2000*

"This is an exceptional addition to the series and is highly recommended for all consumer health collections, hospital libraries, and academic medical centers." —*E-Streams, Mar '00*

"Recommended reference source."
> —*Booklist, American Library Association, Dec '99*

SEE ALSO *Skin Disorders Sourcebook*

Cancer Sourcebook, 1st Edition

Basic Information on Cancer Types, Symptoms, Diagnostic Methods, and Treatments, Including Statistics on Cancer Occurrences Worldwide and the Risks Associated with Known Carcinogens and Activities

Edited by Frank E. Bair. 932 pages. 1990. 1-55888-888-8. $78.

Cited in *Reference Sources for Small and Medium-Sized Libraries*, American Library Association, 1999

"Written in nontechnical language. Useful for patients, their families, medical professionals, and librarians."
— *Guide to Reference Books, 1996*

"Designed with the non-medical professional in mind. Libraries and medical facilities interested in patient education should certainly consider adding the *Cancer Sourcebook* to their holdings. This compact collection of reliable information . . . is an invaluable tool for helping patients and patients' families and friends to take the first steps in coping with the many difficulties of cancer."
— *Medical Reference Services Quarterly, Winter '91*

"Specifically created for the nontechnical reader . . . an important resource for the general reader trying to understand the complexities of cancer."
— *American Reference Books Annual, 1991*

"This publication's nontechnical nature and very comprehensive format make it useful for both the general public and undergraduate students."
— *Choice, Association of College and Research Libraries, Oct '90*

■

New Cancer Sourcebook, 2nd Edition

Basic Information about Major Forms and Stages of Cancer, Featuring Facts about Primary and Secondary Tumors of the Respiratory, Nervous, Lymphatic, Circulatory, Skeletal, and Gastrointestinal Systems, and Specific Organs; Statistical and Demographic Data; Treatment Options; and Strategies for Coping

Edited by Allan R. Cook. 1,313 pages. 1996. 0-7808-0041-9. $78.

"An excellent resource for patients with newly diagnosed cancer and their families. The dialogue is simple, direct, and comprehensive. Highly recommended for patients and families to aid in their understanding of cancer and its treatment."
— *Booklist Health Sciences Supplement, American Library Association, Oct '97*

"The amount of factual and useful information is extensive. The writing is very clear, geared to general readers. Recommended for all levels."
— *Choice, Association of College and Research Libraries, Jan '97*

Cancer Sourcebook, 3rd Edition

Basic Consumer Health Information about Major Forms and Stages of Cancer, Featuring Facts about Primary and Secondary Tumors of the Respiratory, Nervous, Lymphatic, Circulatory, Skeletal, and Gastrointestinal Systems, and Specific Organs

Along with Statistical and Demographic Data, Treatment Options, Strategies for Coping, a Glossary, and a Directory of Sources for Additional Help and Information

Edited by Edward J. Prucha. 1,069 pages. 2000. 0-7808-0227-6. $78.

". . . can be effectively used by cancer patients and their families who are looking for answers in a language they can understand. Public and hospital libraries should have it on their shelves."
— *American Reference Books Annual, 2001*

"Recommended reference source."
— *Booklist, American Library Association, Dec '00*

■

Cancer Sourcebook for Women, 1st Edition

Basic Information about Specific Forms of Cancer That Affect Women, Featuring Facts about Breast Cancer, Cervical Cancer, Ovarian Cancer, Cancer of the Uterus and Uterine Sarcoma, Cancer of the Vagina, and Cancer of the Vulva; Statistical and Demographic Data; Treatments, Self-Help Management Suggestions, and Current Research Initiatives

Edited by Allan R. Cook and Peter D. Dresser. 524 pages. 1996. 0-7808-0076-1. $78.

". . . written in easily understandable, non-technical language. Recommended for public libraries or hospital and academic libraries that collect patient education or consumer health materials."
— *Medical Reference Services Quarterly, Spring '97*

"Would be of value in a consumer health library. . . . written with the health care consumer in mind. Medical jargon is at a minimum, and medical terms are explained in clear, understandable sentences."
— *Bulletin of the Medical Library Association, Oct '96*

"The availability under one cover of all these pertinent publications, grouped under cohesive headings, makes this certainly a most useful sourcebook."
— *Choice, Association of College and Research Libraries, Jun '96*

"Presents a comprehensive knowledge base for general readers. Men and women both benefit from the gold mine of information nestled between the two covers of this book. Recommended."
— *Academic Library Book Review, Summer '96*

"This timely book is highly recommended for consumer health and patient education collections in all libraries." — *Library Journal, Apr '96*

SEE ALSO *Breast Cancer Sourcebook, Women's Health Concerns Sourcebook*

Cancer Sourcebook for Women, 2nd Edition

Basic Consumer Health Information about Specific Forms of Cancer That Affect Women, Including Cervical Cancer, Ovarian Cancer, Endometrial Cancer, Uterine Sarcoma, Vaginal Cancer, Vulvar Cancer, and Gestational Trophoblastic Tumor; and Featuring Statistical Information, Facts about Tests and Treatments, a Glossary of Cancer Terms, and an Extensive List of Additional Resources

Edited by Karen Bellenir. 600 pages. 2001. 0-7808-0226-8. $78.

SEE ALSO *Breast Cancer Sourcebook, Women's Health Concerns Sourcebook*

■

Cardiovascular Diseases & Disorders Sourcebook, 1st Edition

Basic Information about Cardiovascular Diseases and Disorders, Featuring Facts about the Cardiovascular System, Demographic and Statistical Data, Descriptions of Pharmacological and Surgical Interventions, Lifestyle Modifications, and a Special Section Focusing on Heart Disorders in Children

Edited by Karen Bellenir and Peter D. Dresser. 683 pages. 1995. 0-7808-0032-X. $78.

". . . **comprehensive format provides an extensive overview on this subject.**"
— *Choice, Association of College and Research Libraries, Jun '96*

". . . **an easily understood, complete, up-to-date resource. This well executed public health tool will make valuable information available to those that need it most, patients and their families. The typeface, sturdy non-reflective paper, and library binding add a feel of quality found wanting in other publications. Highly recommended for academic and general libraries.** "
— *Academic Library Book Review, Summer '96*

SEE ALSO *Healthy Heart Sourcebook for Women, Heart Diseases & Disorders Sourcebook, 2nd Edition*

■

Caregiving Sourcebook

Basic Consumer Health Information for Caregivers, Including a Profile of Caregivers, Caregiving Responsibilities and Concerns, Tips for Specific Conditions, Care Environments, and the Effects of Caregiving

Along with Facts about Legal Issues, Financial Information, and Future Planning, a Glossary, and a Listing of Additional Resources

Edited by Joyce Brennfleck Shannon. 600 pages. 2001. 0-7808-0331-0. $78.

Colds, Flu & Other Common Ailments Sourcebook

Basic Consumer Health Information about Common Ailments and Injuries, Including Colds, Coughs, the Flu, Sinus Problems, Headaches, Fever, Nausea and Vomiting, Menstrual Cramps, Diarrhea, Constipation, Hemorrhoids, Back Pain, Dandruff, Dry and Itchy Skin, Cuts, Scrapes, Sprains, Bruises, and More

Along with Information about Prevention, Self-Care, Choosing a Doctor, Over-the-Counter Medications, Folk Remedies, and Alternative Therapies, and Including a Glossary of Important Terms and a Directory of Resources for Further Help and Information

Edited by Chad T. Kimball. 638 pages. 2001. 0-7808-0435-X. $78.

■

Communication Disorders Sourcebook

Basic Information about Deafness and Hearing Loss, Speech and Language Disorders, Voice Disorders, Balance and Vestibular Disorders, and Disorders of Smell, Taste, and Touch

Edited by Linda M. Ross. 533 pages. 1996. 0-7808-0077-X. $78.

"**This is skillfully edited and is a welcome resource for the layperson. It should be found in every public and medical library.**" — *Booklist Health Sciences Supplement, American Library Association, Oct '97*

■

Congenital Disorders Sourcebook

Basic Information about Disorders Acquired during Gestation, Including Spina Bifida, Hydrocephalus, Cerebral Palsy, Heart Defects, Craniofacial Abnormalities, Fetal Alcohol Syndrome, and More

Along with Current Treatment Options and Statistical Data

Edited by Karen Bellenir. 607 pages. 1997. 0-7808-0205-5. $78.

"**Recommended reference source.**"
— *Booklist, American Library Association, Oct '97*

SEE ALSO *Pregnancy & Birth Sourcebook*

■

Consumer Issues in Health Care Sourcebook

Basic Information about Health Care Fundamentals and Related Consumer Issues, Including Exams and Screening Tests, Physician Specialties, Choosing a Doctor, Using Prescription and Over-the-Counter Medications Safely, Avoiding Health Scams, Managing Common Health Risks in the Home, Care Options for Chronically or Terminally Ill Patients, and a List of Resources for Obtaining Help and Further Information

Edited by Karen Bellenir. 618 pages. 1998. 0-7808-0221-7. $78.

"Both public and academic libraries will want to have a copy in their collection for readers who are interested in self-education on health issues."
—*American Reference Books Annual, 2000*

"The editor has researched the literature from government agencies and others, saving readers the time and effort of having to do the research themselves. Recommended for public libraries."
—*Reference and User Services Quarterly, American Library Association, Spring '99*

"Recommended reference source."
—*Booklist, American Library Association, Dec '98*

■

Contagious & Non-Contagious Infectious Diseases Sourcebook

Basic Information about Contagious Diseases like Measles, Polio, Hepatitis B, and Infectious Mononucleosis, and Non-Contagious Infectious Diseases like Tetanus and Toxic Shock Syndrome, and Diseases Occurring as Secondary Infections Such as Shingles and Reye Syndrome

Along with Vaccination, Prevention, and Treatment Information, and a Section Describing Emerging Infectious Disease Threats

Edited by Karen Bellenir and Peter D. Dresser. 566 pages. 1996. 0-7808-0075-3. $78.

■

Death & Dying Sourcebook

Basic Consumer Health Information for the Layperson about End-of-Life Care and Related Ethical and Legal Issues, Including Chief Causes of Death, Autopsies, Pain Management for the Terminally Ill, Life Support Systems, Insurance, Euthanasia, Assisted Suicide, Hospice Programs, Living Wills, Funeral Planning, Counseling, Mourning, Organ Donation, and Physician Training

Along with Statistical Data, a Glossary, and Listings of Sources for Further Help and Information

Edited by Annemarie S. Muth. 641 pages. 1999. 0-7808-0230-6. $78.

"Public libraries, medical libraries, and academic libraries will all find this sourcebook a useful addition to their collections."
—*American Reference Books Annual, 2001*

"Recommended reference source."
—*Booklist, American Library Association, Aug '00*

"This book is a definite must for all those involved in end-of-life care." —*Doody's Review Service, 2000*

■

Diabetes Sourcebook, 1st Edition

Basic Information about Insulin-Dependent and Noninsulin-Dependent Diabetes Mellitus, Gestational Diabetes, and Diabetic Complications, Symptoms, Treatment, and Research Results, Including Statistics on Prevalence, Morbidity, and Mortality

Along with Source Listings for Further Help and Information

Edited by Karen Bellenir and Peter D. Dresser. 827 pages. 1994. 1-55888-751-2. $78.

". . . very informative and understandable for the layperson without being simplistic. It provides a comprehensive overview for laypersons who want a general understanding of the disease or who want to focus on various aspects of the disease."
—*Bulletin of the Medical Library Association, Jan '96*

■

Diabetes Sourcebook, 2nd Edition

Basic Consumer Health Information about Type 1 Diabetes (Insulin-Dependent or Juvenile-Onset Diabetes), Type 2 (Noninsulin-Dependent or Adult-Onset Diabetes), Gestational Diabetes, and Related Disorders, Including Diabetes Prevalence Data, Management Issues, the Role of Diet and Exercise in Controlling Diabetes, Insulin and Other Diabetes Medicines, and Complications of Diabetes Such as Eye Diseases, Periodontal Disease, Amputation, and End-Stage Renal Disease

Along with Reports on Current Research Initiatives, a Glossary, and Resource Listings for Further Help and Information

Edited by Karen Bellenir. 688 pages. 1998. 0-7808-0224-1. $78.

"This comprehensive book is an excellent addition for high school, academic, medical, and public libraries. This volume is highly recommended."
—*American Reference Books Annual, 2000*

"An invaluable reference." —*Library Journal, May '00*

Selected as one of the 250 "Best Health Sciences Books of 1999." —*Doody's Rating Service, Mar-Apr 2000*

"Recommended reference source."
—*Booklist, American Library Association, Feb '99*

". . . provides reliable mainstream medical information . . . belongs on the shelves of any library with a consumer health collection." —*E-Streams, Sep '99*

"Provides useful information for the general public."
—*Healthlines, University of Michigan Health Management Research Center, Sep/Oct '99*

■

Diet & Nutrition Sourcebook, 1st Edition

Basic Information about Nutrition, Including the Dietary Guidelines for Americans, the Food Guide Pyramid, and Their Applications in Daily Diet, Nutritional Advice for Specific Age Groups, Current Nutritional Issues and Controversies, the New Food Label and How to Use It to Promote Healthy Eating, and Recent Developments in Nutritional Research

Edited by Dan R. Harris. 662 pages. 1996. 0-7808-0084-2. $78.

"Useful reference as a food and nutrition sourcebook for the general consumer." — *Booklist Health Sciences Supplement, American Library Association, Oct '97*

"Recommended for public libraries and medical libraries that receive general information requests on nutrition. It is readable and will appeal to those interested in learning more about healthy dietary practices." — *Medical Reference Services Quarterly, Fall '97*

"An abundance of medical and social statistics is translated into readable information geared toward the general reader." — *Bookwatch, Mar '97*

"With dozens of questionable diet books on the market, it is so refreshing to find a reliable and factual reference book. Recommended to aspiring professionals, librarians, and others seeking and giving reliable dietary advice. An excellent compilation." — *Choice, Association of College and Research Libraries, Feb '97*

SEE ALSO *Digestive Diseases & Disorders Sourcebook, Gastrointestinal Diseases & Disorders Sourcebook*

■

Diet & Nutrition Sourcebook, 2nd Edition

Basic Consumer Health Information about Dietary Guidelines, Recommended Daily Intake Values, Vitamins, Minerals, Fiber, Fat, Weight Control, Dietary Supplements, and Food Additives

Along with Special Sections on Nutrition Needs throughout Life and Nutrition for People with Such Specific Medical Concerns as Allergies, High Blood Cholesterol, Hypertension, Diabetes, Celiac Disease, Seizure Disorders, Phenylketonuria (PKU), Cancer, and Eating Disorders, and Including Reports on Current Nutrition Research and Source Listings for Additional Help and Information

Edited by Karen Bellenir. 650 pages. 1999. 0-7808-0228-4. $78.

"This book is an excellent source of basic diet and nutrition information." — *Booklist Health Sciences Supplement, American Library Association, Dec '00*

"This reference document should be in any public library, but it would be a very good guide for beginning students in the health sciences. If the other books in this publisher's series are as good as this, they should all be in the health sciences collections." — *American Reference Books Annual, 2000*

"This book is an excellent general nutrition reference for consumers who desire to take an active role in their health care for prevention. Consumers of all ages who select this book can feel confident they are receiving current and accurate information." — *Journal of Nutrition for the Elderly, Vol. 19, No. 4, '00*

"Recommended reference source." — *Booklist, American Library Association, Dec '99*

SEE ALSO *Digestive Diseases & Disorders Sourcebook, Gastrointestinal Diseases & Disorders Sourcebook*

Digestive Diseases & Disorders Sourcebook

Basic Consumer Health Information about Diseases and Disorders that Impact the Upper and Lower Digestive System, Including Celiac Disease, Constipation, Crohn's Disease, Cyclic Vomiting Syndrome, Diarrhea, Diverticulosis and Diverticulitis, Gallstones, Heartburn, Hemorrhoids, Hernias, Indigestion (Dyspepsia), Irritable Bowel Syndrome, Lactose Intolerance, Ulcers, and More

Along with Information about Medications and Other Treatments, Tips for Maintaining a Healthy Digestive Tract, a Glossary, and Directory of Digestive Diseases Organizations

Edited by Karen Bellenir. 335 pages. 1999. 0-7808-0327-2. $48.

"This title would be an excellent addition to all public or patient-research libraries." — *American Reference Books Annual, 2001*

"This title is recommended for public, hospital, and health sciences libraries with consumer health collections." — *E-Streams, Jul-Aug '00*

"Recommended reference source." — *Booklist, American Library Association, May '00*

SEE ALSO *Diet & Nutrition Sourcebook, 1st and 2nd Editions, Gastrointestinal Diseases & Disorders Sourcebook*

■

Disabilities Sourcebook

Basic Consumer Health Information about Physical and Psychiatric Disabilities, Including Descriptions of Major Causes of Disability, Assistive and Adaptive Aids, Workplace Issues, and Accessibility Concerns

Along with Information about the Americans with Disabilities Act, a Glossary, and Resources for Additional Help and Information

Edited by Dawn D. Matthews. 616 pages. 2000. 0-7808-0389-2. $78.

"An excellent source book in easy-to-read format covering many current topics; highly recommended for all libraries." — *Choice, Association of College and Research Libraries, Jan '01*

"Recommended reference source." — *Booklist, American Library Association, Jul '00*

"An involving, invaluable handbook." — *The Bookwatch, May '00*

■

Domestic Violence & Child Abuse Sourcebook

Basic Consumer Health Information about Spousal/ Partner, Child, Sibling, Parent, and Elder Abuse, Covering Physical, Emotional, and Sexual Abuse, Teen Dating Violence, and Stalking; Includes Information about Hotlines, Safe Houses, Safety Plans, and Other

Resources for Support and Assistance, Community Initiatives, and Reports on Current Directions in Research and Treatment

Along with a Glossary, Sources for Further Reading, and Governmental and Non-Governmental Organizations Contact Information

Edited by Helene Henderson. 1,064 pages. 2000. 0-7808-0235-7. $78.

"Because this problem is so widespread and because this book includes a lot of issues within one volume, this work is recommended for all public libraries."
— *American Reference Books Annual, 2001*

■

Drug Abuse Sourcebook

Basic Consumer Health Information about Illicit Substances of Abuse and the Diversion of Prescription Medications, Including Depressants, Hallucinogens, Inhalants, Marijuana, Narcotics, Stimulants, and Anabolic Steroids

Along with Facts about Related Health Risks, Treatment Issues, and Substance Abuse Prevention Programs, a Glossary of Terms, Statistical Data, and Directories of Hotline Services, Self-Help Groups, and Organizations Able to Provide Further Information

Edited by Karen Bellenir. 629 pages. 2000. 0-7808-0242-X. $78.

"Even though there is a plethora of books on drug abuse, this volume is recommended for school, public, and college libraries."
— *American Reference Books Annual, 2001*

"Highly recommended."   — *The Bookwatch, Jan '01*

SEE ALSO *Alcoholism Sourcebook, Substance Abuse Sourcebook*

■

Ear, Nose & Throat Disorders Sourcebook

Basic Information about Disorders of the Ears, Nose, Sinus Cavities, Pharynx, and Larynx, Including Ear Infections, Tinnitus, Vestibular Disorders, Allergic and Non-Allergic Rhinitis, Sore Throats, Tonsillitis, and Cancers That Affect the Ears, Nose, Sinuses, and Throat

Along with Reports on Current Research Initiatives, a Glossary of Related Medical Terms, and a Directory of Sources for Further Help and Information

Edited by Karen Bellenir and Linda M. Shin. 576 pages. 1998. 0-7808-0206-3. $78.

"Overall, this sourcebook is helpful for the consumer seeking information on ENT issues. It is recommended for public libraries."
— *American Reference Books Annual, 1999*

"Recommended reference source."
— *Booklist, American Library Association, Dec '98*

Eating Disorders Sourcebook

Basic Consumer Health Information about Eating Disorders, Including Information about Anorexia Nervosa, Bulimia Nervosa, Binge Eating, Body Dysmorphic Disorder, Pica, Laxative Abuse, and Night Eating Syndrome

Along with Information about Causes, Adverse Affects, and Treatment and Prevention Issues, and Featuring a Section on Concerns Specific to Children and Adolescents, a Glossary, and Resources for Further Help and Information

Edited by Dawn D. Matthews. 350 pages. 2001. 0-7808-0335-3. $78.

■

Endocrine & Metabolic Disorders Sourcebook

Basic Information for the Layperson about Pancreatic and Insulin-Related Disorders Such as Pancreatitis, Diabetes, and Hypoglycemia; Adrenal Gland Disorders Such as Cushing's Syndrome, Addison's Disease, and Congenital Adrenal Hyperplasia; Pituitary Gland Disorders Such as Growth Hormone Deficiency, Acromegaly, and Pituitary Tumors; Thyroid Disorders Such as Hypothyroidism, Graves' Disease, Hashimoto's Disease, and Goiter; Hyperparathyroidism; and Other Diseases and Syndromes of Hormone Imbalance or Metabolic Dysfunction

Along with Reports on Current Research Initiatives

Edited by Linda M. Shin. 574 pages. 1998. 0-7808-0207-1. $78.

"Omnigraphics has produced another needed resource for health information consumers."
— *American Reference Books Annual, 2000*

"Recommended reference source."
— *Booklist, American Library Association, Dec '98*

■

Environmentally Induced Disorders Sourcebook

Basic Information about Diseases and Syndromes Linked to Exposure to Pollutants and Other Substances in Outdoor and Indoor Environments Such as Lead, Asbestos, Formaldehyde, Mercury, Emissions, Noise, and More

Edited by Allan R. Cook. 620 pages. 1997. 0-7808-0083-4. $78.

"Recommended reference source."
— *Booklist, American Library Association, Sep '98*

"This book will be a useful addition to anyone's library."   — *Choice Health Sciences Supplement, Association of College and Research Libraries, May '98*

". . . a good survey of numerous environmentally induced physical disorders . . . a useful addition to anyone's library."
— *Doody's Health Sciences Book Reviews, Jan '98*

"... provide[s] introductory information from the best authorities around. Since this volume covers topics that potentially affect everyone, it will surely be one of the most frequently consulted volumes in the *Health Reference Series*." — *Rettig on Reference, Nov '97*

■

Ethnic Diseases Sourcebook

Basic Consumer Health Information for Ethnic and Racial Minority Groups in the United States, Including General Health Indicators and Behaviors, Ethnic Diseases, Genetic Testing, the Impact of Chronic Diseases, Women's Health, Mental Health Issues, and Preventive Health Care Services

Along with a Glossary and a Listing of Additional Resources

Edited by Joyce Brennfleck Shannon. 664 pages. 2001. 0-7808-0336-1. $78.

■

Family Planning Sourcebook

Basic Consumer Health Information about Planning for Pregnancy and Contraception, Including Traditional Methods, Barrier Methods, Hormonal Methods, Permanent Methods, Future Methods, Emergency Contraception, and Birth Control Choices for Women at Each Stage of Life

Along with Statistics, a Glossary, and Sources of Additional Information

Edited by Amy Marcaccio Keyzer. 520 pages. 2001. 0-7808-0379-5. $78.

SEE ALSO *Pregnancy & Birth Sourcebook*

■

Fitness & Exercise Sourcebook, 1st Edition

Basic Information on Fitness and Exercise, Including Fitness Activities for Specific Age Groups, Exercise for People with Specific Medical Conditions, How to Begin a Fitness Program in Running, Walking, Swimming, Cycling, and Other Athletic Activities, and Recent Research in Fitness and Exercise

Edited by Dan R. Harris. 663 pages. 1996. 0-7808-0186-5. $78.

"A good resource for general readers."
— *Choice, Association of College and Research Libraries, Nov '97*

"The perennial popularity of the topic ... make this an appealing selection for public libraries."
— *Rettig on Reference, Jun/Jul '97*

■

Fitness & Exercise Sourcebook, 2nd Edition

Basic Consumer Health Information about the Fundamentals of Fitness and Exercise, Including How to Begin and Maintain a Fitness Program, Fitness as a

Lifestyle, the Link between Fitness and Diet, Advice for Specific Groups of People, Exercise as It Relates to Specific Medical Conditions, and Recent Research in Fitness and Exercise

Along with a Glossary of Important Terms and Resources for Additional Help and Information

Edited by Kristen M. Gledhill. 646 pages. 2001. 0-7808-0334-5. $78.

■

Food & Animal Borne Diseases Sourcebook

Basic Information about Diseases That Can Be Spread to Humans through the Ingestion of Contaminated Food or Water or by Contact with Infected Animals and Insects, Such as Botulism, E. Coli, Hepatitis A, Trichinosis, Lyme Disease, and Rabies

Along with Information Regarding Prevention and Treatment Methods, and Including a Special Section for International Travelers Describing Diseases Such as Cholera, Malaria, Travelers' Diarrhea, and Yellow Fever, and Offering Recommendations for Avoiding Illness

Edited by Karen Bellenir and Peter D. Dresser. 535 pages. 1995. 0-7808-0033-8. $78.

"Targeting general readers and providing them with a single, comprehensive source of information on selected topics, this book continues, with the excellent caliber of its predecessors, to catalog topical information on health matters of general interest. Readable and thorough, this valuable resource is highly recommended for all libraries."
— *Academic Library Book Review, Summer '96*

"A comprehensive collection of authoritative information."
— *Emergency Medical Services, Oct '95*

■

Food Safety Sourcebook

Basic Consumer Health Information about the Safe Handling of Meat, Poultry, Seafood, Eggs, Fruit Juices, and Other Food Items, and Facts about Pesticides, Drinking Water, Food Safety Overseas, and the Onset, Duration, and Symptoms of Foodborne Illnesses, Including Types of Pathogenic Bacteria, Parasitic Protozoa, Worms, Viruses, and Natural Toxins

Along with the Role of the Consumer, the Food Handler, and the Government in Food Safety; a Glossary, and Resources for Additional Help and Information

Edited by Dawn D. Matthews. 339 pages. 1999. 0-7808-0326-4. $48.

"This book is recommended for public libraries and universities with home economic and food science programs." — *E-Streams, Nov '00*

"This book takes the complex issues of food safety and foodborne pathogens and presents them in an easily understood manner. [It does] an excellent job of covering a large and often confusing topic."
— *American Reference Books Annual, 2000*

"Recommended reference source."
— *Booklist, American Library Association, May '00*

Forensic Medicine Sourcebook

Basic Consumer Information for the Layperson about Forensic Medicine, Including Crime Scene Investigation, Evidence Collection and Analysis, Expert Testimony, Computer-Aided Criminal Identification, Digital Imaging in the Courtroom, DNA Profiling, Accident Reconstruction, Autopsies, Ballistics, Drugs and Explosives Detection, Latent Fingerprints, Product Tampering, and Questioned Document Examination

Along with Statistical Data, a Glossary of Forensics Terminology, and Listings of Sources for Further Help and Information

Edited by Annemarie S. Muth. 574 pages. 1999. 0-7808-0232-2. $78.

"There are several items that make this book attractive to consumers who are seeking certain forensic data. . . . This is a useful current source for those seeking general forensic medical answers."
— *American Reference Books Annual, 2000*

"Recommended for public libraries."
— *Reference & User Services Quarterly, American Library Association, Spring 2000*

"Recommended reference source."
— *Booklist, American Library Association, Feb '00*

"A wealth of information, useful statistics, references are up-to-date and extremely complete. This wonderful collection of data will help students who are interested in a career in any type of forensic field. It is a great resource for attorneys who need information about types of expert witnesses needed in a particular case. It also offers useful information for fiction and nonfiction writers whose work involves a crime. A fascinating compilation. All levels." — *Choice, Association of College and Research Libraries, Jan 2000*

■

Gastrointestinal Diseases & Disorders Sourcebook

Basic Information about Gastroesophageal Reflux Disease (Heartburn), Ulcers, Diverticulosis, Irritable Bowel Syndrome, Crohn's Disease, Ulcerative Colitis, Diarrhea, Constipation, Lactose Intolerance, Hemorrhoids, Hepatitis, Cirrhosis, and Other Digestive Problems, Featuring Statistics, Descriptions of Symptoms, and Current Treatment Methods of Interest for Persons Living with Upper and Lower Gastrointestinal Maladies

Edited by Linda M. Ross. 413 pages. 1996. 0-7808-0078-8. $78.

". . . very readable form. The successful editorial work that brought this material together into a useful and understandable reference makes accessible to all readers information that can help them more effectively understand and obtain help for digestive tract problems."
— *Choice, Association of College and Research Libraries, Feb '97*

SEE ALSO *Diet & Nutrition Sourcebook, 1st and 2nd Editions, Digestive Diseases & Disorders Sourcebook*

Genetic Disorders Sourcebook, 1st Edition

Basic Information about Heritable Diseases and Disorders Such as Down Syndrome, PKU, Hemophilia, Von Willebrand Disease, Gaucher Disease, Tay-Sachs Disease, and Sickle-Cell Disease, Along with Information about Genetic Screening, Gene Therapy, Home Care, and Including Source Listings for Further Help and Information on More Than 300 Disorders

Edited by Karen Bellenir. 642 pages. 1996. 0-7808-0034-6. $78.

"Recommended for undergraduate libraries or libraries that serve the public."
— *Science & Technology Libraries, Vol. 18, No. 1, '99*

"Provides essential medical information to both the general public and those diagnosed with a serious or fatal genetic disease or disorder."
— *Choice, Association of College and Research Libraries, Jan '97*

"Geared toward the lay public. It would be well placed in all public libraries and in those hospital and medical libraries in which access to genetic references is limited." — *Doody's Health Sciences Book Review, Oct '96*

■

Genetic Disorders Sourcebook, 2nd Edition

Basic Consumer Health Information about Hereditary Diseases and Disorders, Including Cystic Fibrosis, Down Syndrome, Hemophilia, Huntington's Disease, Sickle Cell Anemia, and More; Facts about Genes, Gene Research and Therapy, Genetic Screening, Ethics of Gene Testing, Genetic Counseling, and Advice on Coping and Caring

Along with a Glossary of Genetic Terminology and a Resource List for Help, Support, and Further Information

Edited by Kathy Massimini. 768 pages. 2001. 0-7808-0241-1. $78.

■

Head Trauma Sourcebook

Basic Information for the Layperson about Open-Head and Closed-Head Injuries, Treatment Advances, Recovery, and Rehabilitation

Along with Reports on Current Research Initiatives

Edited by Karen Bellenir. 414 pages. 1997. 0-7808-0208-X. $78.

■

Health Insurance Sourcebook

Basic Information about Managed Care Organizations, Traditional Fee-for-Service Insurance, Insurance Portability and Pre-Existing Conditions Clauses, Medicare, Medicaid, Social Security, and Military Health Care

Along with Information about Insurance Fraud

Edited by Wendy Wilcox. 530 pages. 1997. 0-7808-0222-5. $78.

"Particularly useful because it brings much of this information together in one volume. This book will be a handy reference source in the health sciences library, hospital library, college and university library, and medium to large public library."
— *Medical Reference Services Quarterly, Fall '98*

Awarded "Books of the Year Award"
— *American Journal of Nursing, 1997*

"The layout of the book is particularly helpful as it provides easy access to reference material. A most useful addition to the vast amount of information about health insurance. The use of data from U.S. government agencies is most commendable. Useful in a library or learning center for healthcare professional students."
— *Doody's Health Sciences Book Reviews, Nov '97*

■

Health Reference Series Cumulative Index 1999

A Comprehensive Index to the Individual Volumes of the Health Reference Series, Including a Subject Index, Name Index, Organization Index, and Publication Index

Along with a Master List of Acronyms and Abbreviations

Edited by Edward J. Prucha, Anne Holmes, and Robert Rudnick. 990 pages. 2000. 0-7808-0382-5. $78.

"This volume will be most helpful in libraries that have a relatively complete collection of the Health Reference Series."
— *American Reference Books Annual, 2001*

"Essential for collections that hold any of the numerous *Health Reference Series* titles."
— *Choice, Association of College and Research Libraries, Nov '00*

■

Healthy Aging Sourcebook

Basic Consumer Health Information about Maintaining Health through the Aging Process, Including Advice on Nutrition, Exercise, and Sleep, Help in Making Decisions about Midlife Issues and Retirement, and Guidance Concerning Practical and Informed Choices in Health Consumerism

Along with Data Concerning the Theories of Aging, Different Experiences in Aging by Minority Groups, and Facts about Aging Now and Aging in the Future; and Featuring a Glossary, a Guide to Consumer Help, Additional Suggested Reading, and Practical Resource Directory

Edited by Jenifer Swanson. 536 pages. 1999. 0-7808-0390-6. $78.

"Recommended reference source."
— *Booklist, American Library Association, Feb '00*

SEE ALSO Physical & Mental Issues in Aging Sourcebook

Healthy Heart Sourcebook for Women

Basic Consumer Health Information about Cardiac Issues Specific to Women, Including Facts about Major Risk Factors and Prevention, Treatment and Control Strategies, and Important Dietary Issues

Along with a Special Section Regarding the Pros and Cons of Hormone Replacement Therapy and Its Impact on Heart Health, and Additional Help, Including Recipes, a Glossary, and a Directory of Resources

Edited by Dawn D. Matthews. 336 pages. 2000. 0-7808-0329-9. $48.

"Because of the lack of information specific to women on this topic, this book is recommended for public libraries and consumer libraries."
— *American Reference Books Annual, 2001*

"Contains very important information about coronary artery disease that all women should know. The information is current and presented in an easy-to-read format. The book will make a good addition to any library." — *American Medical Writers Association Journal, Summer '00*

"Important, basic reference."
— *Reviewer's Bookwatch, Jul '00*

SEE ALSO Cardiovascular Diseases & Disorders Sourcebook, 1st Edition, Heart Diseases & Disorders Sourcebook, 2nd Edition, Women's Health Concerns Sourcebook

■

Heart Diseases & Disorders Sourcebook, 2nd Edition

Basic Consumer Health Information about Heart Attacks, Angina, Rhythm Disorders, Heart Failure, Valve Disease, Congenital Heart Disorders, and More, Including Descriptions of Surgical Procedures and Other Interventions, Medications, Cardiac Rehabilitation, Risk Identification, and Prevention Tips

Along with Statistical Data, Reports on Current Research Initiatives, a Glossary of Cardiovascular Terms, and Resource Directory

Edited by Karen Bellenir. 612 pages. 2000. 0-7808-0238-1. $78.

"This work stands out as an imminently accessible resource for the general public. It is recommended for the reference and circulating shelves of school, public, and academic libraries."
— *American Reference Books Annual, 2001*

"Recommended reference source."
— *Booklist, American Library Association, Dec '00*

"Provides comprehensive coverage of matters related to the heart. This title is recommended for health sciences and public libraries with consumer health collections."
— *E-Streams, Oct '00*

SEE ALSO Cardiovascular Diseases & Disorders Sourcebook, 1st Edition, Healthy Heart Sourcebook for Women

Immune System Disorders Sourcebook

Basic Information about Lupus, Multiple Sclerosis, Guillain-Barré Syndrome, Chronic Granulomatous Disease, and More

Along with Statistical and Demographic Data and Reports on Current Research Initiatives

Edited by Allan R. Cook. 608 pages. 1997. 0-7808-0209-8. $78.

■

Infant & Toddler Health Sourcebook

Basic Consumer Health Information about the Physical and Mental Development of Newborns, Infants, and Toddlers, Including Neonatal Concerns, Nutrition Recommendations, Immunization Schedules, Common Pediatric Disorders, Assessments and Milestones, Safety Tips, and Advice for Parents and Other Caregivers

Along with a Glossary of Terms and Resource Listings for Additional Help

Edited by Jenifer Swanson. 585 pages. 2000. 0-7808-0246-2. $78.

"This is a good source for general use."
— *American Reference Books Annual, 2001*

■

Kidney & Urinary Tract Diseases & Disorders Sourcebook

Basic Information about Kidney Stones, Urinary Incontinence, Bladder Disease, End Stage Renal Disease, Dialysis, and More

Along with Statistical and Demographic Data and Reports on Current Research Initiatives

Edited by Linda M. Ross. 602 pages. 1997. 0-7808-0079-6. $78.

■

Learning Disabilities Sourcebook

Basic Information about Disorders Such as Dyslexia, Visual and Auditory Processing Deficits, Attention Deficit/Hyperactivity Disorder, and Autism

Along with Statistical and Demographic Data, Reports on Current Research Initiatives, an Explanation of the Assessment Process, and a Special Section for Adults with Learning Disabilities

Edited by Linda M. Shin. 579 pages. 1998. 0-7808-0210-1. $78.

Named "Outstanding Reference Book of 1999."
— *New York Public Library, Feb 2000*

"An excellent candidate for inclusion in a public library reference section. It's a great source of information. Teachers will also find the book useful. Definitely worth reading."
— *Journal of Adolescent & Adult Literacy, Feb 2000*

"Readable . . . provides a solid base of information regarding successful techniques used with individuals who have learning disabilities, as well as practical suggestions for educators and family members. Clear language, concise descriptions, and pertinent information for contacting multiple resources add to the strength of this book as a useful tool." — *Choice, Association of College and Research Libraries, Feb '99*

"Recommended reference source."
— *Booklist, American Library Association, Sep '98*

"This is a useful resource for libraries and for those who don't have the time to identify and locate the individual publications."
— *Disability Resources Monthly, Sep '98*

■

Liver Disorders Sourcebook

Basic Consumer Health Information about the Liver and How It Works; Liver Diseases, Including Cancer, Cirrhosis, Hepatitis, and Toxic and Drug Related Diseases; Tips for Maintaining a Healthy Liver; Laboratory Tests, Radiology Tests, and Facts about Liver Transplantation

Along with a Section on Support Groups, a Glossary, and Resource Listings

Edited by Joyce Brennfleck Shannon. 591 pages. 2000. 0-7808-0383-3. $78.

"A valuable resource."
— *American Reference Books Annual, 2001*

"This title is recommended for health sciences and public libraries with consumer health collections."
— *E-Streams, Oct '00*

"Recommended reference source."
— *Booklist, American Library Association, Jun '00*

■

Medical Tests Sourcebook

Basic Consumer Health Information about Medical Tests, Including Periodic Health Exams, General Screening Tests, Tests You Can Do at Home, Findings of the U.S. Preventive Services Task Force, X-ray and Radiology Tests, Electrical Tests, Tests of Blood and Other Body Fluids and Tissues, Scope Tests, Lung Tests, Genetic Tests, Pregnancy Tests, Newborn Screening Tests, Sexually Transmitted Disease Tests, and Computer Aided Diagnoses

Along with a Section on Paying for Medical Tests, a Glossary, and Resource Listings

Edited by Joyce Brennfleck Shannon. 691 pages. 1999. 0-7808-0243-8. $78.

"A valuable reference guide."
— *American Reference Books Annual, 2000*

"Recommended for hospital and health sciences libraries with consumer health collections."
— *E-Streams, Mar '00*

"This is an overall excellent reference with a wealth of general knowledge that may aid those who are reluctant to get vital tests performed."
— *Today's Librarian, Jan 2000*

Men's Health Concerns Sourcebook

Basic Information about Health Issues That Affect Men, Featuring Facts about the Top Causes of Death in Men, Including Heart Disease, Stroke, Cancers, Prostate Disorders, Chronic Obstructive Pulmonary Disease, Pneumonia and Influenza, Human Immunodeficiency Virus and Acquired Immune Deficiency Syndrome, Diabetes Mellitus, Stress, Suicide, Accidents and Homicides; and Facts about Common Concerns for Men, Including Impotence, Contraception, Circumcision, Sleep Disorders, Snoring, Hair Loss, Diet, Nutrition, Exercise, Kidney and Urological Disorders, and Backaches

Edited by Allan R. Cook. 738 pages. 1998. 0-7808-0212-8. $78.

"This comprehensive resource and the series are highly recommended."
—American Reference Books Annual, 2000

"Recommended reference source."
— Booklist, American Library Association, Dec '98

Mental Health Disorders Sourcebook, 1st Edition

Basic Information about Schizophrenia, Depression, Bipolar Disorder, Panic Disorder, Obsessive-Compulsive Disorder, Phobias and Other Anxiety Disorders, Paranoia and Other Personality Disorders, Eating Disorders, and Sleep Disorders

Along with Information about Treatment and Therapies

Edited by Karen Bellenir. 548 pages. 1995. 0-7808-0040-0. $78.

"This is an excellent new book . . . written in easy-to-understand language."
— Booklist Health Sciences Supplement, American Library Association, Oct '97

". . . useful for public and academic libraries and consumer health collections."
— Medical Reference Services Quarterly, Spring '97

"The great strengths of the book are its readability and its inclusion of places to find more information. Especially recommended." *— Reference Quarterly, American Library Association, Winter '96*

". . . a good resource for a consumer health library."
— Bulletin of the Medical Library Association, Oct '96

"The information is data-based and couched in brief, concise language that avoids jargon. . . . a useful reference source." *— Readings, Sep '96*

"The text is well organized and adequately written for its target audience." *— Choice, Association of College and Research Libraries, Jun '96*

". . . provides information on a wide range of mental disorders, presented in nontechnical language."
— Exceptional Child Education Resources, Spring '96

"Recommended for public and academic libraries."
— Reference Book Review, 1996

Mental Health Disorders Sourcebook, 2nd Edition

Basic Consumer Health Information about Anxiety Disorders, Depression and Other Mood Disorders, Eating Disorders, Personality Disorders, Schizophrenia, and More, Including Disease Descriptions, Treatment Options, and Reports on Current Research Initiatives

Along with Statistical Data, Tips for Maintaining Mental Health, a Glossary, and Directory of Sources for Additional Help and Information

Edited by Karen Bellenir. 605 pages. 2000. 0-7808-0240-3. $78.

"Well organized and well written."
—American Reference Books Annual, 2001

"Recommended reference source."
—Booklist, American Library Association, Jun '00

Mental Retardation Sourcebook

Basic Consumer Health Information about Mental Retardation and Its Causes, Including Down Syndrome, Fetal Alcohol Syndrome, Fragile X Syndrome, Genetic Conditions, Injury, and Environmental Sources

Along with Preventive Strategies, Parenting Issues, Educational Implications, Health Care Needs, Employment and Economic Matters, Legal Issues, a Glossary, and a Resource Listing for Additional Help and Information

Edited by Joyce Brennfleck Shannon. 642 pages. 2000. 0-7808-0377-9. $78.

"Public libraries will find the book useful for reference and as a beginning research point for students, parents, and caregivers."
—American Reference Books Annual, 2001

"The strength of this work is that it compiles many basic fact sheets and addresses for further information in one volume. It is intended and suitable for the general public. The sourcebook is relevant to any collection providing health information to the general public."
— E-Streams, Nov '00

"From preventing retardation to parenting and family challenges, this covers health, social and legal issues and will prove an invaluable overview."
— Reviewer's Bookwatch, Jul '00

Obesity Sourcebook

Basic Consumer Health Information about Diseases and Other Problems Associated with Obesity, and Including Facts about Risk Factors, Prevention Issues, and Management Approaches

Along with Statistical and Demographic Data, Information about Special Populations, Research Updates, a Glossary, and Source Listings for Further Help and Information

Edited by Wilma Caldwell and Chad T. Kimball. 376 pages. 2001. 0-7808-0333-7. $48.

Ophthalmic Disorders Sourcebook

Basic Information about Glaucoma, Cataracts, Macular Degeneration, Strabismus, Refractive Disorders, and More

Along with Statistical and Demographic Data and Reports on Current Research Initiatives

Edited by Linda M. Ross. 631 pages. 1996. 0-7808-0081-8. $78.

∎

Oral Health Sourcebook

Basic Information about Diseases and Conditions Affecting Oral Health, Including Cavities, Gum Disease, Dry Mouth, Oral Cancers, Fever Blisters, Canker Sores, Oral Thrush, Bad Breath, Temporomandibular Disorders, and other Craniofacial Syndromes

Along with Statistical Data on the Oral Health of Americans, Oral Hygiene, Emergency First Aid, Information on Treatment Procedures and Methods of Replacing Lost Teeth

Edited by Allan R. Cook. 558 pages. 1997. 0-7808-0082-6. $78.

"Unique source which will fill a gap in dental sources for patients and the lay public. A valuable reference tool even in a library with thousands of books on dentistry. Comprehensive, clear, inexpensive, and easy to read and use. It fills an enormous gap in the health care literature." — *Reference and User Services Quarterly, American Library Association, Summer '98*

"Recommended reference source."
— *Booklist, American Library Association, Dec '97*

∎

Osteoporosis Sourcebook

Basic Consumer Health Information about Primary and Secondary Osteoporosis and Juvenile Osteoporosis and Related Conditions, Including Fibrous Dysplasia, Gaucher Disease, Hyperthyroidism, Hypophosphatasia, Myeloma, Osteopetrosis, Osteogenesis Imperfecta, and Paget's Disease

Along with Information about Risk Factors, Treatments, Traditional and Non-Traditional Pain Management, a Glossary of Related Terms, and a Directory of Resources

Edited by Allan R. Cook. 584 pages. 2001. 0-7808-0239-X. $78.

SEE ALSO *Women's Health Concerns Sourcebook*

∎

Pain Sourcebook

Basic Information about Specific Forms of Acute and Chronic Pain, Including Headaches, Back Pain, Muscular Pain, Neuralgia, Surgical Pain, and Cancer Pain

Along with Pain Relief Options Such as Analgesics, Narcotics, Nerve Blocks, Transcutaneous Nerve Stimulation, and Alternative Forms of Pain Control, Including Biofeedback, Imaging, Behavior Modification, and Relaxation Techniques

Edited by Allan R. Cook. 667 pages. 1997. 0-7808-0213-6. $78.

"The text is readable, easily understood, and well indexed. This excellent volume belongs in all patient education libraries, consumer health sections of public libraries, and many personal collections."
— *American Reference Books Annual, 1999*

"A beneficial reference." — *Booklist Health Sciences Supplement, American Library Association, Oct '98*

"The information is basic in terms of scholarship and is appropriate for general readers. Written in journalistic style ... intended for non-professionals. Quite thorough in its coverage of different pain conditions and summarizes the latest clinical information regarding pain treatment." — *Choice, Association of College and Research Libraries, Jun '98*

"Recommended reference source."
— *Booklist, American Library Association, Mar '98*

∎

Pediatric Cancer Sourcebook

Basic Consumer Health Information about Leukemias, Brain Tumors, Sarcomas, Lymphomas, and Other Cancers in Infants, Children, and Adolescents, Including Descriptions of Cancers, Treatments, and Coping Strategies

Along with Suggestions for Parents, Caregivers, and Concerned Relatives, a Glossary of Cancer Terms, and Resource Listings

Edited by Edward J. Prucha. 587 pages. 1999. 0-7808-0245-4. $78.

"A valuable addition to all libraries specializing in health services and many public libraries."
— *American Reference Books Annual, 2000*

"Recommended reference source."
— *Booklist, American Library Association, Feb '00*

"An excellent source of information. Recommended for public, hospital, and health science libraries with consumer health collections." — *E-Streams, Jun '00*

∎

Physical & Mental Issues in Aging Sourcebook

Basic Consumer Health Information on Physical and Mental Disorders Associated with the Aging Process, Including Concerns about Cardiovascular Disease, Pulmonary Disease, Oral Health, Digestive Disorders, Musculoskeletal and Skin Disorders, Metabolic Changes, Sexual and Reproductive Issues, and Changes in Vision, Hearing, and Other Senses

Along with Data about Longevity and Causes of Death, Information on Acute and Chronic Pain, Descriptions of Mental Concerns, a Glossary of Terms, and Resource Listings for Additional Help

Edited by Jenifer Swanson. 660 pages. 1999. 0-7808-0233-0. $78.

"Recommended for public libraries."
— *American Reference Books Annual, 2000*

"This is a treasure of health information for the layperson." — *Choice Health Sciences Supplement, Association of College & Research Libraries, May 2000*

"Recommended reference source."
— *Booklist, American Library Association, Oct '99*

SEE ALSO Healthy Aging Sourcebook

■

Podiatry Sourcebook

Basic Consumer Health Information about Foot Conditions, Diseases, and Injuries, Including Bunions, Corns, Calluses, Athlete's Foot, Plantar Warts, Hammertoes and Clawtoes, Clubfoot, Heel Pain, Gout, and More

Along with Facts about Foot Care, Disease Prevention, Foot Safety, Choosing a Foot Care Specialist, a Glossary of Terms, and Resource Listings for Additional Information

Edited by M. Lisa Weatherford. 400 pages. 2001. 0-7808-0215-2. $78.

■

Pregnancy & Birth Sourcebook

Basic Information about Planning for Pregnancy, Maternal Health, Fetal Growth and Development, Labor and Delivery, Postpartum and Perinatal Care, Pregnancy in Mothers with Special Concerns, and Disorders of Pregnancy, Including Genetic Counseling, Nutrition and Exercise, Obstetrical Tests, Pregnancy Discomfort, Multiple Births, Cesarean Sections, Medical Testing of Newborns, Breastfeeding, Gestational Diabetes, and Ectopic Pregnancy

Edited by Heather E. Aldred. 737 pages. 1997. 0-7808-0216-0. $78.

"A well-organized handbook. Recommended."
— *Choice, Association of College and Research Libraries, Apr '98*

"Recommended reference source."
— *Booklist, American Library Association, Mar '98*

"Recommended for public libraries."
— *American Reference Books Annual, 1998*

SEE ALSO Congenital Disorders Sourcebook, Family Planning Sourcebook

■

Prostate Cancer Sourcebook

Basic Consumer Health Information about Prostate Cancer, Including Information about the Associated Risk Factors, Detection, Diagnosis, and Treatment of Prostate Cancer

Along with Information on Non-Malignant Prostate Conditions, and Featuring a Section Listing Support and Treatment Centers and a Glossary of Related Terms

Edited by Dawn D. Matthews. 300 pages. 2001. 0-7808-0324-8. $78.

Public Health Sourcebook

Basic Information about Government Health Agencies, Including National Health Statistics and Trends, Healthy People 2000 Program Goals and Objectives, the Centers for Disease Control and Prevention, the Food and Drug Administration, and the National Institutes of Health

Along with Full Contact Information for Each Agency

Edited by Wendy Wilcox. 698 pages. 1998. 0-7808-0220-9. $78.

"Recommended reference source."
— *Booklist, American Library Association, Sep '98*

"This consumer guide provides welcome assistance in navigating the maze of federal health agencies and their data on public health concerns."
— *SciTech Book News, Sep '98*

■

Reconstructive & Cosmetic Surgery Sourcebook

Basic Consumer Health Information on Cosmetic and Reconstructive Plastic Surgery, Including Statistical Information about Different Surgical Procedures, Things to Consider Prior to Surgery, Plastic Surgery Techniques and Tools, Emotional and Psychological Considerations, and Procedure-Specific Information

Along with a Glossary of Terms and a Listing of Resources for Additional Help and Information

Edited by M. Lisa Weatherford. 374 pages. 2001. 0-7808-0214-4. $48.

■

Rehabilitation Sourcebook

Basic Consumer Health Information about Rehabilitation for People Recovering from Heart Surgery, Spinal Cord Injury, Stroke, Orthopedic Impairments, Amputation, Pulmonary Impairments, Traumatic Injury, and More, Including Physical Therapy, Occupational Therapy, Speech/ Language Therapy, Massage Therapy, Dance Therapy, Art Therapy, and Recreational Therapy

Along with Information on Assistive and Adaptive Devices, a Glossary, and Resources for Additional Help and Information

Edited by Dawn D. Matthews. 531 pages. 1999. 0-7808-0236-5. $78.

"This is an excellent resource for public library reference and health collections."
— *American Reference Books Annual, 2001*

"Recommended reference source."
— *Booklist, American Library Association, May '00*

Respiratory Diseases & Disorders Sourcebook

Basic Information about Respiratory Diseases and Disorders, Including Asthma, Cystic Fibrosis, Pneumonia, the Common Cold, Influenza, and Others, Featuring Facts about the Respiratory System, Statistical and Demographic Data, Treatments, Self-Help Management Suggestions, and Current Research Initiatives

Edited by Allan R. Cook and Peter D. Dresser. 771 pages. 1995. 0-7808-0037-0. $78.

"Designed for the layperson and for patients and their families coping with respiratory illness. . . . an extensive array of information on diagnosis, treatment, management, and prevention of respiratory illnesses for the general reader." *— Choice, Association of College and Research Libraries, Jun '96*

"A highly recommended text for all collections. It is a comforting reminder of the power of knowledge that good books carry between their covers." *— Academic Library Book Review, Spring '96*

"A comprehensive collection of authoritative information presented in a nontechnical, humanitarian style for patients, families, and caregivers." *— Association of Operating Room Nurses, Sep/Oct '95*

■

Sexually Transmitted Diseases Sourcebook, 1st Edition

Basic Information about Herpes, Chlamydia, Gonorrhea, Hepatitis, Nongonoccocal Urethritis, Pelvic Inflammatory Disease, Syphilis, AIDS, and More

Along with Current Data on Treatments and Preventions

Edited by Linda M. Ross. 550 pages. 1997. 0-7808-0217-9. $78.

■

Sexually Transmitted Diseases Sourcebook, 2nd Edition

Basic Consumer Health Information about Sexually Transmitted Diseases, Including Information on the Diagnosis and Treatment of Chlamydia, Gonorrhea, Hepatitis, Herpes, HIV, Mononucleosis, Syphilis, and Others

Along with Information on Prevention, Such as Condom Use, Vaccines, and STD Education; And Featuring a Section on Issues Related to Youth and Adolescents, a Glossary, and Resources for Additional Help and Information

Edited by Dawn D. Matthews. 538 pages. 2001. 0-7808-0249-7. $78.

Skin Disorders Sourcebook

Basic Information about Common Skin and Scalp Conditions Caused by Aging, Allergies, Immune Reactions, Sun Exposure, Infectious Organisms, Parasites, Cosmetics, and Skin Traumas, Including Abrasions, Cuts, and Pressure Sores

Along with Information on Prevention and Treatment

Edited by Allan R. Cook. 647 pages. 1997. 0-7808-0080-X. $78.

". . . comprehensive, easily read reference book." *—Doody's Health Sciences Book Reviews, Oct '97*

SEE ALSO *Burns Sourcebook*

■

Sleep Disorders Sourcebook

Basic Consumer Health Information about Sleep and Its Disorders, Including Insomnia, Sleepwalking, Sleep Apnea, Restless Leg Syndrome, and Narcolepsy

Along with Data about Shiftwork and Its Effects, Information on the Societal Costs of Sleep Deprivation, Descriptions of Treatment Options, a Glossary of Terms, and Resource Listings for Additional Help

Edited by Jenifer Swanson. 439 pages. 1998. 0-7808-0234-9. $78.

"This text will complement any home or medical library. It is user-friendly and ideal for the adult reader." *—American Reference Books Annual, 2000*

"Recommended reference source." *—Booklist, American Library Association, Feb '99*

"A useful resource that provides accurate, relevant, and accessible information on sleep to the general public. Health care providers who deal with sleep disorders patients may also find it helpful in being prepared to answer some of the questions patients ask." *—Respiratory Care, Jul '99*

■

Sports Injuries Sourcebook

Basic Consumer Health Information about Common Sports Injuries, Prevention of Injury in Specific Sports, Tips for Training, and Rehabilitation from Injury

Along with Information about Special Concerns for Children, Young Girls in Athletic Training Programs, Senior Athletes, and Women Athletes, and a Directory of Resources for Further Help and Information

Edited by Heather E. Aldred. 624 pages. 1999. 0-7808-0218-7. $78.

"Public libraries and undergraduate academic libraries will find this book useful for its nontechnical language." *—American Reference Books Annual, 2000*

"While this easy-to-read book is recommended for all libraries, it should prove to be especially useful for public, high school, and academic libraries; certainly it should be on the bookshelf of every school gymnasium." *—E-Streams, Mar '00*

Substance Abuse Sourcebook

Basic Health-Related Information about the Abuse of Legal and Illegal Substances Such as Alcohol, Tobacco, Prescription Drugs, Marijuana, Cocaine, and Heroin; and Including Facts about Substance Abuse Prevention Strategies, Intervention Methods, Treatment and Recovery Programs, and a Section Addressing the Special Problems Related to Substance Abuse during Pregnancy

Edited by Karen Bellenir. 573 pages. 1996. 0-7808-0038-9. $78.

"A valuable addition to any health reference section. Highly recommended."
— *The Book Report, Mar/Apr '97*

". . . a comprehensive collection of substance abuse information that's both highly readable and compact. Families and caregivers of substance abusers will find the information enlightening and helpful, while teachers, social workers and journalists should benefit from the concise format. Recommended."
— *Drug Abuse Update, Winter '96/'97*

SEE ALSO *Alcoholism Sourcebook, Drug Abuse Sourcebook*

■

Transplantation Sourcebook

Basic Consumer Health Information about Organ and Tissue Transplantation, Including Physical and Financial Preparations, Procedures and Issues Relating to Specific Solid Organ and Tissue Transplants, Rehabilitation, Pediatric Transplant Information, the Future of Transplantation, and Organ and Tissue Donation

Along with a Glossary and Listings of Additional Resources

Edited by Joyce Brennfleck Shannon. 600 pages. 2001. 0-7808-0322-1. $78.

■

Traveler's Health Sourcebook

Basic Consumer Health Information for Travelers, Including Physical and Medical Preparations, Transportation Health and Safety, Essential Information about Food and Water, Sun Exposure, Insect and Snake Bites, Camping and Wilderness Medicine, and Travel with Physical or Medical Disabilities

Along with International Travel Tips, Vaccination Recommendations, Geographical Health Issues, Disease Risks, a Glossary, and a Listing of Additional Resources

Edited by Joyce Brennfleck Shannon. 613 pages. 2000. 0-7808-0384-1. $78.

"This book is recommended for any public library, any travel collection, and especially any collection for the physically disabled."
—*American Reference Books Annual, 2001*

Women's Health Concerns Sourcebook

Basic Information about Health Issues That Affect Women, Featuring Facts about Menstruation and Other Gynecological Concerns, Including Endometriosis, Fibroids, Menopause, and Vaginitis; Reproductive Concerns, Including Birth Control, Infertility, and Abortion; and Facts about Additional Physical, Emotional, and Mental Health Concerns Prevalent among Women Such as Osteoporosis, Urinary Tract Disorders, Eating Disorders, and Depression

Along with Tips for Maintaining a Healthy Lifestyle

Edited by Heather E. Aldred. 567 pages. 1997. 0-7808-0219-5. $78.

"Handy compilation. There is an impressive range of diseases, devices, disorders, procedures, and other physical and emotional issues covered . . . well organized, illustrated, and indexed." —*Choice,*
Association of College and Research Libraries, Jan '98

SEE ALSO *Breast Cancer Sourcebook, Cancer Sourcebook for Women, 1st and 2nd Editions, Healthy Heart Sourcebook for Women, Osteoporosis Sourcebook*

■

Workplace Health & Safety Sourcebook

Basic Consumer Health Information about Workplace Health and Safety, Including the Effect of Workplace Hazards on the Lungs, Skin, Heart, Ears, Eyes, Brain, Reproductive Organs, Musculoskeletal System, and Other Organs and Body Parts

Along with Information about Occupational Cancer, Personal Protective Equipment, Toxic and Hazardous Chemicals, Child Labor, Stress, and Workplace Violence

Edited by Chad T. Kimball. 626 pages. 2000. 0-7808-0231-4. $78.

"Highly recommended." — *The Bookwatch, Jan '01*

■

Worldwide Health Sourcebook

Basic Information about Global Health Issues, Including Malnutrition, Reproductive Health, Disease Dispersion and Prevention, Emerging Diseases, Risky Health Behaviors, and the Leading Causes of Death

Along with Global Health Concerns for Children, Women, and the Elderly, Mental Health Issues, Research and Technology Advancements, and Economic, Environmental, and Political Health Implications, a Glossary, and a Resource Listing for Additional Help and Information

Edited by Joyce Brennfleck Shannon. 614 pages. 2001. 0-7808-0330-2. $78.